U.S.News
& WORLD REPORT

Best Hospitals

2018 EDITION

EXCLUSIVE RANKINGS

▶ Get **Expert Care** in Cancer, Cardiology, Neurology, Orthopedics and More

▶ The Best **Children's Hospitals**

Plus: The Top Hospitals in **Your State**

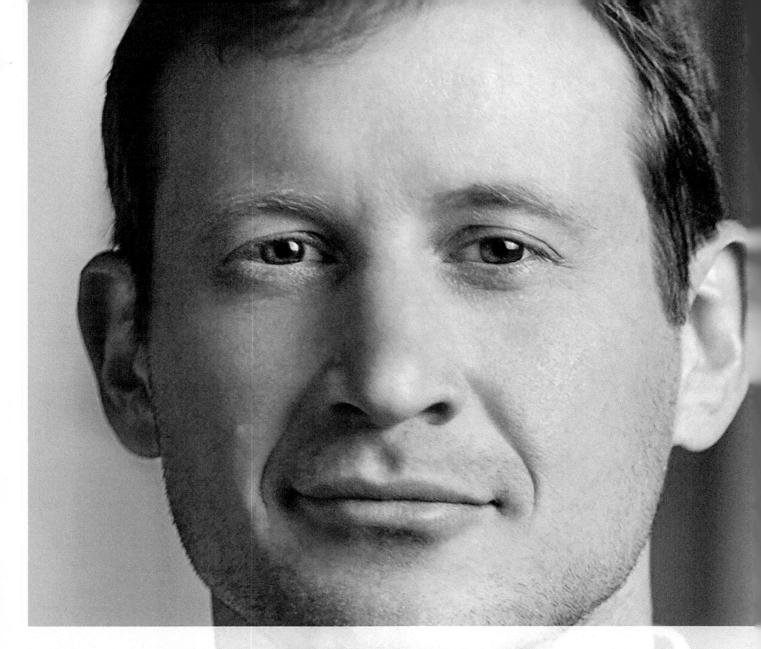

"My team has what it takes, ~~cancer~~"

Brian Ross | Cancer Survivor

With MD Anderson's expert team, Brian Ross defeated cancer. The exact outcome
we work for diligently, every day, for every patient. Let us fight for you.
To make an appointment today, call 1-855-894-0145 or visit MakingCancerHistory.com.

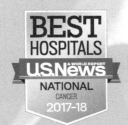

Ranked number one in the
nation for cancer care by
U.S. News & World Report.

THE UNIVERSITY OF TEXAS
MD Anderson
~~Cancer~~ Center

Making Cancer History®

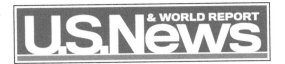

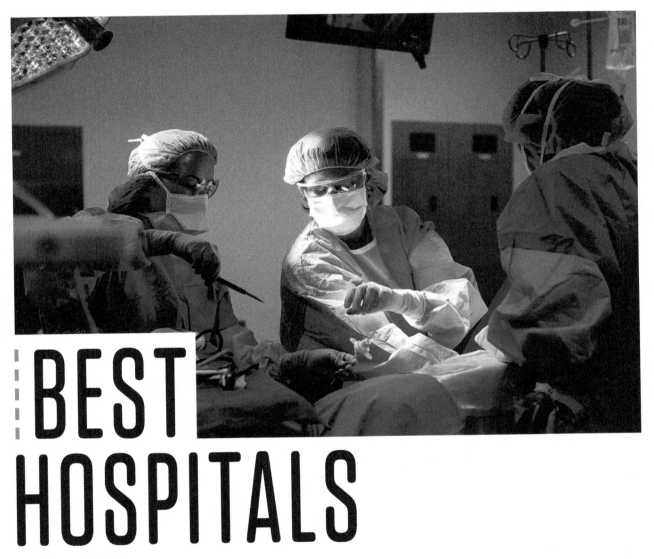

BEST HOSPITALS

2018 EDITION

Northwestern Memorial Hospital
BRETT ZIEGLER FOR USN&WR

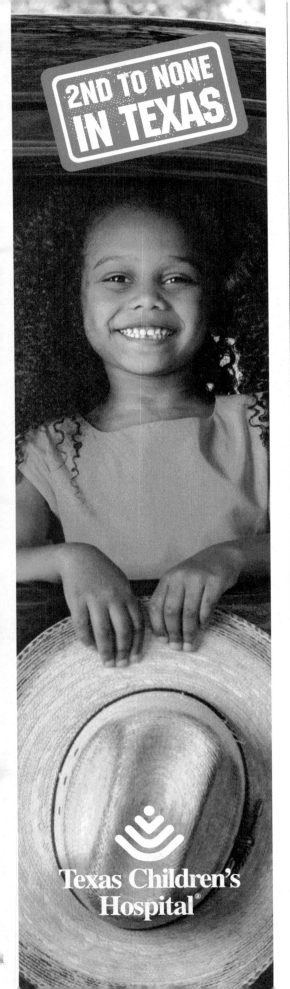
CONTENTS

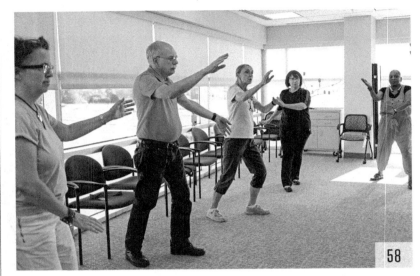

58

CONTENTS CONTINUED ON PAGE 4 ▶

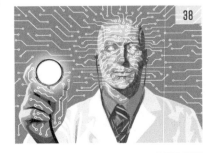

38

Yee Haw! 4th in the nation!

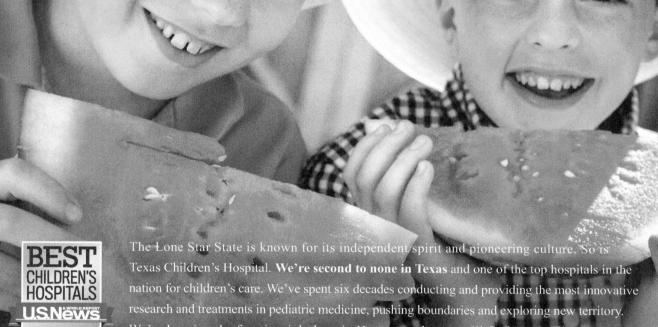

The Lone Star State is known for its independent spirit and pioneering culture. So is Texas Children's Hospital. **We're second to none in Texas** and one of the top hospitals in the nation for children's care. We've spent six decades conducting and providing the most innovative research and treatments in pediatric medicine, pushing boundaries and exploring new territory. We're keeping the frontier right here in Houston, where you'll find extraordinary care whenever you need it.

BEST CHILDREN'S HOSPITALS
U.S.News & WORLD REPORT
HONOR ROLL
2017-18

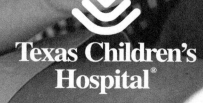

Texas Children's Hospital®

CONTENTS

THE U.S. NEWS RANKINGS

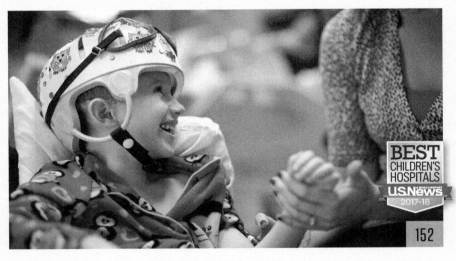

BEST CHILDREN'S HOSPITALS
U.S.News & WORLD REPORT
2017-18

152

RYAN KURTZ – CINCINNATI CHILDREN'S HOSPITAL

AMAZING
THINGS
ARE
HAPPENING
HERE

NEW YORK'S #1 HOSPITAL. 17 YEARS IN A ROW.

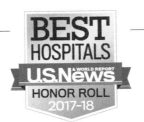

BEST HOSPITALS
U.S.News & WORLD REPORT
HONOR ROLL
2017-18

Our deepest thanks to the volunteers, staff, nurses, and doctors from Columbia and Weill Cornell for the expertise and commitment that make this honor possible.

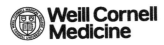 Weill Cornell Medicine | 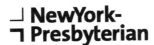 NewYork-Presbyterian | 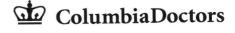 ColumbiaDoctors

@ USNEWS.COM

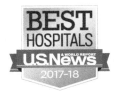

NUTRITION & LIFESTYLE

BEST DIETS

A look at some of the most popular and most researched diets, with reviews by a panel of health experts. Discover the top diets for weight loss, diabetes management and heart health, as well as the best plant-based and commercial diets.
usnews.com/bestdiets

EAT + RUN

Doing what it takes to stay in shape can be tough to manage. We serve up expert advice daily.
usnews.com/eat-run

INSURANCE

BEST MEDICARE ADVANTAGE PLANS

State-by-state ratings of Medicare Advantage and Medicare Part D plans, plus tips on choosing one of these plans vs. original Medicare.
usnews.com/medicare

HEALTH INSURANCE GUIDE

Your marketplace: a state-by-state guide. Plus answers to frequently asked questions.
usnews.com/healthinsurance

MEDICAL CARE

HEALTH CARE OF TOMORROW

Health reform, technological innovation and big data are transforming hospitals and care delivery. U.S. News explores how the industry is adapting.
usnews.com/
healthcareoftomorrow

BEST HOSPITALS HONOR ROLL

A VISUAL TOUR OF THE TOP 20

See the best of the Best Hospitals – 20 medical centers that lead the pack in a host of specialties, procedures and conditions, excelling in both breadth and depth of care.
usnews.com/hospitalphototour

BEST HOSPITALS

IN SPECIALTIES, PROCEDURES & CONDITIONS

We've evaluated more than 4,000 hospitals in up to nine common procedures and conditions, including hip replacement, knee replacement, heart bypass surgery, and COPD, as well as 16 medical specialties, including cancer care.
usnews.com/best-hospitals

SENIOR CARE

BEST NURSING HOMES

We've analyzed government data and published ratings of nearly 16,000 facilities.
usnews.com/nursinghomes

PHARMACIST PICKS

TOP RECOMMENDED HEALTH PRODUCTS

Which over-the-counter products do pharmacists prefer? Check out Top Recommended Health Products.
usnews.com/tophealthproducts

PHYSICIAN SEARCH TOOL

DOCTOR FINDER

A searchable directory of more than 800,000 doctors, created with Doximity, a professional network for physicians. Patients can find and research doctors who have the training, expertise and hospital affiliation they need. With free registration, physicians can expand or update the profile patients see.
usnews.com/doctors

BEST HOSPITALS
2018 EDITION

Executive Committee Chairman and Editor-in-Chief Mortimer B. Zuckerman
Co-Chairman Eric Gertler
Editor and Chief Content Officer Brian Kelly
Executive Editor Anne McGrath
Managing Editor & Chief, Health Analysis Ben Harder
Health Rankings Editor Avery Comarow
Art Director Rebecca Pajak
Director of Photography Avijit Gupta
Photography Editor Brett Ziegler
Deputy Editors Elizabeth Whitehead, Michael Morella
Associate Editor Lindsay Cates
Research Manager Myke Freeman
Contributors Linda Childers, Stacey Colino, Elizabeth Gardner, Mariya Greeley, Katherine Hobson, Beth Howard, Linda Marsa, Courtney Rubin, Barbara Sadick, Arlene Weintraub

USNEWS.COM/HEALTH

Executive Editor, Consumer Advice Kimberly Castro
Managing Editor Katy Marquardt
Assistant Managing Editors Angela Haupt (Health), Nathan Hellman (Consumer Advice)
Senior Editors Dennis Kelly (Health), Lindsay Lyon (Consumer Advice)
Reporters Ruben Castaneda, Lisa Esposito, Anna Medaris Miller, Michael Schroeder
Senior Health Services Researcher Geoff B. Dougherty
Research Manager Anna George
Analysts Zach Adams, Anwesha Majumder, Greta Martin
Contributing Analysts Keri Calkins, Carolyn K. Hulme-Lowe, Michael Marrone
Senior Product Manager Anne Roberts

HOSPITAL DATA INSIGHTS

Vice President, Insights Evan Jones
Director, Business Development Marsha Proulx
Senior Product Manager Laura Kovach
Product Manager Sabine Schulz
Manager, Marketing and Product Services Taylor Suggs
Analyst Ji Lee
Sales Associate Manny Plummer

TECHNOLOGY

Senior Director of Engineering Matt Kupferman
Director of Software Development Jerome Gipe
Senior Systems Manager Cathy Cacho
Software Technical Lead Corey Hutton
Developers Yasin Yaqoobi, Marc Simon
Project Manager Derrick Stout
Quality Assurance Sandy Sathyanarayanan
Digital Production Michael A. Brooks (Manager); Michael Fingerhuth

President and Chief Executive Officer William D. Holiber

ADVERTISING

Publisher and Chief Advertising Officer Kerry Dyer
Vice President, Advertising Ed Hannigan
Vice President, Marketing and Advertising Strategy Alexandra Kalaf
Director, Integrated Media Solutions Peter Bowes
West Coast Sales Director Peter Teese
Financial Sales Manager Heather Levine
Health Care Manager Colin Hamilton
Sales Manager Dan DeMonte
Senior Account Executives Anthony Patterson, Shannon Tkach, Ivy Zenati
Account Executives Julie Izzo, Eddie Kelly, Samantha Stefanacci
Managing Editor, BrandFuse Jada Graves
Web Designer, BrandFuse Sara Hampt
Director of Programmatic, Data and Revenue Partnerships Joseph Hayden
Programmatic Analyst Liam Kristinnsson
Senior Manager of Ad Technology and Platforms Teron Samuel
Senior Manager, Sales Strategy Tina Lopez
Manager, Sales Strategy Gary DeNardis
Sales Planners Spencer Vastoler, Michael Zee
Marketing Coordinator Brielle Schwartz
Director of Advertising Operations Cory Nesser
Senior Manager, Client Success Katina Sangare
Account Managers James Adeleye, Jennifer Fass, Katie Harper, Gabby Iwunze
Ad Operations Tessa Gluck (Manager), Samantha Seigerman
Director of Advertising Services Phyllis Panza
Business Operations Karolee Jarnecki
Administration Judy David, Anny Lasso, Carmen Caraballo

Vice President, Specialty Marketing Mark W. White
Director of Specialty Marketing Abbe Weintraub

Chief Operating Officer Karen S. Chevalier
Chief Product Officer Chad Smolinski
Chief Financial Officer Neil Maheshwari
Senior Vice President, Education, News/Opinion, Money Chris DiCosmo
Senior Vice President, Strategic Development and General Counsel Peter M. Dwoskin
Senior Vice President, Technology Yingjie Shu
Senior Vice President, Human Resources Jeff Zomper

Additional copies of the 2018 edition of U.S. News & World Report's Best Hospitals guidebook are available for purchase at (800) 836-6397 or online at usnews.com/hospitalbook. To order custom reprints, please call (877) 652-5295 or email usnews@wrightsmedia.com. For all other permissions, email permissions@usnews.com.

Morristown Medical Center. Top Rated. Again. Again. Again. Again. And Again.

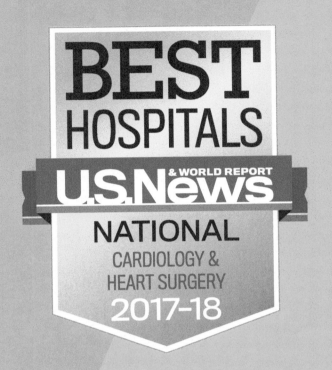

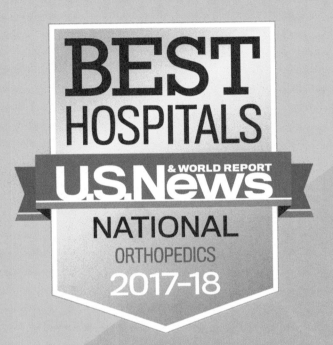

U.S. News & World Report has named Morristown Medical Center a top hospital in the entire country for Cardiology & Heart Surgery **SIX YEARS** in a row.

We've also been ranked a top hospital for Orthopedics **FOUR YEARS** in a row.

We give our best. You get the best.

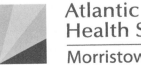

Because these partners give,

Children's Miracle Network Hospitals® provide the best care for kids like Zion.

Thank you to our top corporate partners for raising funds that save and improve the lives of local kids. Since becoming a CMN Hospitals partner, each has raised more than $20 million, totalling more than $2 billion, collectively, for member children's hospitals across North America.

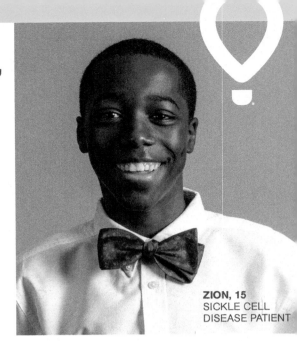

ZION, 15
SICKLE CELL
DISEASE PATIENT

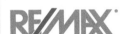   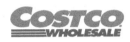

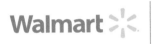   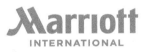

Children's Miracle Network Hospitals celebrates the anniversaries of partners who do so much for the kids.

30 YEARS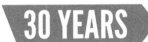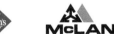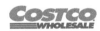

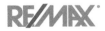 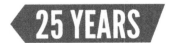 **25 YEARS**

20 YEARS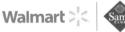

  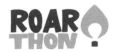 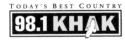 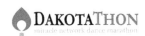

CMNHospitals.org

▶ CHAPTER 1 ◀

ON MEDICINE'S FRONT LINES

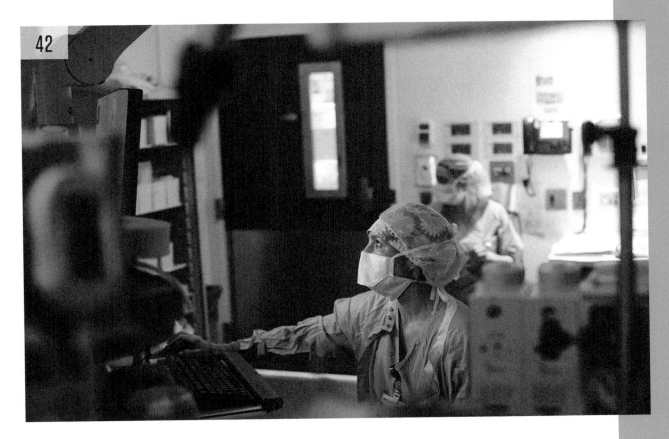

42

10 HEALTH CARE TRENDS THAT WILL AFFECT YOU

A LIFESAVING CHAIN

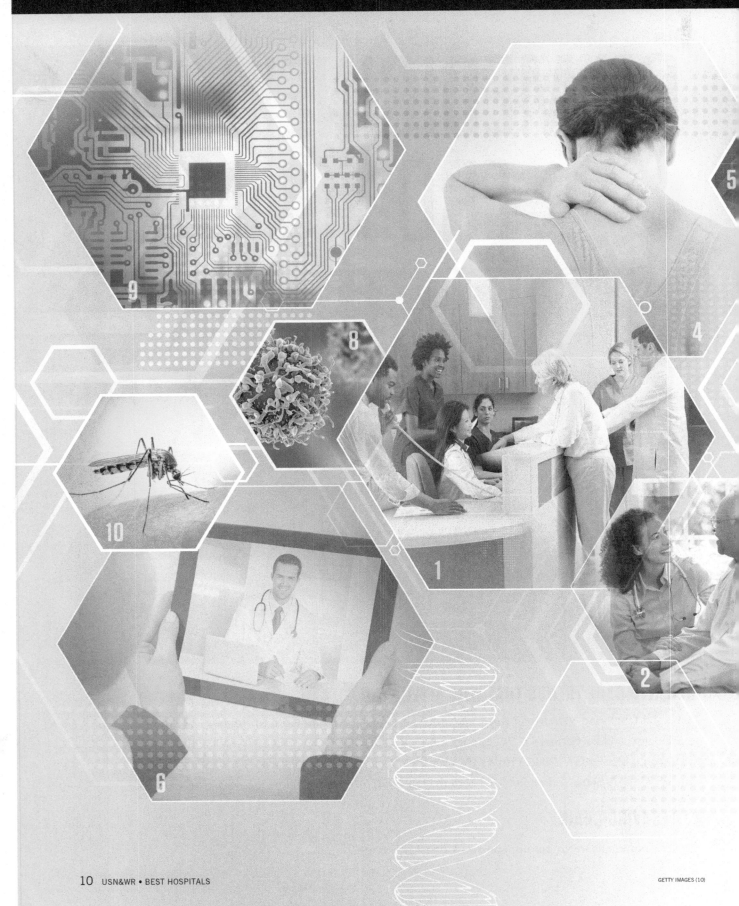

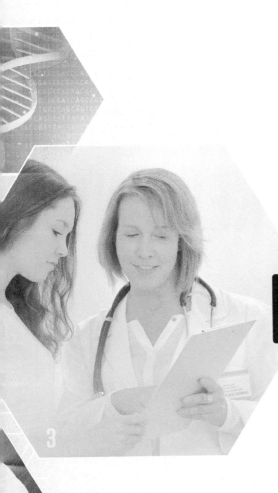

10 HEALTH CARE TRENDS
THAT WILL AFFECT YOU

Smarter, more personalized, and more prevention-oriented medicine is coming your way: supercomputers acting as doctors' superassistants combing masses of data to speed diagnosis, identify risk factors, and find the best ways to head off trouble or treat it; immunotherapies and other treatments tailored to your DNA; STEM cells harnessed to relieve what ails you. Miss the days of house calls? Get set for the new world of home care 2.0, where hospital patients sleep in their own beds and the chronically ill can be monitored in real time via wireless devices. Keep reading to find out what lies ahead.

ILLUSTRATION BY **ALICIA BUELOW** FOR USN&WR

1. GOOD DOCTORING WILL MEAN KEEPING YOU WELL

By Beth Howard

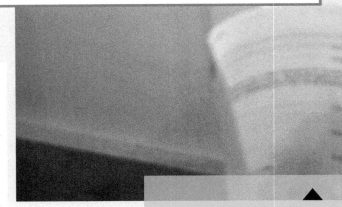

Eric M. Weil, a primary care doctor at Massachusetts General Hospital in Boston, was worried about a patient – a recovering alcoholic who had previously been hospitalized due to his drinking. Now a close family member had died. "If he's ever going to start drinking, it's going to be now," Weil remembers thinking.

But Weil didn't have to leave his patient's fate to chance. Staffers of his practice reached out with a customized support plan. They called the man frequently, making sure that he was eating and taking his medications, and that family members were providing support. "I felt comfortable knowing that people on my team were taking care of him," Weil says. His patient weathered the crisis.

Looking after patients' mental and behavioral health needs at the doctor's office is one of the ways that hospitals are embracing the emerging concept of population health. Based on the idea of taking responsibility for the well-being of an entire group of patients – Medicare patients, say, or those in a particular health plan or geographic area – population health emphasizes prevention, better management of chronic disease, and a payment model that rewards keeping people well and out of the hospital.

That might include deploying nurse practitioners to frail patients' homes rather than exposing them to infections in the emergency room. And it might entail keeping close tabs on patients with complex conditions, tackling psychological issues with coaching and peer support, and even addressing factors like hunger and the lack of healthy foods (box, Page 16). "Health care doesn't just happen in the exam room," reasons Weil. "It's all the other minutes of the day where bad stuff happens."

Nurse care coordinator Christine Duchesneau, left, talks with Gladys Ramos at the Phyllis Jen Center for Primary Care before Ramos sees her doctor.

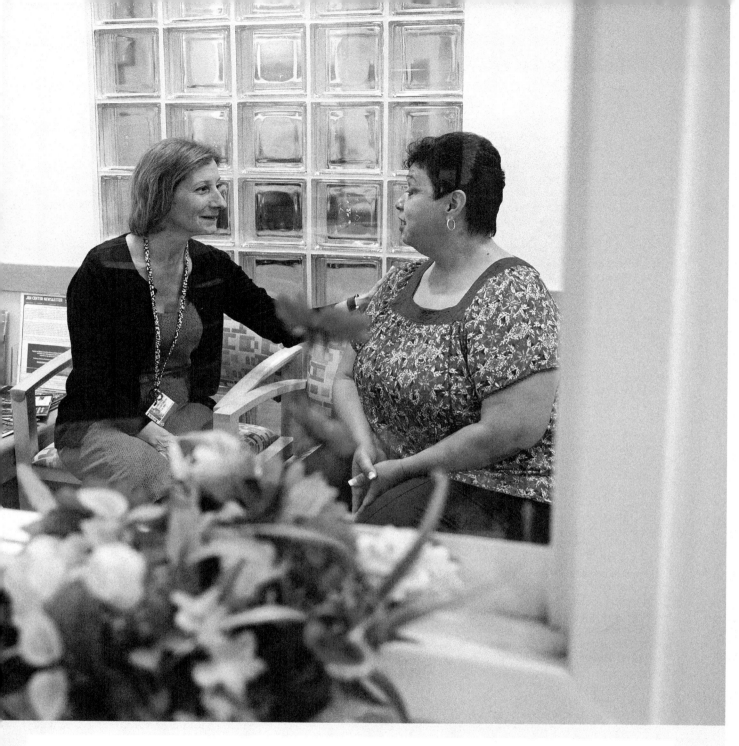

Besides Partners HealthCare System, which Mass General is part of, scores of systems are adopting the population health approach, from Christiana Care Health System in Delaware to Hennepin County Medical Center in Minnesota and San Francisco General Hospital. While the momentum has primarily been due to incentives in the Affordable Care Act, experts predict the trend will stick if it delivers on the promise to improve care and save money. According to an American Hospital Association survey, 85 percent of responding executives reported a strong commitment to the model or have it in their vision statement.

Few are as far along as Partners, which started down this route more than 10 years ago. Here are some of the ways that providers are taking action – and how those steps might affect you:

They're putting a team on the case

The sickest 5 percent of the population accounts for roughly half of health care costs, so getting a better handle on these people is paramount. At the Phyllis Jen Center, a primary care practice at Brigham & Women's Hospital, another Partners facility, a team of nurses, doctors, psychologists, and social and community health workers huddle each day to coordinate the care of medically complicated patients like Marie Josee

Sam, 75, who battles diabetes, COPD, arthritis and a painful spinal condition. "My doctors all know each other," she says. "They have conferences over me." If she has an issue, she can call her nurse care coordinator, Christine Duchesneau.

The team closely monitors Sam and other patients, troubleshooting problems before they become a crisis. They handle everything from cajoling people to wear compression stockings and inspecting their food stores to sending out the mobile observation team to provide treatment in the home. "We can do a number of bedside laboratory tests, X-rays, EKGs and ultrasounds," says nurse practitioner Dana Sheer, director of advanced clinical programs. "And we can run an IV for things like steroids, IV antibiotics."

The proactive monitoring and coordination is working. Partners' data show a 20 percent lower rate of hospitalization where it's been implemented. And for every $1 spent on "extras" like home visits and increased staffing, Partners has saved $2.65. Likewise, when FirstHealth of the Carolinas began embedding diabetes educators in primary care offices, implementing group medical visits in which a doctor talks with several patients together, and providing medications for free to patients temporarily while they linked up with assistance programs, the diabetes mortality rate dropped from 40.8 to 22.8 per 100,000 people over four years.

Much of this closer attention will happen remotely. Virtual visits (story, Page 32) should make follow-up more convenient for patients who need to be seen frequently. Erica Jensen of Wilmington, Massachusetts, 24, checked in virtually with her Brigham & Women's endocrinologist to stay on top of her Type 1 diabetes during her pregnancy two years ago and has continued to do so since. "Sometimes it's hard taking time off work," says Jensen. "And you push that appointment back as far as you can."

Similarly, liver and kidney transplant patients can interact from home with their caregivers at Dallas-based Children's Health. And at Banner Health in Phoenix, patients with five or more chronic ailments such as heart failure and hypertension receive a tablet and tools like a blood pressure cuff and scale to transmit their health signals from home in real time. A pilot program showed the approach resulted in fewer hospitalizations, shorter hospital stays, and 34.5 percent lower costs.

They're building in mental health care

Research shows that mental and behavioral health issues figure into some 70 percent of primary care visits, and untreated, issues such as depression, anxiety or sub-

> "
> -------------------
> **Mental and behavioral health issues figure into 70% of primary care visits.**

stance abuse often worsen physical health and interfere with other treatments. People with depression, say, tend to stop taking their medications regularly.

A growing number of systems, including Partners, Utah-based Intermountain Healthcare, Montefiore Health System in the Bronx, and Cleveland Clinic Children's Hospital, are responding by adding screening and teaming doctors with social workers, addiction specialists, psychiatrists and behavioral care managers. "If I have patients who need mental health services, I now can go down the hall and introduce them to a mental health or addiction specialist or a social worker," says Timothy Ferris, chairman and CEO of the Massachusetts General Physicians Organization.

People who get this kind of attention are twice as likely as those who don't to have their problems resolve, and much faster, statistics show. Having mental health workers in the primary care clinics of Intermountain cost the health system $22 a year for each patient, for example, but health savings added up to $115 per patient.

Surprisingly, the approach also reduces the overall cost of an individual's care. "It really is pretty amazing," says Brent Forester, chief of the division of geriatric psychiatry at the Partners-affiliated McLean Hospital. "By treating depression, you can impact general outcomes in a huge way."

They're making use of big data

Population health hinges on the adroit use of data to spot patterns and measure outcomes. What does that mean for patients? Those with chronic conditions like diabetes may become part of a registry of similar patients targeted for more frequent interaction with the system, including alerts for overdue tests or less-than-optimal test results, plus coaching. The goal, says Weil, "is to prevent admission to the hospital by moving farther upstream and taking steps that would make bad outcomes less likely later on."

The data also help to chart the best course of action. For instance, information collected on similar patients based on characteristics like age, sex and health status may point to a specific treatment option. Since outcomes that patients report – such as pain and mobility after a knee operation – are a part of the equation, patients fill out lots of questionnaires and surveys, often on iPads in the waiting room.

They're engaging patients in getting results

Successfully making that move upstream requires patients to take a bigger role in their own care. So many systems offer a growing array of programs and tools to help patients stay healthy, from smartphone apps that remind them to take their medications to 24/7 access to

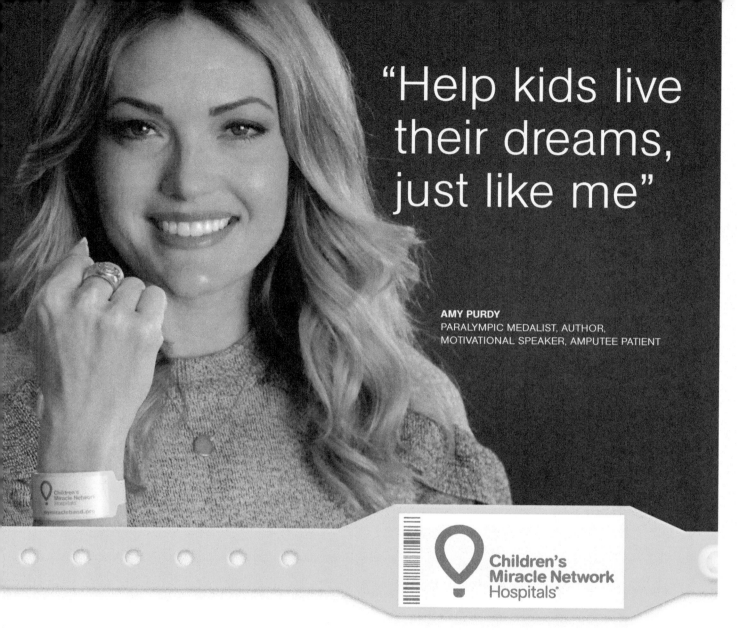

"Help kids live their dreams, just like me"

AMY PURDY
PARALYMPIC MEDALIST, AUTHOR,
MOTIVATIONAL SPEAKER, AMPUTEE PATIENT

Children's Miracle Network Hospitals

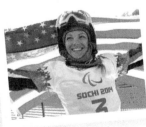

"As a kid, I wanted to explore every inch of the world — on a snowboard, when possible. But then I contracted bacterial meningitis. My kidneys shut down. My spleen burst. Both of my legs were amputated below the knees. Everyone told me I would never snowboard again. But, I didn't give up on my dreams. I medaled in the Paralympics. I'm a motivational speaker, published author, Dancing with the Stars runner up and training to compete in the next Paralympic Games. Help kids live their dreams – just like me."

PUT YOUR MONEY WHERE THE MIRACLES ARE.

Give Today to your children's hospital

Speedway has supported the drive of kids like Amy since 1991—raising more than $90 million for local Children's Miracle Network Hospitals.

CMNHospitals.org

health coaches who help them set and meet fitness goals. Jersey City Medical Center's Health Navigator program lets patients earn rewards and discounts by accessing interactive programs on medical conditions, picking up their prescriptions on time, keeping appointments with providers, and making healthy choices, such as ordering a salad instead of fries at a local restaurant or taking exercise and yoga classes in the community.

Other health systems are finding novel ways to serve the needs of their patients. At Eskenazi Health in Indianapolis, for instance, care coordinators monitor and coach elderly people with dementia, delirium and depression and family caregivers through home and clinic visits and telephone calls. Nurses also drop in to address medical needs. The result: at least a 50 percent drop in depression scores and fewer preventable hospital and ER visits. The Geisinger Health System in Pennsylvania has launched an initiative to analyze the DNA of every patient (story, Page 28). One payoff: Members of a family found to have mutations associated with fatal cardiac arrhythmias are now being closely monitored, and some have received pacemakers. "Overall we've found that about 3 to 4 out of 100 patients have a medically actionable condition," says President and CEO David Feinberg.

There is much more to be done before population health fulfills its promise. But, says Ferris: "We're starting to see real progress in changing the way health care is delivered." ●

PRESCRIBING A BAG OF GROCERIES

For ProMedica, the lightbulb went on about seven years ago. While working in the community to try and prevent obesity, "we realized that hunger is a health issue," says Randy Oostra, president and CEO of the health system, which serves parts of Ohio and Michigan.

So ProMedica focused on getting sustenance to people in need. It teamed up with community partners to collect unserved food from a local casino for food banks and provide meals to kids during the summer at local schools and other sites. And it began screening patients for hunger. Today ProMedica is also helping patients find housing, transportation, child care and even jobs.

While some health systems have been addressing nonmedical "social determinants of health" for years, there's recently been a new surge of interest, says Pamela Riley, assistant vice president for delivery system reform at the Commonwealth Fund. Evidence continues to mount that such factors are crucial to health. Poor housing conditions are associated with a host of diseases and condi-

tions, from low birth weight to Type 2 diabetes. The unemployed are more likely to develop heart disease and arthritis. The shift to paying providers for improving people's health – and keeping them out of the hospital – adds incentive. There's not "an asterisk in our mission statement that we only care for you when you're within our walls," Oostra says.

Food insecurity is often the first action item. At Boston Medical Center, the Grow Clinic helps children who are failing to grow and thrive get access to nutritional assistance and other social services, says Megan Sandel, a pediatrician and associate director of the clinic. The hospital has a preventive food pantry where families can fill "prescriptions" for several days of healthful groceries.

BMC is also participating in a study to see whether referring patients to housing services can get them into stable housing, reduce emergency room visits, and get families in the door for well-child visits and immunizations. Montefiore Health System in the Bronx, meantime, is working with govern-

ment and community groups to study whether dealing with the source of roach and rodent infestations, rather than just using pesticides, can improve health outcomes. Pests can exacerbate asthma, explains Marina Reznik, an attending physician at Children's Hospital at Montefiore and the principal investigator. ProMedica and other health systems are also steering people to affordable transportation, child care subsidies and even on-campus legal assistance. "Needs related to housing, food and safety can all be ameliorated by a certain level of access to legal expertise," says Ellen Lawton, co-director of the National Center for Medical-Legal Partnership at George Washington University. The group says 294 institutions are finding ways to provide legal services within the clinic or hospital.

Someday, experts predict, a prescription for housing, financial counseling, or a ride to the hospital will be as routine as one for a drug. "In time," says Sandel, such moves "will all be health interventions."

–Katherine Hobson

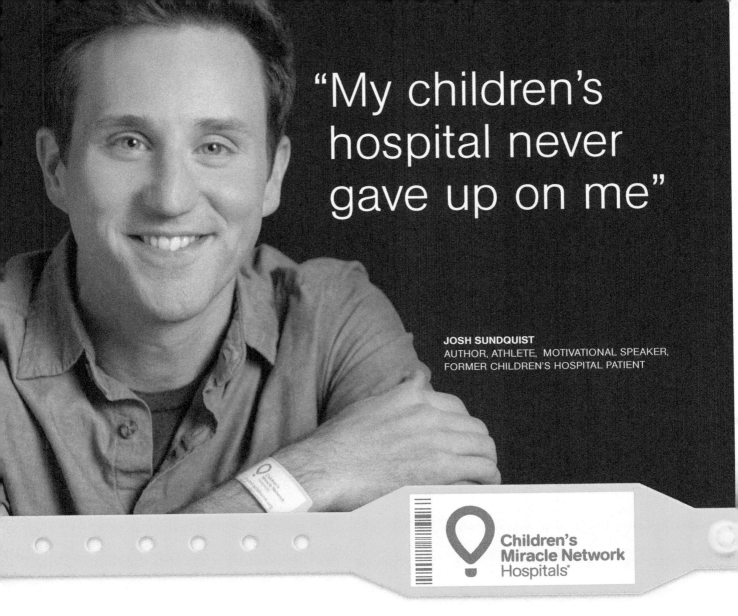

"My children's hospital never gave up on me"

JOSH SUNDQUIST
AUTHOR, ATHLETE, MOTIVATIONAL SPEAKER, FORMER CHILDREN'S HOSPITAL PATIENT

Children's Miracle Network Hospitals®

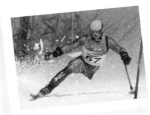

I was 9 when I lost my leg to bone cancer. I had a 50 percent chance to live. After chemotherapy treatments at my children's hospital and the amputation, I had beaten the odds. But would I ever be as active as I once was? Fast forward 20 years: I've competed in the Paralympics and now play on the U.S. Amputee Soccer Team. My successes are because of my children's hospital. They never gave up on me.

PUT YOUR MONEY WHERE THE MIRACLES ARE.

Give Today to your children's hospital

Josh was supported in his fight by Dairy Queen® franchisees and fans who have raised more than $125 million for children's hospitals since 1984.

CMNHospitals.org

2. YOU'LL GET CARE AT HOME

By Mariya Greeley

"Are you okay? What were you doing? You had a little spike," the nurse on the phone said to Brittany Jackson. Jackson, 31, recently had developed a rare form of heart failure after giving birth. Her cardiologist at the University of Pittsburgh Medical Center recommended remote monitoring to help manage her condition, and sensors had wirelessly reported an increased heart rate to nurses at UPMC while she was at a well-child visit for her infant. Jackson's weight, blood pressure and blood oxygen level are also transmitted to the call center once a day. If anything points to a problem, she gets a call.

UPMC's program is one example of the innovative approaches hospitals are employing to keep people out of the hospital. Such home health care programs typically focus on managing people with chronic diseases and treating acutely ill patients who may need to avoid the hospital because of the risk of infection, say. These days, more doctors are even making house calls thanks in large part to Medicare's Independence at Home Demonstration, which has been testing primary care at home for people with multiple chronic conditions and functional limitations. Many children's hospitals, including Cincinnati Children's, Boston Children's and Children's Hospital of Philadelphia, provide home care for acutely ill youngsters.

The value to patients "is largely peace of mind," says Joseph Kvedar, vice president of Connected Health at Partners HealthCare. It's more comfortable and less stressful to be cared for at home, and these programs have been shown to reduce trips to the ER. Geisinger Health Plan found a 23 percent lower hospitalization rate in heart failure patients using remote monitoring – and savings of about $216 per heart failure patient per month between 2008 and 2012. A Brigham and Women's pilot program of home visits and telemonitoring lowered costs and improved the patient experience while maintaining quality.

Another big advantage of ongoing remote checks, Kvedar notes, is that it keeps people more engaged in their care. Jackson says monitoring has helped her recognize which behaviors – what she eats, say – affect her condition.

Until reimbursement practices change, these programs won't exactly be moneymakers. Patients and insurers "don't pay a dime" now for UPMC's monitoring, says Ravi Ramani, director of the Integrated Heart Failure Program there. But reducing admissions is a key benefit, he notes. And there is hope that payment will eventually be possible as the system emphasizes value rather than volume of services.

Acute care is the focus of Hospital at Home, a model developed by Bruce Leff, professor of medicine at John Hopkins and director of its Center for Transformative Geriatric Research. Presbyterian Healthcare Services in New Mexico, Kaiser Permanente in California, Atrius Health in Massachusetts and 11 Veterans Affairs hospitals have found success implementing the HaH model, which involves an initial visit to set up the hospital equipment followed by a few days of intensive medical services in the home. Nurses visit between one and three times a day and a physician stops by once a day, or more if necessary. Once a patient is "discharged" from the acute phase of the program, visits continue less frequently during a recovery phase. New York's Mount Sinai Health System is currently testing a program based on HaH that entails about three days of acute care followed by up to 30 days of transitional care. Results so far: higher patient satisfaction, lower costs and fewer complications. "Being at home is a lot better," says Lydia Cepeda, who was able to sleep in her own bed in Manhattan and look after her teenage son while being treated for cellulitis.

Jackson's remote monitoring was set to last 90 days. But Ramani says UPMC is getting a lot of requests to extend the program as a safety net. For her part, Jackson would consider continuing if UPMC allowed it. "It's good to know you have something like that to keep you out of the hospital," she says. ●

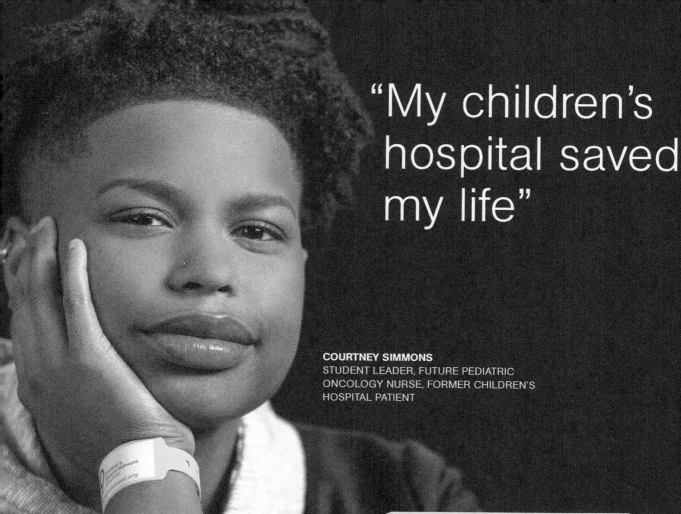

"My children's hospital saved my life"

COURTNEY SIMMONS
STUDENT LEADER, FUTURE PEDIATRIC
ONCOLOGY NURSE, FORMER CHILDREN'S
HOSPITAL PATIENT

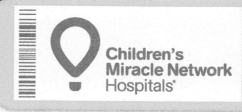

Children's
Miracle Network
Hospitals

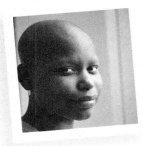

Before my 17th birthday, I lost my sister and my mom to cancer. Then I got it too. I had 30 weeks of chemotherapy and several surgeries to remove the tumor and repair my damaged bones. Thanks to my children's hospital, I'm cancer-free. They never gave up on me. I am now studying to be a pediatric oncology nurse and I started a Dance Marathon at my university to help my local children's hospital.

PUT YOUR MONEY WHERE THE MIRACLES ARE.

Give Today to your children's hospital

Over the last 25 years, RE/MAX agents and offices have raised $157 million to help kids get the same excellent care Courtney received at her Children's Miracle Network Hospital.

CMNHospitals.org

PAYING
FASHION
FORWARD

When 8-year-old Sasha Bogosian met Kristen Bell, she gifted her a pair of jeans. They were much more than a fashionable gesture. Sasha, who has Cerebral Palsy, hand-painted them. Sasha has turned what began as art therapy to manage her physical challenges, into a fundraiser for the art therapy program at her children's hospital.

Kristen, an actress, philanthropist and mom, immediately put on the jeans, recognizing their significance. A spokesperson for Children's Miracle Network Hospitals,® Kristen understands that Medicaid and insurance programs do not cover the full cost of providing care for kids. Children's hospitals rely on donations to fund life-saving treatments and programs, research and charitable care for kids — more than 10 million across the country.

"I've been very fortunate in my life and I feel a real internal obligation to give back," Kristen says. "Also, even though I am so lucky to have two healthy,

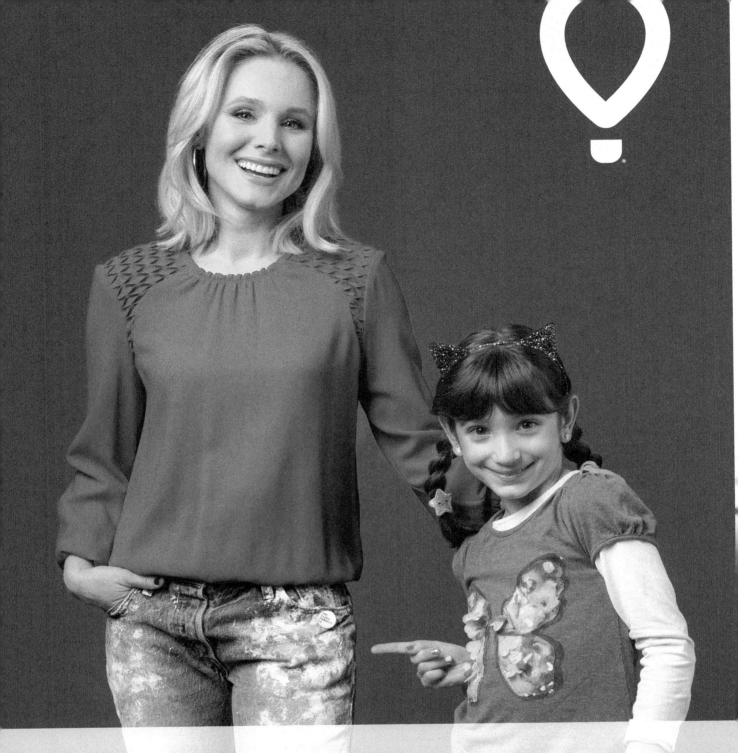

thriving children, I understand that there is nothing worse for a parent than having your child be sick or hurt, even in a minor way. It's so important that Children's Miracle Network Hospitals are there to help families in their times of greatest need."

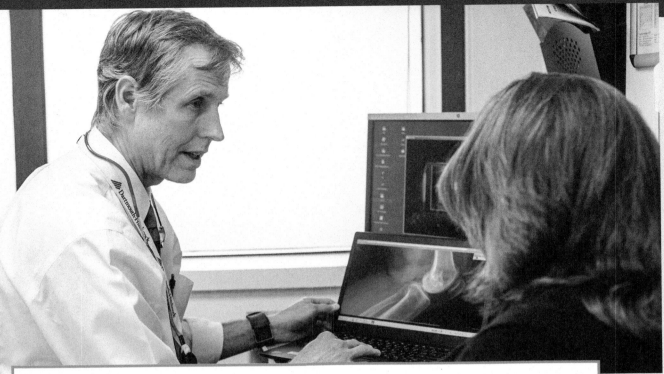

3. YOU AND YOUR DOCTOR WILL BE PARTNERS

By Barbara Sadick

After Michael Michael was diagnosed with colon cancer, he underwent three rounds of chemotherapy – without success – at Massachusetts General Hospital. Then he and his wife were faced with a major decision. They sat down with Michael's oncologist, and were encouraged to talk honestly about their values as a family and how they would like to spend the time they had left together. Their doctor explained each of what he believed were their options, laying out the risks and benefits. Michael could participate in a clinical trial or try radiation treatments, neither of which would likely prolong his life and both of which probably would make him more miserable. Or he could stop treatment. In that conversation, "our focus shifted to his remaining quality of life," says Carol Michael. "My husband wanted to finish the play he was writing." They chose to tap Mass General's palliative care service, whose doctor would keep Michael out of pain and alert so he could spend his time writing at home. He died there five months later, in 2010.

The Michaels' experience was an early example of "shared decision-making," a partnership of patients and their physicians at the core of recent efforts to improve care quality and safety. The concept of formally making the patient an active partner in choosing a medical path began spreading widely in the aftermath of a 2001 Institute of Medicine report bluntly pointing out that the health system "has fallen far short in its ability to translate knowledge into practice" and calling for patient-centered care "ensuring that patient values guide all clinical decisions." In 2017, the definition was expanded to include families as well as patients.

What does this mean for people grappling with a diagnosis? The traditional next steps – you go see a clinician who often unilaterally prescribes treatment based on what is known to work for patients with similar conditions – are giving way to conversations in which the doctor explains, probes and listens while you ask questions and explore which course of action best meets your needs. If as a physician "you don't

▲

Dartmouth-Hitchcock orthopedic surgeon Michael Sparks shares the decision-making with Kerry McNally, who has a bone disorder.

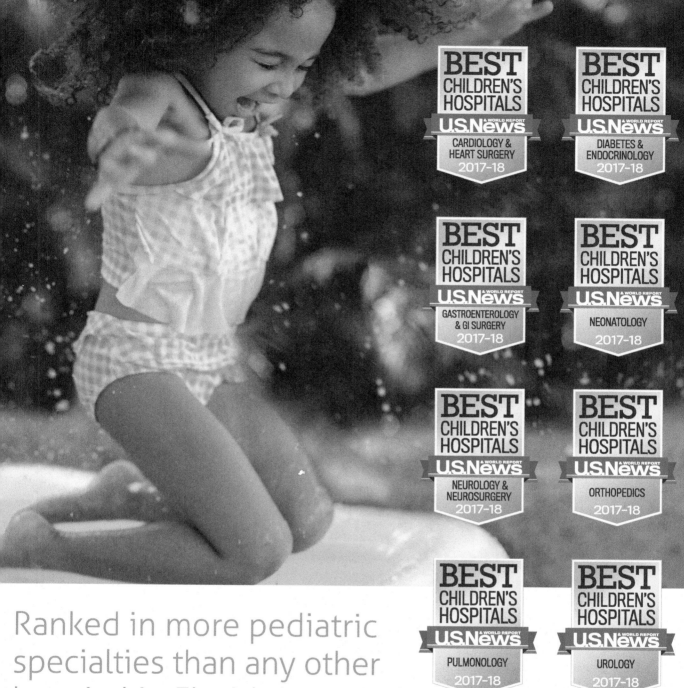

Ranked in more pediatric specialties than any other hospital in Florida

Nicklaus Children's Hospital has more programs listed in *U.S.News & World Report's* 2017-18 pediatric rankings than any other hospital in Florida. In five of these categories, no other program in Florida ranks higher. What's more, our neurology and neurosurgery, and neonatology programs are among the top 15 in the nation. That means, you have world-class pediatric care right here in your own backyard. And through our network of outpatient and urgent care centers, chances are, we are only a few blocks away. It's great to be a leader, but even better to lead with compassion, innovation and extraordinary care. Nicklaus Children's Hospital. For Health. For Life.

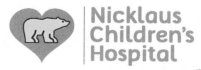

For Health. For Life.

know what matters to a patient and what that patient is going through, you cannot possibly know if you are practicing the best medicine," says Albert G. Mulley, Jr., managing director of Global Health Care Delivery Science at Dartmouth and a leader in the field of patient-centered care. Services free to patients at Dartmouth-Hitchcock Medical Center include web-based and paper educational materials about treatments, counseling by health coaches who help families weigh their choices in light of their values, and assistance with end-of-life planning.

Shared decision-making isn't necessary or even possible if there is one treatment, and it is needed urgently. But a man facing early prostate cancer, for example, might be offered surgery and/or radiation or the choice to wait and see. In deciding what course to take, he may weigh whether it is more important to avoid the risks of surgery so he can remain sexually active or to be surer of living cancer-free.

Hospitals doing the most thorough job of involving patients have buy-in from the top, notes cardiologist Steven Horowitz, medical director of Planetree, the patient-centered care system at Stamford Hospital in Connecticut. There, he says, every new staff member, from doctors to cleaning staff, participates in a full-day orientation to better understand – and learn to improve – the patient experience. A council that includes patients and family members meets regularly to review current procedures from the patient's viewpoint.

For patient-centered care to take hold everywhere, financial incentives will have to change, experts note. The traditional payment model rewards physicians for rapid-fire visits and quantity of procedures, not quality of care. Instead, the system ought to pay them for "the kind of in-depth communication required to learn what is most important to a patient," says Mulley. That may be possible if the shift from a fee-for-service model to one focused on value plays out as planned. ●

SELF-SERVICE MEDICINE

One huge influence on patients' engagement in their care: technology that lets them do everything from run their own electrocardiogram on a smartphone and track medication use from smart pillboxes to hold their own stress-busting mindfulness session. Mobile technologies can put patients managing conditions like diabetes and high blood pressure "in the driver's seat," and even allow for quick diagnosis of routine ailments like a urinary tract infection, notes Andrew Ellner, director of Global Primary Care and Executive Education at Harvard Medical School's Center for Primary Care. "These technologies give the convenience of self-service, much in the way banking has changed in the last decade."

"One in 2 Americans suffers from a chronic disease that requires a certain level of monitoring in addition to seeing a physician periodically," says Ash-

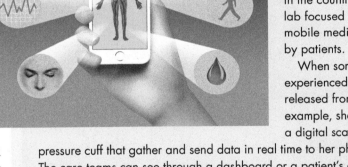

ish Atreja, the chief technology and engagement officer and director of the Sinai AppLab at the Icahn School of Medicine at Mount Sinai. It's one of the first medical centers in the country to have its own lab focused on developing mobile medical apps for use by patients.

When someone who has experienced heart failure is released from the hospital, for example, she might be given a digital scale and a blood pressure cuff that gather and send data in real time to her physician's office. The care teams can see through a dashboard or a patient's electronic medical record if anything looks off, and an alert sounds for both patient and health care staff when an emergency arises.

Other new apps and devices suggest possible diagnoses and guide patients to the right specialist based on their symptoms, monitor blood glucose levels and guide diabetic patients to adjust their medical dosage, help smokers give up the habit, and provide hypnotherapy. It's possible to diagnose and monitor sleep apnea using a wearable device, and there are even apps that can help people recover from traumatic brain injury.

It's still too early to be sure which solutions truly improve results – and which will work best for which patients. Neither doctors nor health care systems yet know how to choose the best approaches and make them available, Atreja says. "What we do know," he says, "is that in the future, a person's first connection to health care – finding a doctor, making an appointment, and having access to telemedicine – will be through a mobile platform."–B.S.

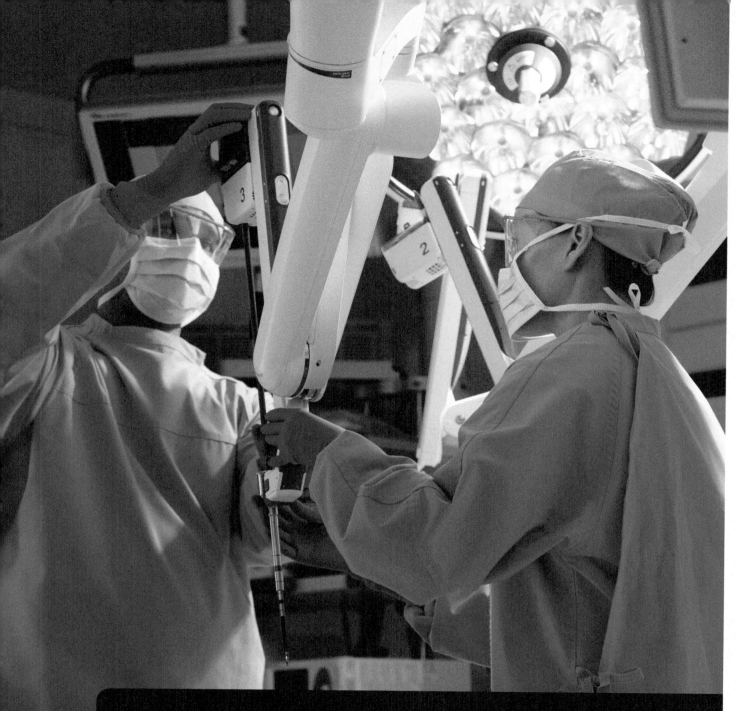

FOR SOME ELITE SOLDIERS, THIS IS A PATH TO VICTORY.

As a surgeon and officer on the U.S. Army health care team, you'll work in cutting-edge facilities boasting the latest in surgical technology, like the da Vinci robotic surgical system, which allows doctors to perform less invasive laparoscopic surgery. Thanks to our Health Professions Scholarship Program, you may also be eligible to receive full tuition assistance, plus a monthly stipend of more than $2,200. But more importantly, you'll be protecting the Army's greatest assets: Soldiers and their families.

To see the benefits of being at the forefront of Army medicine call 800-431-6691 or visit healthcare.goarmy.com/ha84

4. EXPECT A NEW RX FOR PAIN

By Lindsay Cates

Esty Gorman suffered "horrific" headaches for three years, undergoing MRI scans, epidural injections, physical therapy, massage therapy and acupuncture in search of relief. Percocet alone numbed the pain, and she "hit her lowest point" when, after being turned away from surgery, she faced a life taking pain medication – especially since her father, a doctor who suffered from chronic pain, had died after overdosing on demerol. Then, at a workshop on pain, she tried expressive writing, jotting down her stressors and then ripping the paper up. "I could feel my body relaxing," Gorman says. Although writing is not a proven treatment, within six months she was pain-free.

An estimated 100 million Americans suffer from pain, and the go-to treatment typically has been a prescription for opioids. Indeed, prescriptions for hydrocodone and oxycodone have quadrupled since 1999. Now, with drug overdose the leading cause of accidental death in the U.S., and opioid addiction driving the epidemic, medicine is aggressively turning to new approaches. Emerging trends focus on improving physical and emotional health and counseling patients to realize their own role in relieving their pain, says Bhiken Naik, an anesthesiology and neurosurgery professor at the University of Virginia Health System.

The workshop Gorman attended, led by David Hanscom, a spine surgeon at Swedish Medical Center in Seattle, explored the link between anger and anxiety and pain; she realized that her headaches had started six months after a breakup and had worsened the longer she went without answers. Centers for Disease Control and Prevention guidelines published in 2016 recommend that physicians turn to cognitive behavioral therapy, exercise and patient education first, along with nonopioid medications.

Pain specialists add that massage, physical therapy and stretching techniques, along with ultrasound therapy, heating pads, cryotherapy, and applying low-voltage electrical currents help many people. "Even a simple, regular walking regimen can greatly improve overall health and pain control," says Peter Staats, a pain specialist at Premier Pain Centers in New Jersey.

While opioids still can be a safe option, they increasingly are being used ultracautiously and as a last resort. Instead, there's a growing focus on the possibility of a psychological component to pain that needs attention. "It's a huge part of treatment," says Stephen Esper, a professor in the University of Pittsburgh Medical Center's department of anesthesiology. Because pain and certain emotions are tightly intertwined, he says, as long as anxiety and anger pathways are fired up, they will keep the pain circuits firing, too. Negative emotions can amplify the experience of pain, Staats says, and a positive outlook can ease it.

Hanscom recommends a combination of sleep, exercise, meditation and expressive writing to steer patients away from opioids or surgery. "Sleep was totally key," says Deborah Gray, 53, whose chronic neck pain has disappeared since she attended a workshop and began using guided imagery and hypnotherapy to fall asleep. At UPMC, instead of walking out with a prescription for opioids, patients might leave with a "prescription for wellness" giving a phone number for a wellness coach who might help with, say, a daily exercise routine. UVA and UPMC are both expanding their Enhanced Recovery After Surgery programs to treat surgery pain using as little opioid medication as possible. This includes combining opioids and nonopiods, getting patients on their feet immediately after surgery, and not having them fast for as long beforehand. It's all about keeping the body as functional as possible, says Jennifer Holder-Murray, a colon and rectal surgery professor at UPMC.

The latest research focuses on neuromodulation or "electroceuticals," devices smaller than a piece of spaghetti that are placed under the skin and emit electrical pulses to interrupt pain signals sent to the brain. Spinal cord stimulation is already being used to treat chronic lower back pain, but newer research is looking into more targeted approaches. Stimulating the vagus nerve through the skin in the neck, for example, can potentially ease pain from rheumatoid arthritis and headaches. Similarly, small electrodes can be strategically placed prior to knee surgery, or in the shoulder after a stroke, to greatly reduce pain. ●

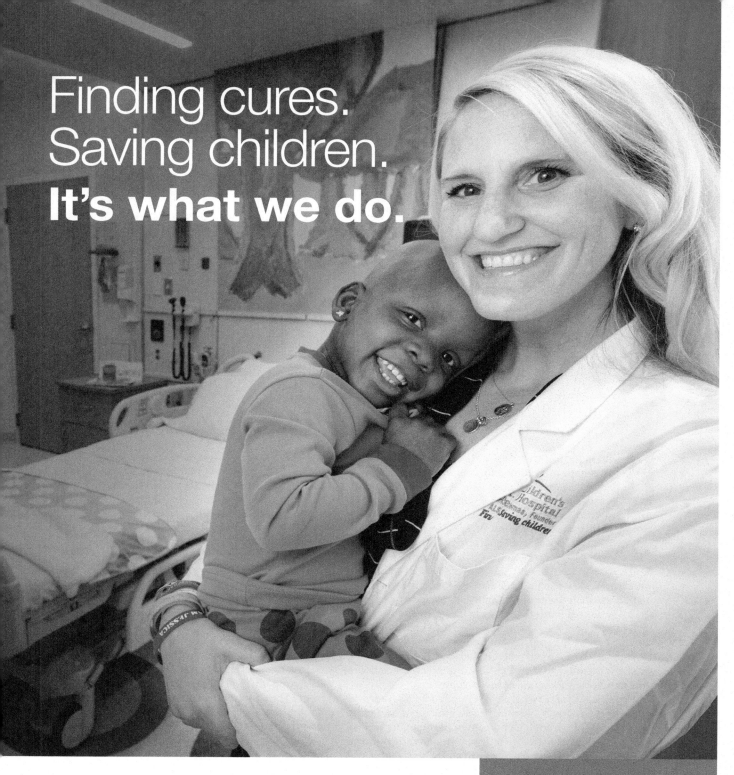

Finding cures.
Saving children.
It's what we do.

St. Jude Children's Research Hospital is dedicated to accelerating progress against childhood cancer and other life-threatening diseases through research and treatment.

At St. Jude, renowned scientists and clinicians work together to save the lives of children around the globe. We've created more clinical trials for cancer than any other children's hospital in the U.S., and we have the only National Cancer Institute–designated Comprehensive Cancer Center devoted solely to children.

Learn more at **stjude.org**.

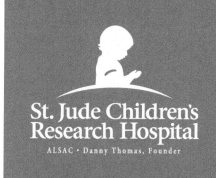

St. Jude Children's
Research Hospital
ALSAC • Danny Thomas, Founder

5. YOUR DNA WILL POINT THE WAY

By Elizabeth Gardner

Barbara Barnes is alive today because she contributed her genetic information to a research project. On her doctor's recommendation, the 58-year-old Hazleton, Pennsylvania, homemaker gave a blood sample in April 2016 to a growing biobank called the MyCode Community Health Initiative. Based at Geisinger Health System in Danville, Pennsylvania, its goal is to help health care professionals develop more targeted, effective treatments for patients. Barnes' DNA joined that of over 150,000 volunteers who are notified if genetic changes are found in their information associated with conditions that can then be treated. Geisinger alerted Barnes that she carried a gene putting her at high risk for breast and ovarian cancer. As a precaution, she decided to have her ovaries removed. Surgeons found a malignancy the size of a golf ball that had caused no symptoms. "MyCode literally saved my life," she says. Her physicians are now monitoring a suspicious breast lump.

It's not just cancer risk that MyCode can flag, says David Ledbetter, Geisinger's executive vice president and chief scientific officer. About 3.5 percent of participants receive some type of alert for 27 genetic conditions ranging from cardiomyopathy (abnormal heart muscle) to high cholesterol to malignant hypothermia (a life-threatening reaction to certain anesthesia drugs). "They all have clinically actionable options available," he says. "Doctors will treat patients more aggressively and patients will comply better with treatment when they know they have a genetic condition that puts them at high risk."

Welcome to personalized medicine, where analyzing your genome and your microbiome – the bacteria that live in and on your body – will increasingly help your doctor pinpoint optimal ways to treat your illnesses and keep you healthier. The National Institutes of Health believes that the ability to customize patient treatments can be such a game-changer that last year it launched the All of Us Research Program to pull together data from 1 million or more participants nationwide, covering their lifestyle, environment and genetics, to accelerate research into personalized disease prevention and treatment. Enrollment is scheduled to start later this year or early next. As research evolves, you can expect to see more recommendations based on your specific profile: the best strategies to treat your cancer, which drugs you should take or avoid, and which diseases you are most at risk to develop if you don't take care of yourself.

Ten years ago, full genome sequencing was an eight-figure proposition. Now it's down to four figures and still falling. Someday it will be so inexpensive as to be a routine part of every patient's care, says Keith Stewart, director of the Mayo Clinic's Center for Individualized Medicine.

The field is changing so fast that the limited genome sequencing used commonly today, which analyzes only the 1.5 percent of genetic material that has an identified function, might be inadequate in 10 years as more is understood about apparently "useless" DNA. "It might be more efficient to sequence it again the next time you have a question," Stewart says. He estimates that Mayo used genetic information to treat 12,000 patients last year. About half had cancer and the other half had rare diseases or more common ailments like high cholesterol, irritable bowel disease, and peripheral neuropathy.

Analyzing the genomes of tumors from material obtained

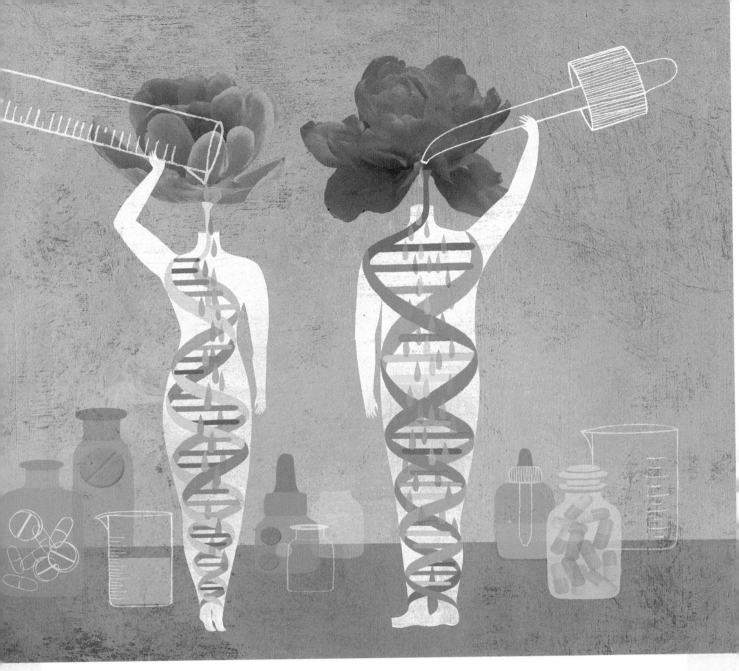

during biopsies is becoming common, because some of the new generation of targeted drugs are extremely effective against tumors with certain genetic profiles but don't work well otherwise. For example, mutations in the "EGFR" gene can dramatically affect whether a lung cancer patient will respond to several different drugs, including Tarceva and Iressa. Patients whose tumors have the right genes can benefit immensely while others can be spared time, money and debilitating treatments that can't help them. Increasingly, a tumor's genetic profile will matter more than its location in the body: In May the FDA gave its first approval to a cancer drug, Keytruda, to treat cancers based on their biomarkers rather than their location in the body.

In general, a small blood sample or cheek swab yields enough genetic material to do gene tests, and turnaround time can be as little as two days or as much as several weeks depending on what's being ordered. Costs can range from under $100 to over $2,000, according to the NIH. Since insurance coverage can vary, patients may want to check in advance with their provider if their physician recommends a genetic test. But Howard McLeod, medical director of the Personalized Medicine Institute at Moffitt Cancer Center in Tampa, Florida, notes that once a cancer treatment is known to vary in effectiveness depending on genetics, insurers may not pay for the treatment until testing has confirmed that the patient will benefit.

Now, personalized medicine is extending beyond genes to the microbiome. Researchers know that the trillions of microbes in your body – in your stomach and intestines, on your skin, in your mouth and nose – have intricate relationships with your cells and can impact the course of diseases. One initiative, the NIH's Human Microbiome Project, is currently targeting three areas: how changes in the microbiome impact the development of inflammatory bowel disease and

Type 2 diabetes, and how the mother's microbiome interacts with the baby's during pregnancy and birth. However, it may be a few years before work in the lab translates to practical applications.

For the average person, personalized medicine's most immediate benefit may be in pharmacogenomics – the study of how variations in an individual's genes affect the body's response not just to cancer drugs but also to other medications. Of the 2,000 drugs on the market, about 170 are known to differ in their effects depending on the patient's genes, says Lynn Dressler, director of personalized medicine at Mission Health in Asheville, North Carolina, one of a handful of community hospital systems in the U.S. with a formal personalized medicine program including pharmacogenomics.

About 30 noncancer drugs in that group may be ineffective or even have serious side effects for people with certain gene variations, like the anti-platelet drug Plavix, which can lead to a higher risk of heart attacks if it is not effective. The same is true of some antidepressants, anti-anxiety medications, anti-seizure drugs and painkillers. One Mission Health pa-

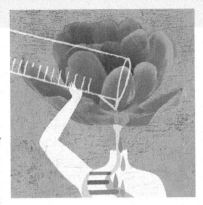

tient who did not get good pain relief after spinal fusion surgery was hesitant about another surgery until she had pharmacogenomics testing. A better option was found and her pain was greatly reduced after her second procedure.

This testing can also benefit pediatric patients. The Inova Health System in Virginia, for example, recently started giving all newborns a seven-gene test called MediMap that flags potential problems with 24 different drugs, including the narcotic painkiller codeine.

The FDA maintains a list of drugs with pharmacogenomic labeling information that can be searched on www.FDA.gov/drugs. If you've experienced significant side effects taking any of these medications or found them to be ineffective, consider asking your doctor about being tested. Mayo's Keith Stewart used this screening to discover that some of his genes render certain cholesterol drugs (and higher doses of antidepressants) potentially toxic. His cholesterol is fine, but that could change, and "having that information in my back pocket is handy." Someday it could save a lot of trial and error. ●

A PERSONAL RISK PROFILE

Discoveries surrounding the genome and microbiome are generating new businesses. Companies are offering cutting-edge tools directly to consumers for purposes ranging from predicting your risk of hereditary diseases to measuring how fast your chromosomes are aging or determining which diet and exercise regimen will help you lose weight (story, Page 87).

At least two companies offer genome and microbiome analysis as part of a personalized medicine service aimed at well-heeled healthy people who will spare no expense to stay that way. Health Nucleus, co-founded by noted biochemist and geneticist J. Craig Venter, offers a $25,000 head-to-toe "platinum" assessment that lasts eight hours and comes with comprehensive reports, follow-up consultations and an app. In May the company introduced

a more economical $7,500 service that provides full-body imaging, heart monitoring, blood tests, and whole genome sequencing, with a microbiome analysis for an extra $500. Both promise to help people assess their risk for cancer, dementia and cardiovascular disease. Arivale, founded by DNA sequencing pioneer Leroy Hood, offers a less elaborate assessment and coaching program aimed at goals like weight loss or "optimal aging" for $3,500. Tests include analysis of specific genes, gut microbiome, and blood and saliva.

The potential benefits of these services are clear. In a recent article, Hood wrote, "In this brave new world of heath care, we will be able to identify the earliest markers of disease and reverse them before the disease can develop."

Still, consumers need to do their homework. The FDA has sent warning letters to makers of genetic testing products who market to consumers without completing the agency's required review process for tests that promise a clinical benefit. The testing company 23andMe received such a warning in 2013; in April it won agency authorization for its Genetic Health Risk direct-to-consumer test that identifies predispositions to certain diseases including Parkinson's and late-onset Alzheimer's disease.

Comprehensive screening can have downsides, of course. If a test finds a possible cancer risk, say, the patient may have a biopsy for something that would never have caused trouble, notes oncologist John Deeken of Virginia's Inova Health System. Still, Deeken says, "If these tests are done well and patients are fully informed of what the results might mean, I think they will be part of the future." –E.G.

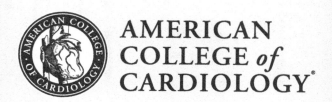

THE HEART OF QUALITY PATIENT CARE

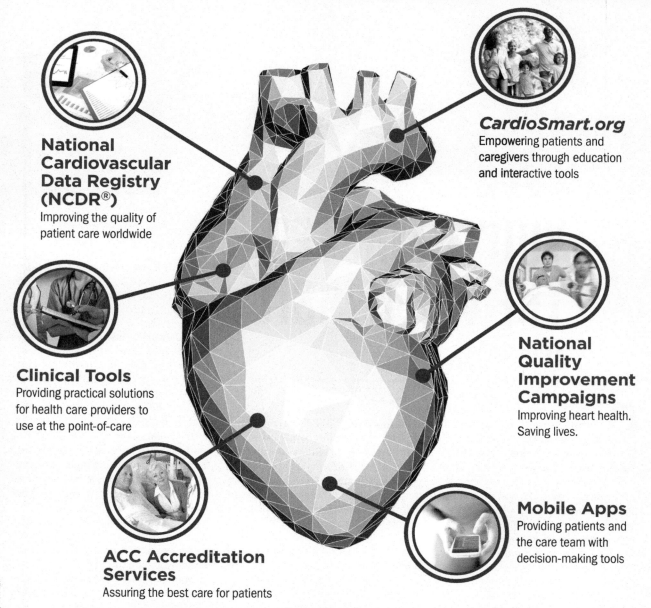

National Cardiovascular Data Registry (NCDR®)
Improving the quality of patient care worldwide

Clinical Tools
Providing practical solutions for health care providers to use at the point-of-care

ACC Accreditation Services
Assuring the best care for patients

CardioSmart.org
Empowering patients and caregivers through education and interactive tools

National Quality Improvement Campaigns
Improving heart health. Saving lives.

Mobile Apps
Providing patients and the care team with decision-making tools

The American College of Cardiology is committed to supporting patients and health care providers by ensuring the right care is delivered to the right patient, every time. Visit **CVQuality.ACC.org** to learn more about the American College of Cardiology's Quality Improvement for Institutions program.

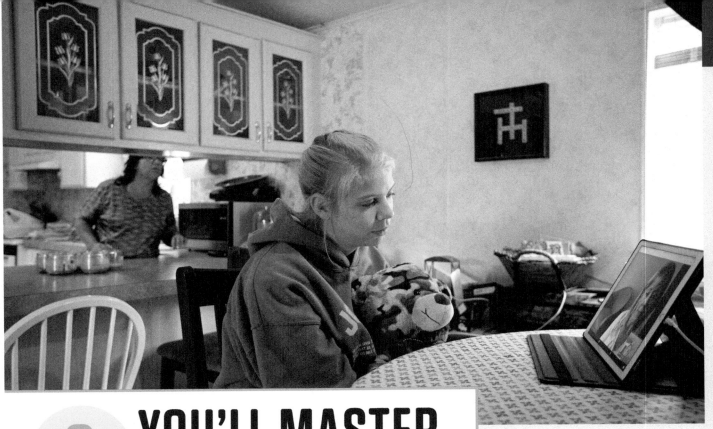

6. YOU'LL MASTER THE VIDEO VISIT

By Elizabeth Gardner

Savanna Edwards has been visiting Nemours Children's Hospital in Orlando three to four times a year to treat her arthritis and amplified pain disorder. Her hometown 200 miles away lacks the specialized services she requires, which include help from a psychologist to manage the pain. Edwards, 16, has been able to get that support twice a month courtesy of Nemours' telehealth service. "It took a little doing" to get their insurer to cover the visits, says her mother, Leslie, but the treatment has "done wonders" for Savanna, who participates in dance and leads an active life. She still travels to the pain clinic twice a year.

"Video visits are the future," says Peter Rasmussen, a neurosurgeon and medical director of distance health at the Cleveland Clinic, whose physicians will conduct up to 40,000 telehealth

visits this year. While the technology is used for many different purposes – urgent care, remote patient monitoring, and routine check-ins on homebound patients, to name a few – it holds particular promise for making the expertise at top medical centers available to people at a distance.

Rasmussen, for example, uses the service routinely to see new patients and people seeking second opinions, as long as he can access their current radiology images if needed. (One exception is headache patients, who still require an initial assessment in person.) Doctors also now do post-surgery checks remotely, a big boon for patients from around the world who used to have to return to Cleveland for the 10-minute follow-ups.

Similarly, New York-Presbyterian

started offering telehealth services last year through its 10 New York City hospitals and has already racked up more than 2,800 encounters. "Not everyone can fight their way into Manhattan to see our world-class physicians," says Daniel Barchi, chief information officer. "And for our existing patients, what's so special about a 10-minute office visit that you have to take half a day off and spend an hour in transit, and then pay for parking?"

The technology also allows NYP to share resources. Most hospitals lack 24/7 psychiatrist coverage, for example, and NYP patients have sometimes waited up to 24 hours in the emergency room to be seen. Now, they can see a psychiatrist via telehealth within two hours on average; emergency psych visits account for 20 percent of the system's telehealth visits.

Many insurers now cover remote visits, says Roy Schoenberg, CEO of American Well, a provider of telehealth services that offers visits to its

▲
Savanna Edwards "meets" twice a month with psychologist Beth Long of Nemours Children's Hospital.

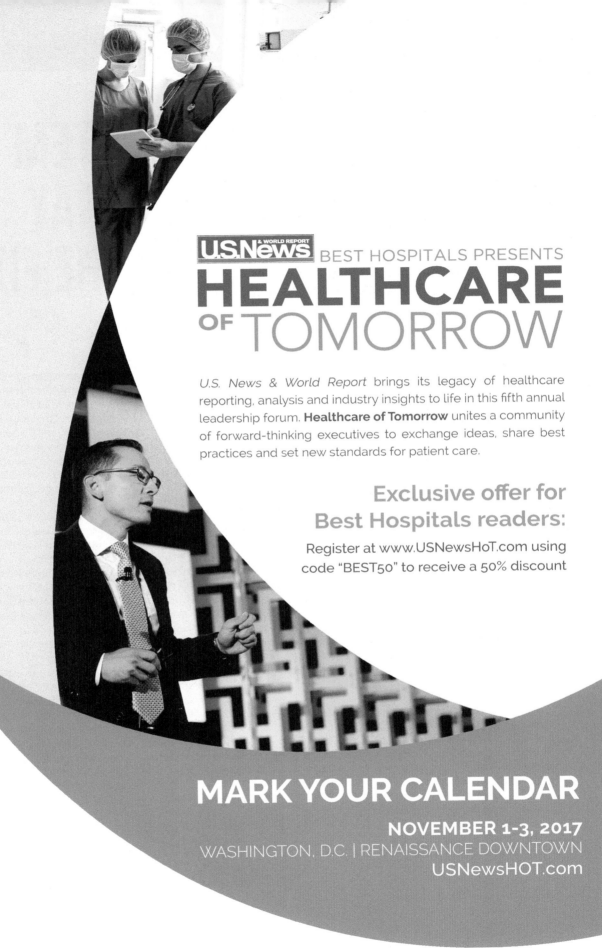

U.S. News & WORLD REPORT BEST HOSPITALS PRESENTS

HEALTHCARE
OF TOMORROW

U.S. News & World Report brings its legacy of healthcare reporting, analysis and industry insights to life in this fifth annual leadership forum. **Healthcare of Tomorrow** unites a community of forward-thinking executives to exchange ideas, share best practices and set new standards for patient care.

Exclusive offer for Best Hospitals readers:

Register at www.USNewsHoT.com using code "BEST50" to receive a 50% discount

MARK YOUR CALENDAR

NOVEMBER 1-3, 2017
WASHINGTON, D.C. | RENAISSANCE DOWNTOWN
USNewsHOT.com

own staff of physicians and also provides a platform for use by other providers, including the Cleveland Clinic, Nemours and New York-Presbyterian. "Three years ago it was a luxury," he notes, "but it's now grown to the point where if you're a payer and not covering telehealth, you risk losing customers." Schoenberg says 85 million people have access to American Well services through more than 40 insurers. Other telehealth providers include Teladoc, Doctor on Demand, and MDLIVE.

Patients without coverage sometimes choose to pay out of pocket because they save so much on travel. New York-Presbyterian charges $99 for an urgent care visit and $800 for a second opinion from one of its specialists, which includes a full review of the patient's records and a detailed report.

Telehealth is a particular blessing for children, says Shayan Vyas, medical director for telehealth at Nemours, because it expands the availability of scarce specialists like Richard Finkel, an expert in pediatric spinal muscle atrophy. The crippling condition leads to early death, and families have relocated to Orlando to have access to his expertise, Vyas says. "For them to be able to see him from anywhere without even getting in the car is amazing."

Finkel uses telehealth to pre-screen patients for clinical trials and other treatments, saving them a long – and potentially wasted – trip. The news was good for Camille Callais, 3, who qualifies to receive a new drug that slows the disease. The family will have to make the 640-mile trip from Mandeville, Louisiana, several times a year for the injections. But dad Brandon has been able to consult with Finkel from home to discuss Camille's care. ●

7. YOUR STEM CELLS MAY HOLD THE FIX

By Stacey Colino

Believe it or not, the cure to what ails you could already be inside you. Welcome to the dawning world of stem cell therapy, in which researchers are exploring the possibilities of growing new body parts and healing old ones by using patients' own stem cells. The idea is that these unspecialized cells (which can also be harvested from a donor) can be induced to develop into heart or lung or brain cells, say, and be injected to replace those damaged by disease or injury. While bone marrow stem cell therapies for certain cancers date back several decades, the approach is now being used or studied for a wide array of diseases and injuries.

"Stem cells could be the new antibiotics," says Joshua Hare, director of the Interdisciplinary Stem Cell Institute at the University of Miami Miller School of Medicine. "When you put the pieces of the puzzle together, stem cells could touch just about every area of medicine."

For the record: The cells Hare is talking about are not taken from embryos, a practice mired in controversy. They come from an adult's body tissue, usually the bone marrow, fat or skin. These "master cells" operate as a kind of internal repair system because they can replicate in a continuous fashion to replenish other cells or morph into cells with specialized functions.

Recently, headlines have cast a shadow over stem cell therapy by drawing attention to private clinics offering unproven interventions – and sometimes unfortunate outcomes. For example, an article in the New England Journal of Medicine this spring described three women who experienced vision loss after injections of stem cells derived from their fat tissue for age-related macular degeneration. At this point, most stem cell therapies are experimental, and patients should be looking for rigorous research. But "if you take stem cells from a patient and re-inject them back into the patient, there's no regulation of that," explains Donald Zack, director of the Johns Hopkins Center for Stem Cell and Ocular Regenerative Medicine, which is preparing to test whether

Stem cells could touch just about every area of medicine.

such therapies can treat conditions like glaucoma, macular degeneration and retinitis pigmentosa.

Among the most established therapies to date are those for musculoskeletal problems such as arthritis of the knees, hips and shoulders; meniscus tears; and Achilles tendonitis. Stem cells from a patient's bone marrow or belly fat are injected into an injured joint in an outpatient procedure that lasts about 45 minutes. "It's not a panacea, but it offers another opportunity to delay a joint replacement," says Laith Jazrawi, chief of the division of sports medicine at NYU Langone Medical Center. Delay is good "because there's a longevity issue with joint replacement."

"I didn't want that type of surgery," says Mike Barnet, 62, an avid cyclist and squash player from Margate, New Jersey, who'd been advised to have both knees replaced for bone-on-bone arthritis and a torn meniscus in his right one. He contacted Jazrawi, and a few weeks after an injection into his right knee of stem cells from his pelvic bone, the knee was free of pain and swelling. That was two and a half years ago. "I might need a knee replacement down the road," says Barnet, "but I'm hoping that this will be a long-term fix."

At the Cleveland Clinic, researchers are conducting trials to see if stem cells can address stress urinary incontinence. "We're trying to regenerate the muscle cells, so the sphincter muscle can close and prevent leakage," explains Courtenay Moore, a physician at the Clinic's Glickman Urological Institute. Early findings have shown that after a single injection into the urethra, over two-thirds of women improved by more than 50 percent, compared to a 75 to 80 percent cure rate for surgery. "Three of the women I've injected run on the treadmill at my gym," Moore reports. "And they run faster than me!"

Precisely how stem cell therapies work is still being uncovered. What's emerging is a realization that "they teach the body to heal from within," explains Atta Behfar, a cardiologist and director of the cardiac regenerative medicine program at the Mayo Clinic. Stem cells delivered into a heart injured by a heart attack don't "serve as the brick and mortar to repair the heart," he says. "It's the proteins and other substances they secrete that tell your body to heal."

Research on stroke, for example, has suggested that when stem cells are injected into the brain, they set off a release of factors that contribute to the recovery process, notes Lawrence Wechsler, chairman of the department of neurology at the University of Pittsburgh School of Medicine. (Mayo Clinic researchers in Florida are investigating whether the healing power might extend to brain cancer. In rodents, the effects of stem cells range from a shrinking of the tumors to complete remission. This is noteworthy because few drugs can cross the blood-brain barrier. Stem cells injected into the carotid artery get through, "act as Trojan horses and begin to kill cancer cells," says Alfredo Quinones-Hinojosa, chair of neurosurgery and director of Mayo Clinic's Brain Tumor Stem Cell Research Laboratory in Jacksonville.)

Not surprisingly, results aren't always dramatic. That was the case for Kate Brock of Gambrills, Maryland, 57, whose 2010 stroke left her right side semiparalyzed. In 2013, she had stem cells injected into her brain at Pittsburgh. She gained mobility and strength in her arm, but it didn't last. "The only thing that really changed a lot," says Brock, is that "my legs work better together."

Besides targeted injections, intravenous infusion of stem cells from a healthy donor is being studied as a way to deal with the frailty associated with aging. Preliminary findings from the University of Miami indicate that the therapy

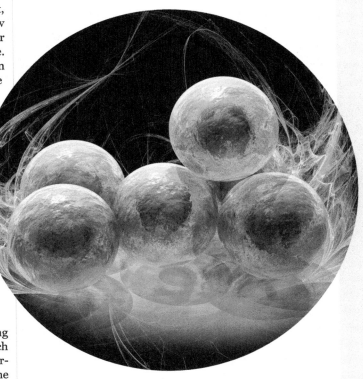

significantly reduces systemic inflammation, improves immune function, and boosts physical performance. "Look, I don't want to exaggerate these effects – I can't leap over buildings," says Phillip George, a retired plastic surgeon whose aches and pains, especially after playing golf, led him to participate in the frailty program. "But I have more energy and I feel much more comfortable." Six weeks after treatment, he performed dramatically better on pulmonary function tests and increased his distance on a six-minute walking test. His need for anti-inflammatory drugs is down by 90 percent.

With the field still developing, it's vital that people investigate a treatment's safety and efficacy for their condition. "There's a lot of excitement about stem cells," says Zack, "but we have to do this in a smart way." What that means, he says, is that a treatment should be based on science, not simply hope or beliefs. ●

8.

T CELLS TAKE ON CANCER

By Linda Childers

When cancer patients first meet Joshua Brody, director of the lymphoma immunotherapy program at the Icahn School of Medicine at Mount Sinai Hospital in New York, one of the first things they ask about is "the Jimmy Carter cure."

For those diagnosed with an advanced cancer, former President Carter's story is nothing short of a bombshell. When Carter announced in August 2015 that he had melanoma that had spread to his liver and brain, the prognosis seemed grim. Yet seven months later, he revealed that his treatment in Atlanta – a drug called Keytruda designed to rally the body's immune response rather than attack the cells directly, as chemotherapy does – had sent him into remission. "Immunotherapy is one of the greatest advances in cancer treatment in the last 40 years," says Brody.

The push is on to take full advantage. In the last seven years, immunotherapy drugs have been approved for melanoma, lung cancer, head and neck cancer, Hodgkin's lymphoma, and kidney and bladder cancer. In May, the Food and Drug Administration extended Keytruda's approval, OK'ing it to treat cancers of various types that share a certain genetic glitch that seems to make them vulnerable to the drug. Some 500 open immunotherapy trials are listed currently on clinicaltrials.gov, and an estimate last year by the Parker Institute for Cancer Immunotherapy in San Francisco put the number of drugs in the research pipeline at more than 1,500.

How do the new drugs work? The earliest to receive FDA approval, which also include Yervoy for metastatic melanoma, Opdivo for several cancers, and Tecentriq for bladder cancer, work by targeting proteins that normally interfere with immune function. The immune system has mechanisms, or "checkpoints," that prevent it from attacking the body's own cells; the checkpoints "act much like the brakes on a car," explains Brody. The drugs, known as checkpoint inhibitors, release the brakes, so to speak. Another promising approach helps the immune system recognize cancer cells and destroy them. Vaccines hold promise to both treat and prevent cancer. Gardasil, for instance, protects against cervical cancer by spurring the body to fight off HPV infections.

"I was told the type of cancer I had was incurable and that chemo wouldn't prolong my life," says Sergei German of Queens, New York, who learned four years ago that a lump in his neck was follicular lymphoma. German came to Mount Sinai to see if he could enter a trial Brody was leading to test whether administering two immune stimulants into a patient's tumor, combined with radiotherapy, could lead to tumor regression.

Elated to find that he qualified, German began coming in daily for two weeks for injections of immune stimulants directly into his tumor. The idea: Awaken his immune system to the cancer cells at the site and in effect teach his system to recognize and kill cancer cells in other parts of his body. He also had low-dose radiotherapy. His tumors began shrinking, and a month after the treatment ended, German found out he was in remission. Unlike traditional chemotherapy and radiation, which often result in patients becoming ill or losing their hair, German's treatment caused no side effects other than several slight fevers. That was it. Today, at 57, he comes in for a checkup every four months and says he feels great.

On the other hand, immunotherapy has a rather large downside: It doesn't work for most people, and researchers aren't sure why. In the case of the drug for advanced bladder cancer approved by the FDA last year, just 15 percent of people were helped in clinical trials; several immunotherapies

> ❝ ---
> ## Immunotherapy is one of the greatest advances in cancer treatment.

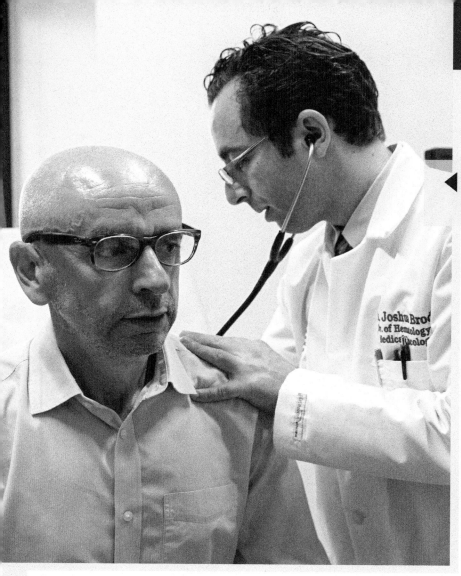

have been approved in recent months based on tumors shrinking in 15 to 25 percent of recipients. Still, doctors say, when treatment does work, the results are often dramatic, with remissions lasting years in people who otherwise would have had weeks or months to live.

"I have one patient with stage 4 bladder cancer, and through the use of combined immunotherapies, he has no detectable signs of cancer," says Matthew Galsky, a professor of medicine and director of genitourinary medical oncology at Mount Sinai.

In addition to checkpoint inhibitors,

a type of immunotherapy showing promise is chimeric antigen receptor T-cell therapy, in which T cells, a key part of the immune system, are genetically modified in the lab to target the person's specific cancer. "CAR T-cell therapy involves engineering patients'

own immune cells to recognize and attack their tumors," says Carl June, director of translational research and a professor of pathology and laboratory medicine in the Perelman School of Medicine and the Abramson Cancer Center of the University of Pennsylvania. The cells are extracted from the blood, then "genetically engineered and multiplied in a lab before being put back into a patient's bloodstream, where they work as hunters to destroy cancer cells."

The hope, June says, is that the patient's system will gain a lasting ability to fight the cancer. Though a few people have died from cerebral edema after treatment, halting one CAR T-cell trial at another institution, the first such therapy to come up for approval, developed by the Penn team with Novartis, got the nod from an FDA advisory panel in July. In 2014, Novartis announced that 27 of 30 patients with

acute lymphoblastic leukemia who had not responded to traditional chemotherapy were in remission after treatment, and subsequent results have been similarly encouraging.

At Duke University, Matthias Gromeier and his colleagues have developed a way to battle brain cancer that involves treating the tumor with an engineered poliovirus to activate the immune system. In the spring of last year, the approach received the FDA's "breakthrough therapy designation," which will facilitate development and review. Early clinical trials of the therapy have found a 20 percent three-year survival rate in people with glioblastoma, compared to a historical 4 percent survival rate.

As was true for German, who was able to manage his treatment-related fevers with over-the-counter medications, immunotherapy drugs often are well tolerated. But some patients do experience troubling or dangerous side effects such as colitis, skin rashes and endocrine disorders including thyroid abnormalities and adrenal insufficiency. One recent study found that 30 percent of patients experienced "interesting, rare or unexpected" side effects, with a quarter of the reactions described as severe, life-threatening or requiring hospitalization. This summer the FDA paused three trials of Keytruda combined with other drugs for multiple myeloma, given a worrisome number of deaths. Commonly, though, reactions can be controlled with corticosteroids and antihistamines that tame the inflammatory reaction, experts say.

Despite the currently low response rate, immunotherapy is the future of cancer treatment, June predicts. "We're at the beginning stages," he says, "similar to where Microsoft was when they released Windows 1.0." ●

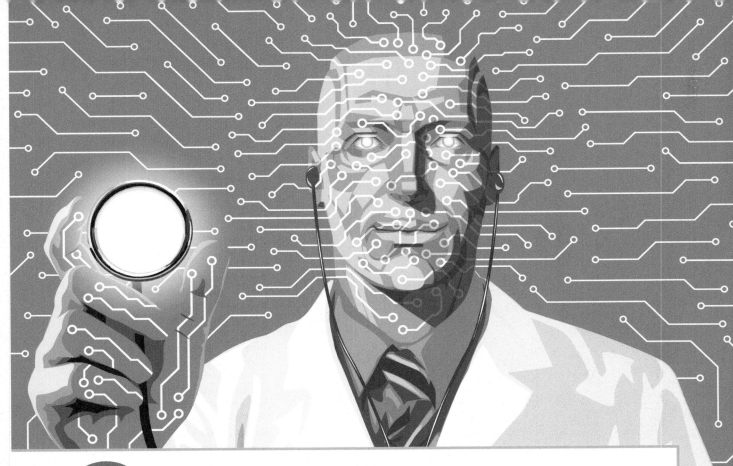

9. A SMART COMPUTER WILL "TREAT" YOU

By Arlene Weintraub

Just six months after El Camino Hospital in Silicon Valley implemented artificial intelligence technology, the rate at which patients suffered dangerous falls dropped 39 percent. The key, alongside additional fall prevention strategies, was a software program that predicts which individuals are most likely to fall by combing over electronic health records for risk factors and merging the data discovered there with real-time tracking of patients.

"Every time a patient pushes a call light or hits a bathroom or bed alarm, it's recorded," says Cheryl Reinking, chief nursing officer at El Camino. The software takes that information and compares the rate at which a patient is requesting assistance to data such as what surgeries he's had or which medications have been prescribed.

These data are all processed through "machine learning" – a form of artificial intelligence whereby computers take in new information and perform tasks based on it without being reprogrammed to do so. In this case, the program "learns" if a person may be more likely to fall based on his behavior and treatments. "Then it pushes an alert to the nurse saying 'your patient in room 2308 is at risk right now for falling,'" Reinking says, after which that individual might be moved closer to the nursing station or monitored via video.

The ability of computer systems to assume tasks for humans has improved efficiency in virtually every industry, from manufacturing to transportation. Now hospitals are getting into the game, deploying AI to take on challenges from diagnosing patients more quickly in the emergency room and streamlining communication between doctors to lessening the risk of complications so patients can go home sooner – and avoid being readmitted. One big way in which patients will benefit directly is in AI's ability to help clinicians make diagnoses. IBM brought AI into the mainstream of medical care a few years back, when it offered its "Jeopardy!"-winning system Watson to cancer centers to help oncologists determine the best treatments for patients. Physicians can now plug patient diagnoses into IBM's Watson for Oncology and instantly receive treatment recommendations based on patient data and information pulled from reams of medical journal articles.

Since Watson's initial baby steps, AI has quickly demonstrated its potential to be a game-changer in many areas of health care. Other technology developers, for example, are focusing on software that can read CT scans and other medical images and then suggest the most likely diagnosis by reviewing similar images stored in patient databases. And these programs can accurately process these tasks far faster than human technicians. AI's potential is so promising that some experts predict it will eventually be every doctor's and nurse's go-to assistant.

James Shoemaker, a physician with Elkhart Emergency Physicians in Elkhart, Indiana, can attest to its value. Shoemaker uses a program called VisualDx, which allows him to input medical images along with patient symptoms and immediately pull up a list of possible diagnoses. One parent brought in a child with a bad rash that turned out to be a rare disorder called Stevens-Johnson syndrome, he recalls. "I had an idea it could be that," Shoemaker says. The program "reinforced my diagnosis and helped me figure out the next step."

New York University's Langone Medical Center is developing one AI system to predict which patients are likely to develop the dangerous condition sepsis and another that alerts doctors to cases of heart trouble. "If you're admitted to the ER for pneumonia, the people who are treating you may not think about the fact that you also have congestive heart failure," says Michael Cantor, an internist and associate professor in the hospital's departments of population health and medicine. The system will go through each patient's record when they're admitted and automatically alert cardiologists to anyone who has heart failure, so they can advise on how to avoid treatments that might exacerbate that condition.

Artificial intelligence is also being employed to improve efficiencies. Several hospitals are experimenting with

technology to optimize schedules for surgeries and imaging tests by predicting how long each procedure that's scheduled in a particular day will take. Partners HealthCare, which includes Brigham and Women's and Massachusetts General hospitals in Boston, announced in May that it will work with General Electric over the next 10 years to incorporate AI into virtually every area of patient care, including developing applications to cut down on unnecessary biopsies and streamline administrative tasks for doctors.

These are all tasks that people traditionally do, but sometimes machines do them better, says Michael Williams, president of the University of

son said the organization is constantly reviewing technologies that promise to improve cancer prevention and patient care, and that "while a variety of approaches have been examined, a final approach using this technology to benefit patients has not been determined at this time."

Rob Merkel, general manager of oncology and genomics for Watson Health, says the company is making headway in the market with Watson for Oncology, which IBM developed with Memorial Sloan Kettering Cancer Center in New York. And he cites research the firm did with MD Anderson that he believes shows Watson's potential. "We demonstrated 95 percent con-

AI has quickly demonstrated its potential to be a game-changer.

North Texas Health Science Center. "Reducing ER wait times, improving surgical workflows – those are key to improving the patient experience, and AI has a real role to play."

If there's anything that's holding back the widespread adoption of AI in hospitals, it's nagging doubts that the technology will produce a good return on investment. A 2017 survey by HIMSS Analytics and Healthcare IT News found that 35 percent of health care organizations plan to adopt AI within two years, but 15 percent of respondents said they couldn't make a business case for doing so. And more than 20 percent said they thought the technology was still underdeveloped.

The field of AI in health care suffered a setback in February, when the University of Texas MD Anderson Cancer Center put its partnership with IBM on hold after an internal audit reported that the institution's effort to incorporate Watson into patient care ultimately failed to meet its goal. In an email, a spokeswoman for MD Ander-

cordance with what Watson would recommend as a treatment option versus what an MD Anderson physician would recommend," he says.

Meanwhile, the University of Pittsburgh Medical Center is funding a project aimed at using AI to get treatment ideas for individual cancer patients by comparing genomic information from their tumors to molecular data housed in the Cancer Genome Atlas – an interactive database maintained by the National Institutes of Health containing data on 10,000 tumor samples of 33 cancer types.

So could AI someday even substitute for doctors? Peter Slavin, president of Mass General, believes people will always be essential to delivering high-quality care – but that machines will become increasingly vital to making that care better. Improvements in computing power and the ability of computer programs to emulate neural networks in the brain unlock enormous possibilities for the use of AI in medicine, Slavin says. "We haven't really even begun to see its impact." ●

10. A HOTTER CLIMATE COULD MAKE YOU SICK

By Beth Howard

Leaving aside the debate over who or what is to blame, 16 of the 17 hottest years on record have occurred since 2001 – and 2016 was the hottest ever. While the consequences of melting ice caps or vanishing species may seem remote, the health effects of a warming planet are already being felt, experts warn. The Centers for Disease Control and Prevention launched a Climate and Health Program in 2009 to address the issue, although its future is uncertain. A CDC conference on the subject that had been scheduled for this past January was cancelled before the inauguration of President Donald Trump.

The growing menace of mosquito-borne infections like last year's Zika outbreak, skyrocketing rates of allergies and asthma, and illness and deaths from heat waves and catastrophic "superstorms" are a few of the ways that climate change wreaks havoc. "There are so many pathways through which climate affects health that when you add them all up, I view this as the greatest environmental public health crisis of our times," says Jonathan Patz, professor of environ-mental public health at the University of Wisconsin–Madison and director of its Global Health Institute. These are some of the health effects physicians and scientists are most worried about:

Air quality

Studies have shown that the changing climate has altered weather patterns, which in turn are changing the location and concentrations of ground-level ozone and fine particulate matter from vehicle exhaust and industrial pollution. Result: a greater risk of cancer and of worsening respiratory ailments like chronic obstructive pulmonary disease and asthma. Some particulates can pass into the bloodstream and raise the potential for heart attacks and strokes. In addition, "pollutants can have harmful effects on other parts of the body, affecting pregnancy, child development and the central nervous system," says Janice Nolen, assistant vice president of national policy for the American Lung Association. According to the ALA, 4 in 10 Americans now live in counties that have unhealthy levels of ozone or particle pollution.

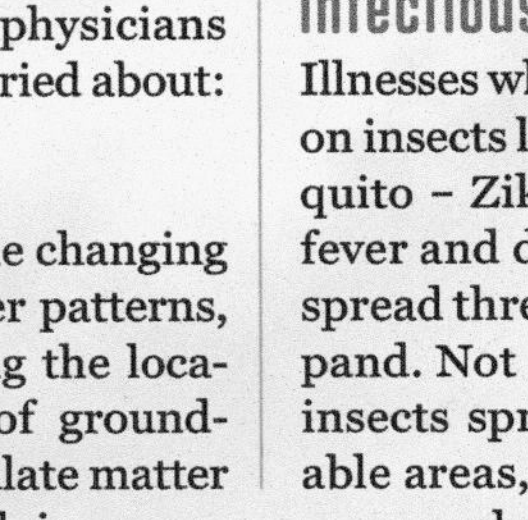

What's more, says Patz, warmer temperatures plus more carbon dioxide in the air lead to an increase in ragweed pollen, which is dangerous for asthmatics. Research from the University of Massachusetts–Amherst shows that plants growing in an environment with high levels of CO_2 boost pollen levels by 50 percent. And an Italian study of 12 European cities found that for every degree Celsius the temperature jumped (about 2 degrees Fahrenheit), hospitalizations from respiratory- and asthma-related illnesses in the elderly rose by 4.5 percent.

Infectious diseases

Illnesses whose transmission depends on insects like the Aedes aegypti mosquito – Zika virus, as well as yellow fever and dengue – are a more widespread threat as warmer latitudes expand. Not only does the reach of the insects spread into once uninhabitable areas, but also the reproductive cycle accelerates so that more mosquitoes are born each year. In addition, the incubation period of the virus inside the insects shortens, and when mosquitoes bite they are more likely to be infectious. As a result of the Zika virus, a new CDC report shows, pregnant women who are infected are having babies with birth defects at a rate 20 times higher than during the pre-Zika years. National Institutes of Health scientists are racing to test vaccines against the viral illness along with effective ways to eradicate mosquitoes, while health officials in

Florida and the Gulf Coast brace for more cases. It's not just mosquitoes: Ticks responsible for transmitting Lyme disease and other harmful microbes have also expanded their range. Long term, scientists expect warmer temperatures to lead to the emergence of new pathogens.

Heat waves and extreme weather events

When heat spikes to the high 90s and into the triple digits, people who work outside and vulnerable populations – children, the elderly, those battling chronic illnesses – are at heightened risk of heat stroke and even heart attack and death in many cases. Extreme heat also exacerbates chronic conditions like asthma, heart disease, respiratory illnesses and diabetes. Over 700 people died during a 1995 Chicago summer heat wave, and scientists believe more such deaths can be expected in coming years. A recent analysis in the journal Nature Climate Change predicts that Persian Gulf cities will be too hot for humans to live in by the end of the century.

Changing weather patterns also cause more tornadoes, hurricanes, floods and serious droughts. Beyond the obvious danger of injuries and drownings, the disruption and displacement caused by these events can result in long-lasting psychological trauma. A 2015 study of more than 100,000 New Jersey residents who had experienced significant damage to their homes in the wake of 2012's Superstorm Sandy found that 30 months after the storm, 27 percent were still experiencing moderate to severe mental health distress and 14 percent reported symptoms suggestive of post-traumatic stress disorder. "You can't call these severe climate events acts of God anymore," says Patz. "They can be attributed to greenhouse gases that we are emitting into the atmosphere."

Food production and nutrition

A warming planet might seem to be a plus for growing foods, but the stress on plants from heat actually decreases crop yields and quality. "There are 15 different mechanisms by which climate change can hurt food production, from the impact of carbon dioxide on the growth of plants to changes in the actual nutrient content," says Samuel Myers, a senior research scientist in environmental health at the Harvard T.H. Chan School of Public Health and director of the Planetary Health Alliance, a consortium of universities and other groups focused on research and policy surrounding health and the changing environment. Myer's research on foods grown at levels of carbon dioxide expected by 2050 found that staples like grains and legumes lost significant nutritional value. Population-wide deficiencies in zinc and iron, for example, would likely increase the incidence of infectious disease and of maternal and neonatal deaths, respectively, he says.

Despite these threats, many scientists remain hopeful. The new administration's skeptical positions on climate change notwithstanding, many cities and states are forging ahead with plans to go greener. Around 30 states now have established standards requiring power companies to boost their reliance on renewable energy sources, and scores of cities have committed to reducing their carbon footprint. But recognizing the climate challenge as a health crisis may have an even more powerful impact. Says Patz: "People always care about their health and the health of their children." ●

THE HOSPITAL EFFECT

Last year, a Yale University study showed that greenhouse gases emitted from hospitals and health systems accounted for almost 10 percent of the national total. At the same time, medical incinerators spew out harmful chemicals like dioxin due to the PVC plastic in many medical products. "Of all people who should understand the connection between health and climate, it should be the health care community," says Gary Cohen, co-founder and president of Health Care Without Harm, a group focused on making the industry environmentally sustainable.

There are encouraging signs. Through the Healthy Hospitals Initiative, some 1,400 systems have pledged to reduce energy use and waste and choose less toxic products. One standout: Gundersen Health System in Wisconsin, which offsets its fossil fuel use by producing clean energy locally through a subsidiary, using wind and solar power, for example, and converting manure into fuel. –B.H.

Matched with a Stranger

Four Chicago-area residents needed kidney transplants but did not have matching donors. At Northwestern Memorial Hospital, they got the organs they required from willing strangers through a kidney transplant chain.

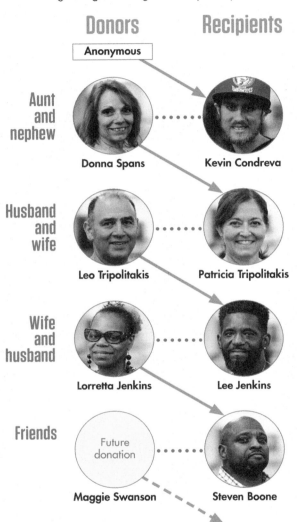

Donors   **Recipients**

Anonymous

Aunt and nephew
Donna Spans — Kevin Condreva

Husband and wife
Leo Tripolitakis — Patricia Tripolitakis

Wife and husband
Lorretta Jenkins — Lee Jenkins

Friends
Maggie Swanson — Steven Boone
Future donation

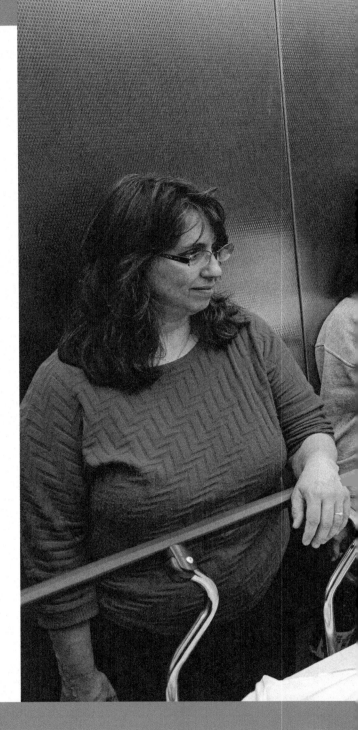

A LIFESAVING

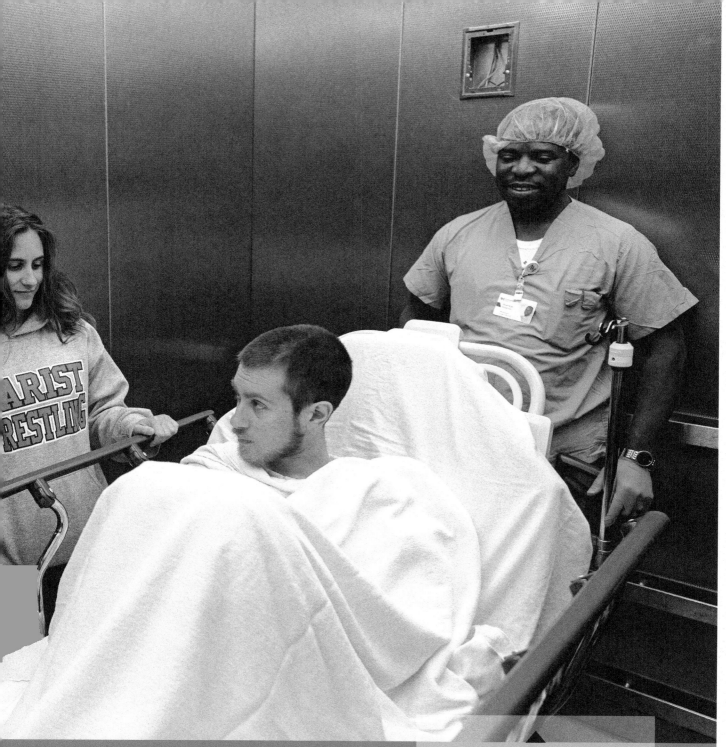

CHAIN

U.S. News sits in as surgeons carry out an eight-person kidney exchange

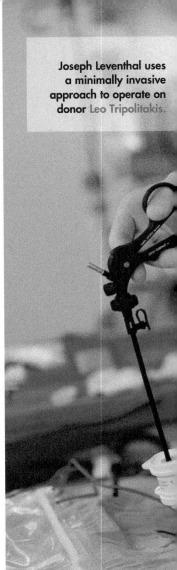

By Michael Morella

CHICAGO – Today, Kevin Condreva will receive a new kidney at Northwestern Memorial Hospital. All told, his transplant will involve surgery on eight people.

Condreva, 22, and his aunt, Donna Spans, 63, are two links in a transplant "chain" that by the end of the day tomorrow will give a new lease on life to four people from the Chicago area. Condreva is actually undergoing his second transplant; he was just 15 when he first noticed blood in his urine and was diagnosed with IgA nephropathy, a common kidney disease that damages the organ's ability to filter waste from the blood. When he was 17, his mom was his donor, but the disease came back. That kidney failed, too.

Now Spans, who is not a match for her nephew, is preparing for surgery here as well – ready to trade one of her kidneys to a stranger so that Condreva can receive one from another stranger and be freed from nightly dialysis. She and the other members of the group won't know who donates to whom as they head into surgery, but Spans' kidney will go to Patricia Tripolitakis, 51, who has polycystic kidney disease. Her husband, Leo, 51, is donating to Lee Jenkins, 53, whose wife, Lorretta, 46, is giving a kidney to Steven Boone, 46. Condreva's donor, a good Samaritan who prefers to remain anonymous, turned up as a match for him just a few weeks ago and set the chain in motion. Later this year, Maggie Swanson, a friend of

Photography by Brett Ziegler

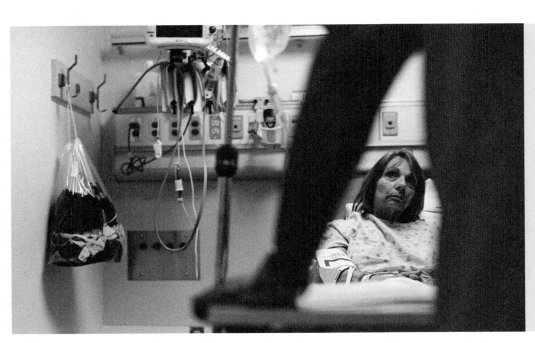

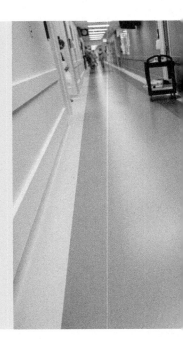

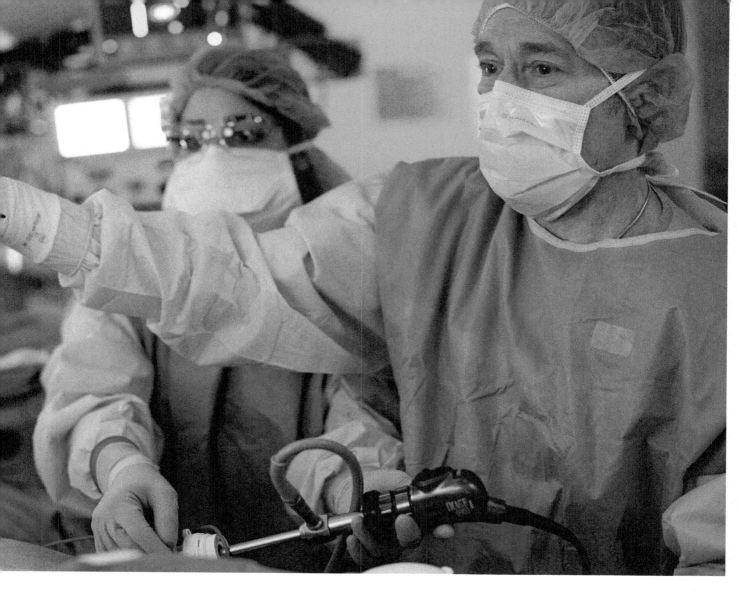

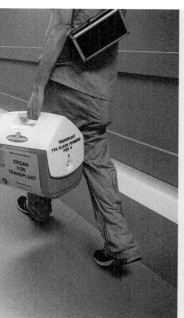

Surgery Starts

▶ **Donna Spans** (far left) preps for surgery. The nurse from Tinley Park, Illinois, is giving up a kidney so her nephew can be healthy and end his nightly dialysis. Her kidney is transported to the blood bank for testing before going to **Patricia Tripolitakis,** Leo's wife and a real estate broker from Homer Glen. "I call them all heroes, all these donors," Patricia says.

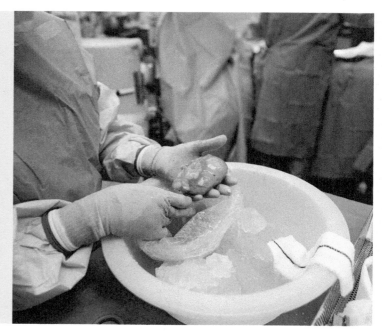

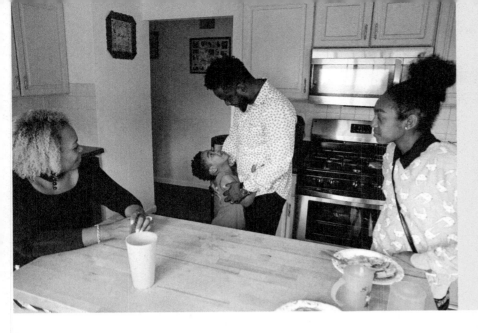

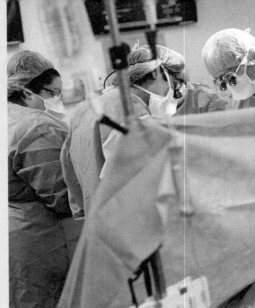

Boone's who wanted to help him but wasn't a match, will donate a kidney to someone else in need – potentially starting a new chain.

Such "paired exchanges," first performed in the U.S. at Rhode Island Hospital in 2000, have taken off in the last seven years or so as a way to shorten what can otherwise be a long wait for a healthy kidney. Some 97,000 people are now on the waiting list maintained by the United Network for Organ Sharing, a nonprofit that manages the federal organ transplant system; the average wait time is generally about three to five years. That's too long for many people: About 12 die each day as they hope for a kidney to turn up. A swap like this one effectively fast-tracks the process. At Northwestern, the period between joining the exchange program and surgery typically varies from about two to six months depending on the difficulty of matching.

Today, 20 to 30 percent of living donor kidney transplants here are done through the paired exchange program, mostly in four- to eight-person swaps. Each week, clinicians run a computer program to explore potential matches from among the incompatible pairs in the system. "There are actually multiple potential solutions that we can look through," says John Friedewald, a transplant nephrologist and medical director of the kidney transplant program. Northwestern also participates in the UNOS kidney paired donation program, which includes roughly 250 paired donors and candidates across the country. The National Kidney Registry, another nonprofit organization, facilitates hundreds of exchanges a year nationwide. In 2015, the NKR organized the longest swap to date, a 70-person chain involving teams at 26 hospitals.

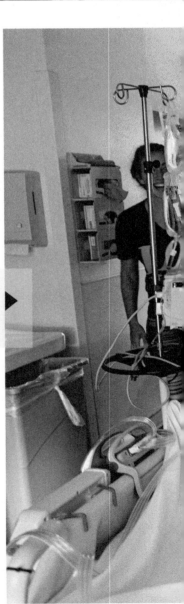

With her new kidney working fine, **Patricia Tripolitakis** pays a visit to her recovering husband, **Leo.**

By about 7:30 a.m., Condreva's donor and Spans are in separate operating rooms. Surgeons use a minimally invasive approach, making a series of incisions about the size of a centimeter through which they insert instruments and a tiny camera to guide their work; the kidneys are extracted through a slightly larger cut. The minimally invasive technique has "made the idea of donating a less scary undertaking" because it's safer than open surgery and recovery is much more rapid, says Joseph Leventhal, who directs the kidney and pancreas transplant programs and is performing several of this week's procedures.

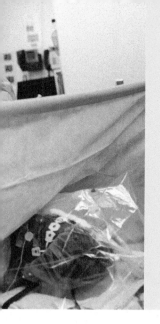

Husbands and Wives

▶ Lorretta and Lee Jenkins relax with their kids at home in Bolingbrook. Lee, a forklift operator diagnosed with chronic kidney disease in 2011, gets his new organ from Leo Tripolitakis. At right, Lorretta recovers after surgery to remove her kidney, which goes to Steven Boone (not pictured). He's been on dialysis since 2013.

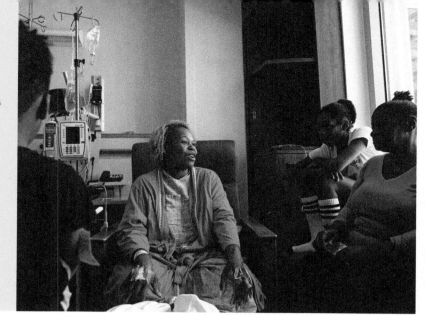

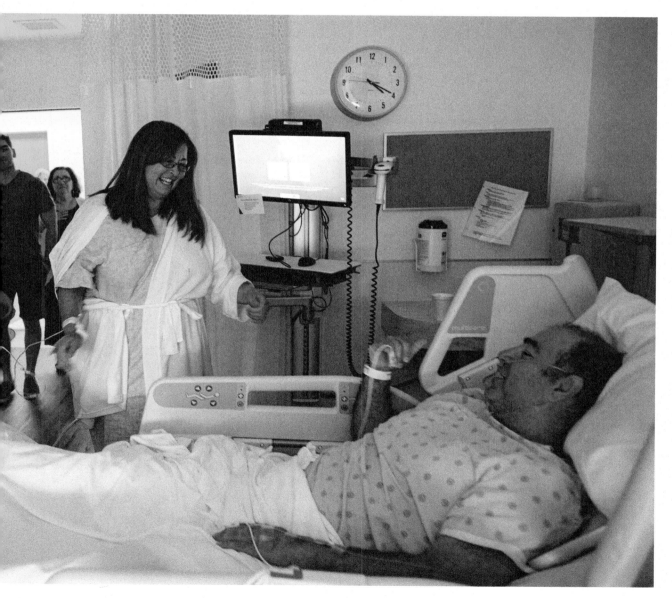

By late morning, Condreva and Patricia Tripolitakis are sedated and in the OR. Their surgeons make a long incision across their lower abdomens and patch each new kidney into its blood supply and the ureter, the tube that moves urine from the kidney to the bladder. Before long, the transplanted organs are working fine. Later that day, Condreva and Tripolitakis are up and moving gingerly around the hospital floor.

A match depends largely on blood type and the presence of antibodies, proteins in a recipient's immune system that guard against foreign viruses and bacteria and can cause the system to reject a kidney even from a donor whose blood type matches. Such was the case for Condreva and Spans, who both have Type A blood and initially were a match. They became incompatible because Condreva developed resistance to his aunt – likely a result of several blood transfusions and the transplant from his mom, Patricia, who is Spans' sister.

After Condreva's doctors at Northwestern determined that his aunt could not be his donor, "that forced the issue of swap," says Spans, who was eager to help her nephew by way of giving to another recipient. ("I think God wants more than one person to get a kidney," she reflected the night before surgery.) Condreva "was very hard to find a match for, so this was sort of a needle in the haystack," Friedewald says. But early this summer, when the altruistic donor approached Northwestern and was determined to be an answer for Condreva, that kidney was the first domino that allowed the other matches to be made. U.S. News visited Northwestern Memorial in late June to attend the surgeries – and the celebration days later when the donors and recipients met. ●

Lorretta and Lee Jenkins are back on their feet. "I just feel like a new man," Lee says.

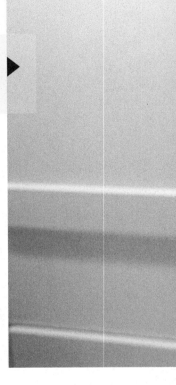

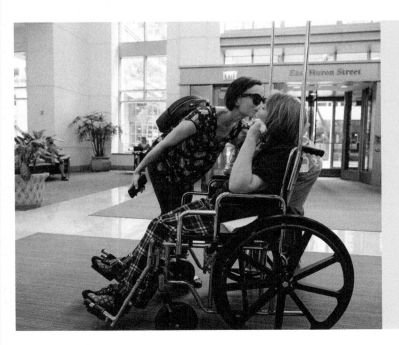

The Recovery

▶ Donna Spans checks out of the hospital and is greeted by her daughter, Michelle. Kevin Condreva, Spans' nephew, meets with surgeon Felicitas Koller and learns that his new kidney is functioning well. A week later, donors and recipients return for a checkup and meet for the first time. "Thank you just seems too small to express our gratitude," says Steven Boone (seated, far left).

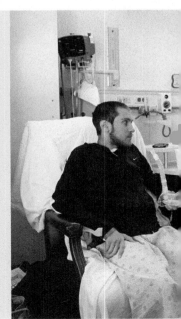

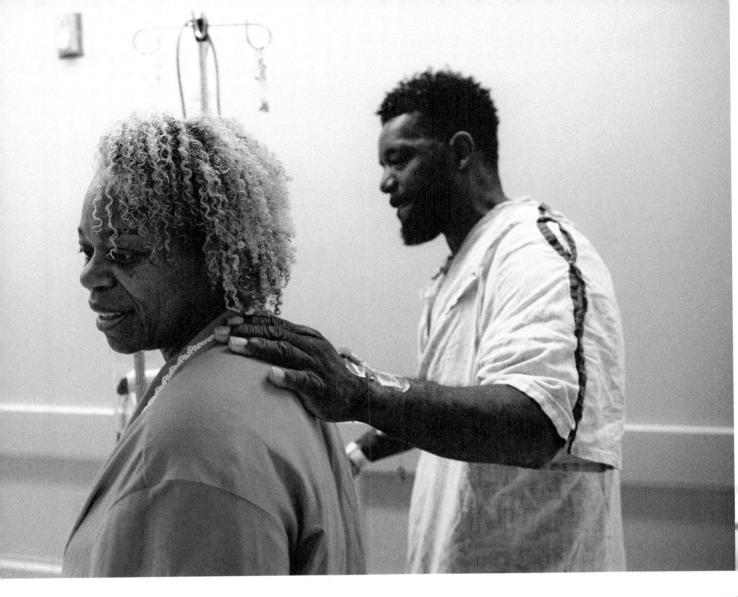

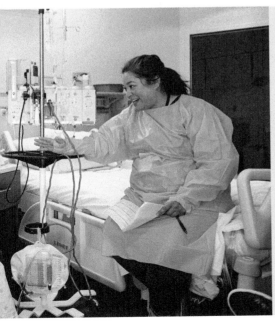

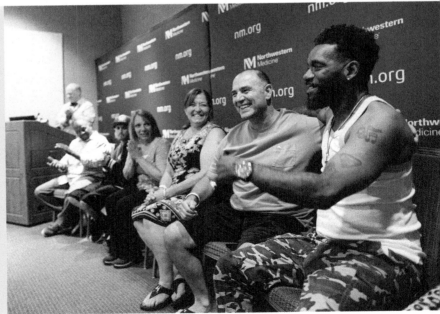

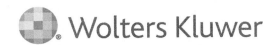
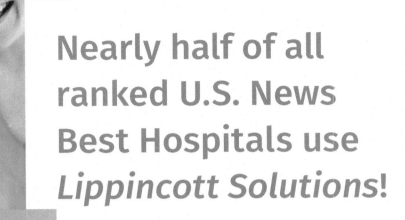

▶ CHAPTER 2 ◀

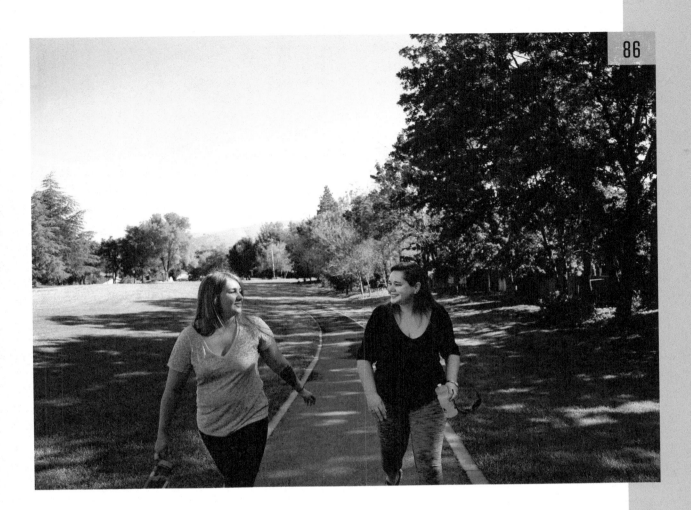

86

PATIENT POWER

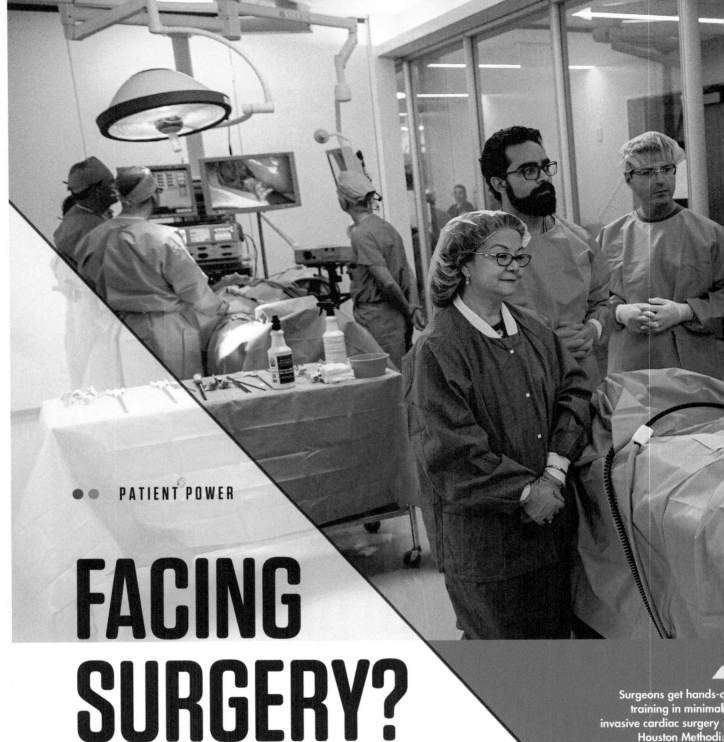

Surgeons get hands-on
training in minimally
invasive cardiac surgery
Houston Methodist

FACING SURGERY?

Experts advise asking if a minimally invasive
procedure would be an option for you

By Linda Marsa

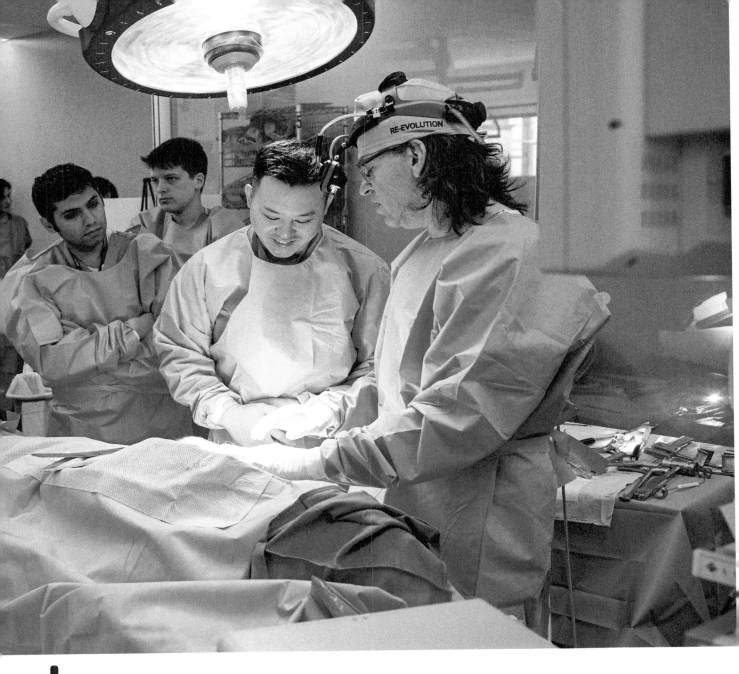

Last year defense attorney Charles LoPresti of Pittsburgh faced the worst adversary of his life: pancreatic cancer. His only chance for a cure was the Whipple procedure, a highly complex surgery that removes part of the pancreas, the gallbladder and surrounding lymph nodes. But instead of cutting him open, the traditional practice, surgeons at the University of Pittsburgh Medical Center removed his tumor plus 24 lymph nodes through a 2-inch incision. He went home three days later and was back in court within the month. "My recovery was very fast," says LoPresti, who vacationed in Italy with his wife this summer. "I feel better than I have in years."

LoPresti's experience is becoming more common as surgeons adopt minimally invasive or laparoscopic surgical techniques, which many consider the biggest technical advance in the field in several decades. These procedures are a stark contrast to conventional operations, which typi-

cally entail inches-long incisions that can leave patients debilitated for weeks and susceptible to infections and other postoperative woes. In fact, complications from surgery cost about $25 billion annually, a 2013 Harvard study showed, resulting in an average hospital payment increase of $39,000 per surgical patient. Less invasive techniques can greatly lessen the number of costly – and potentially deadly – side effects.

Minimally invasive surgical incisions can be under half an inch long; the team inserts thin instruments and a high-resolution fiber optic video camera through the tiny "keyhole" openings. The camera transmits images of the internal organs onto a monitor as a guide.

"Visualization is way better" than with open techniques, says Paul Wetter, chairman of the Society of Laparoendoscopic Surgeons and an emeritus professor at the University of Miami Miller School of Medicine. "You have a camera right inside [and] can see things you'd miss otherwise."

In spite of the advantages, you can't make the assumption that surgeons even "at a big brand name hospital" will be doing these procedures, warns Marty Makary, a surgeon and professor of health policy at Johns Hopkins who has researched the issue. Most patients who are good candidates for these procedures but don't have them were never told of the choice, he has found. Partly, he says, that's because surgeons who aren't skilled in the procedures may "downplay the options." In addition, insurers now pay the same or less for minimally invasive procedures, which works against a switch. In a value-based system, that may change "to reward hospitals that do better, safer, more effective care," says Makary.

In the meantime, experts strongly advise patients faced with surgery to ask about a minimally invasive option. Not everyone is a good candidate: People who have extensive scar tissue from previous procedures or have another underlying medical condition may not be suitable for minimally invasive surgery. But studies show that more than 80 percent of all common operations, including hysterectomy, colon removal, prostate surgery and appendectomy, can be done through keyhole incisions, Makary says.

That awareness, plus growing familiarity with the technology, has even made it standard for operations once considered too difficult to do without opening up a patient. Surgeons now routinely replace leaky heart valves by threading replacement parts through the femoral artery, or patch damaged arteries with bypass grafts without stopping the heart and cracking open the chest. When Clay Barker, a 28-year-old nursing student from Victoria, Texas, donated a kidney to his ailing mother in March, surgeons at Houston Methodist Medical Center removed his organ through a 3-inch incision. "I had virtually no pain afterwards," Barker marvels.

Besides lower rates of pain and infection, the technique results in less trauma to nerves, muscles and tissues; and shorter hospital stays. "People are often back to their normal life in less than a week," says Wetter.

One 2014 Hopkins study that looked at complications for four common procedures – appendectomy, hysterectomy, lung lobectomy and colectomy – found that serious complications such as infections, sepsis, pneumonia and death were substantially lower for all four types of operations performed this way. And the savings can be substantial – from $280 million to $340 million a year, according to a Hopkins study.

If the choice is not available at your hospital, a second opinion elsewhere is a good idea. Pick a surgeon who has done your procedure frequently; studies consistently show that complication rates drop considerably with a rise in surgeons' number of cases. For a routine operation like a

> ## "
> # Over 80% of common operations can be done through keyhole incisions.

hysterectomy, you'd want to see at least one or two a week, experts say. A high-volume academic center is a good place to look, advises Scott Melvin, vice chairman of clinical surgery at Montefiore Medical Center in New York.

Integrated health systems like Kaiser Permanente, the not-for-profit HMO with nearly 12 million members in eight states and the District of Columbia, have been leaders in adopting minimally invasive techniques; besides being better for patients, reducing complications curbs costs. Payment at Kaiser Permanente involves a set amount for each member rather than a fee for every service provided, so the emphasis is on preventing disease and the need for treatment. Moreover, within such organizations where doctors are salaried employees, the organization can decide on surgical policy and hire surgeons who are already trained.

Patients at Kaiser Permanente are referred to a well-practiced surgeon. For example, about 90 percent of gastric cancer procedures are done through keyhole incisions, and in Northern California, all are performed at two hospitals "to maximize their volumes," says Robert Pearl, until recently executive director and CEO of The Permanente Medical Group. "We want to make sure the surgeon and the surgical team – nurses, anesthesiologists – have enough experience to optimize their skills."

Other institutions are looking at ways to better prepare surgeons for 21st-century technologies. "It's hard for surgeons to leave busy practices and be away from their own operating rooms to learn these complex techniques, which are not something that can be picked up in a weekend course," says Brian Dunkin, head of surgical endoscopy at Houston Methodist Hospital and medical director of the Methodist Institute for Technology, Innovation and Education, an educational and research institute.

Training centers like the Methodist Institute are attempting to fill this gap by devising longitudinal educational programs that combine hands-on sessions with

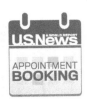

U.S. NEWS APPOINTMENT BOOKING

usnews.com/health | A Booking Service from *U.S. News & World Report*

From U.S. News to Your Office

Appointment Booking lets U.S. News visitors request or book appointments with your providers directly from our website.

Why Appointment Booking?

- 5 million monthly website visitors
- 85% of those surveyed use Find a Doctor to research or book an appointment
- Shared Analytics for Trackable ROI

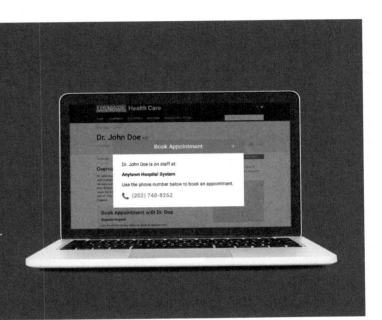

January Weekly Appointment Booking Calls

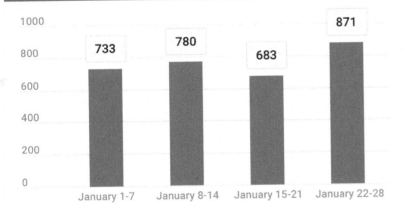

Steps to Success

1. Select your Physicians
2. Update your Physician Profiles
3. Choose where to route your calls
4. See new patients

Colin Hamilton
Healthcare Director, US News Health Solutions Group
✉ chamilton@usnews.com
☎ Phone: 212-916-8729
📱 Mobile: 646-784-4162

Marsha Proulx
Director, Business Development, Healthcare
✉ mproulx@usnews.com
☎ Phone: 202-955-2060
📱 Mobile: 443-285-1561

For more information or to request a demo, contact us

mentoring afterward. In a recent pilot program, for example, selected surgeons came to the Houston campus for four days of classes in which they practiced doing laparoscopic colon surgery on a cadaver under the watchful eyes of expert coaches. Then they were joined by members of their surgical teams, including nurses and technicians, to do two similar surgeries. When surgeons returned home, the teaching surgeons at Houston Methodist guided them remotely by videoconference in the OR. "It's a simple concept," says Dunkin of the telementoring. "But there's a lot of science validating that it works."

At the University of Pittsburgh Medical Center, surgical residents as well as practicing physicians from all over the country are being trained in the next generation of minimally invasive techniques: robotic or computer-assisted surgery. Instead of bending over an operating table, surgeons sit in front of a console nearby with a magnified 3-D screen that gives them a much better view than regular laparoscopic or open incisions. They operate by moving two controllers that manipulate robotic arms equipped with tiny surgical instruments so intricate they can sew together a grape peel. Computer software takes the place of actual hand movements, making movements very precise.

Robotic technology has its downsides. For one thing, it's expensive – robots cost about $2 million, and their use adds anywhere from $1,500 to $2,000 per patient. Experts think prices will tumble within the next few years as more companies enter the market. Also, because surgeons don't get the tactile stimulation they get when they're cutting directly into tissue, there's a risk of injuring adjacent organs or nicking blood vessels or nerves. And so far, research has not found that robotic surgery improves outcomes.

At UPMC, surgeons first practice on a simulator, akin to how pilots learn to fly, and then gain experience working on lifelike bioartificial organs before they move on to assisting in real surgeries. The learning curve is shorter than it is with regular laparoscopic procedures, says Herbert Zeh, chief of gastrointestinal surgical oncology at UPMC, because robotics provide that "all-important 3-D vision and improved dexterity." The next generation of robots will help surgeons even more: The technology will rely on the science of haptics to simulate for the doctors at the controls the sense of touch that they lose by not holding the instruments, and allow them to overlay scans taken just before the patient enters the OR on the real-time images of his or her anatomy. Such augmented reality will guide surgeons in ways that are unimaginable today, predicts Zeh. "That's the future," he says. "And it's going to happen." ●

THE CASE FOR ASKING TWICE

Before you let yourself be wheeled into the OR, it's smart to ask: Do I really need this? There may be other ways of treating what ails you. Up to 20 percent of operations are unnecessary for some conditions, according to a 2013 USA Today review of government records and medical databases; they range from cardiac stent and pacemaker implants to spinal surgeries, knee replacements, hysterectomies and cesarean sections. One study of more than 140,000 heart catheterization procedures, which include diagnostic angiograms and angioplasties to clear clogged arteries, found that nearly 12 percent didn't need to be done and 38 percent were borderline questionable.

Physical therapy can be as effective as surgery in relieving back and joint pain. And sometimes medication is the right answer. Hysterectomies,

for instance, are often performed on women who have ovarian cysts or suffer from heavy menstrual bleeding. But taking oral contraceptives can lessen the intensity and duration of menstrual bleeding and prevent the formation of ovarian cysts. Even appendicitis can be controlled with antibiotics in 80 percent of cases, according to a 2015 Finnish study.

A second opinion would have been life-changing for one patient USA Today highlighted: Jonathan Stelly, 38. At age 23, Stelly was in peak condition, playing semipro baseball and talking to scouts from the big leagues. But then a couple of fainting spells prompted him to see a cardiologist. The doctor told him he needed a pacemaker.

Stelly complied, even though the implant meant an end to strenuous athletics and a career in baseball. Months

later, when he consulted another doctor, he discovered the real source of his troubles. "My thyroid was out of whack," says the Denver MBA student, who now takes pills for his thyroid and has turned off the pacemaker. "I never needed the surgery."

Such stories are not unusual. In a 2017 study of nearly 300 patients who had come to the Mayo Clinic for a second opinion, researchers found that up to 88 percent of them were given an entirely new or refined diagnosis that completely altered their care.

Another benefit of double-checking the facts is that it can help you be sure of getting care from the right surgeon. Complex and demanding procedures need to be performed by specialists who handle them routinely. Look for nearby centers of excellence such as a teaching hospital connected to a medical school. You want a surgeon who does a high volume of your operation every year. –L.M.

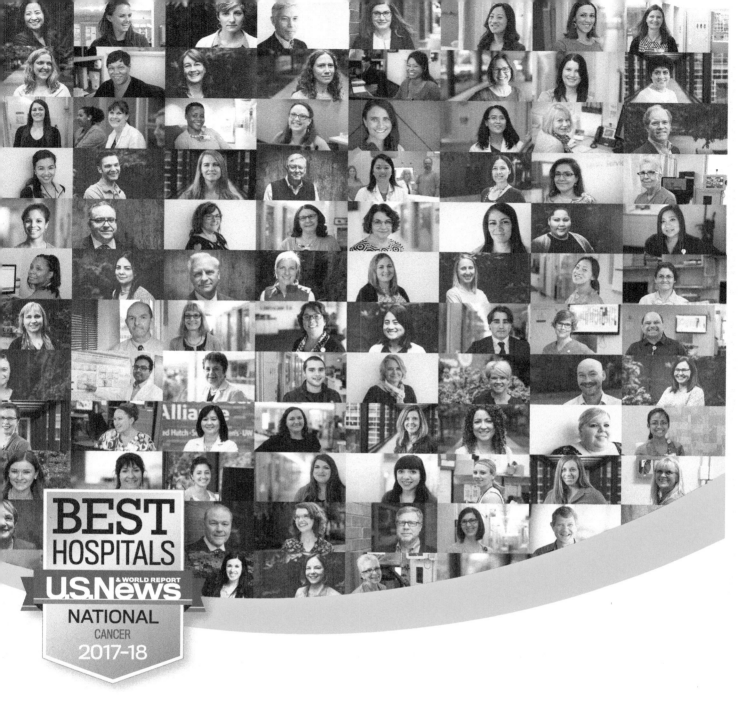

Top 10 in the nation, 12 years running.

Since 2005, Seattle Cancer Care Alliance has ranked among the top 10 cancer hospitals in the nation. And this year, our #5 ranking is a distinction that is a true reflection of our staff. The doctors and nurses, who treat our patients with an unwavering commitment and dedication. The researchers, who face each complex and unanswered question with relentless determination. And every staff member, who works tirelessly to deliver personalized and compassionate care.

Learn more about what makes us #1 to our patients at **SeattleCCA.org**.

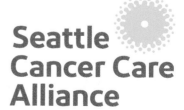

Seattle Cancer Care Alliance

Fred Hutch · Seattle Children's · UW Medicine

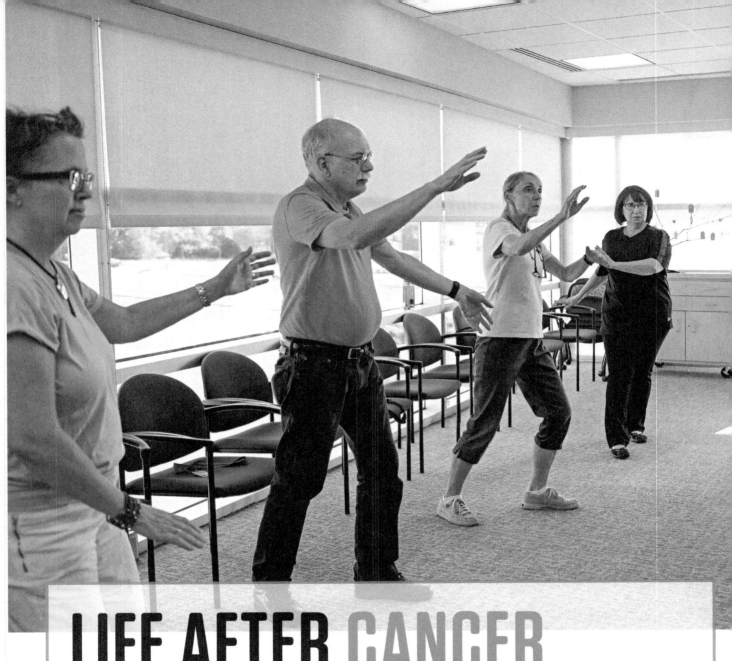

LIFE AFTER CANCER

Hospitals are stepping up post-treatment support for survivors

By Linda Marsa

Anne Macy, 51, has been battling cancer for almost half of her life. Diagnosed at age 28 with Hodgkin's lymphoma, the real estate broker from Lansdale, Pennsylvania, has been hit with two other cancers since that first one was cured. What has helped her cope with all the

turmoil with her sanity intact? The unflagging support of Linda Jacobs, the "angel on my shoulder" who has checked in with Macy regularly to answer questions, see how she's feeling physically and emotionally, and offer support and the occasional gentle prodding needed to get her through all the tests and follow-up that come with a cancer diagnosis.

Jacobs, a nurse practitioner and clinical professor of nursing who directs

the development of cancer survivorship programs at the Hospital of the University of Pennsylvania's Abramson Cancer Center, may have even saved Macy's life. When the protocol for ongoing surveillance of Hodgkin's lymphoma survivors changed, Jacobs alerted her that she needed a breast MRI. That test revealed MALT lymphoma in Macy's breast, and a follow-up PET scan uncovered a tumor behind her ear. "I can't imagine getting through these

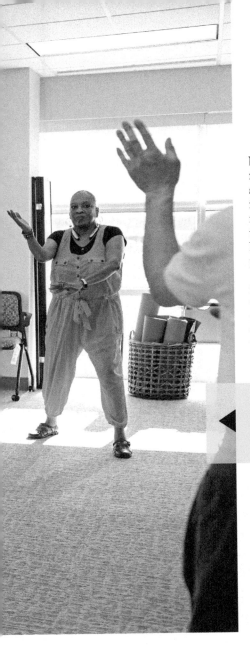

A tai chi class is one of the many cancer survivorship supports offered to OSUCCC–James patients.

What's more, the graying of the baby-boom generation is expected to dramatically boost the number of elderly survivors, who often suffer from other ills exacerbated by their cancer treatments. Experts are predicting a "silver tsunami" of survivors with complex health issues who will benefit from practical and moral support.

Their challenges are many and varied. Patients have to deal not only with the symptoms of their disease and the ravages of chemotherapy and radiation, but also with emotional turmoil like anxiety, feelings of hopelessness, and changes in self-image. Some peo-ple struggle with permanent cognitive damage, memory loss, personality changes, and damage to the heart, for example. Many must also grapple with financial difficulties.

"In the past, we knew very little about what happened to cancer patients after treatment ended," notes Julia Rowland, director of the National Cancer Institute's Office of Cancer Survivorship. "We now know that cancer has the capacity to affect all aspects of survivors' lives," she says, and have "a profound and lasting impact on their psychological and social health."

The survivorship movement has its roots in pediatric oncology. Many long-term survivors of childhood cancers reach adulthood with disabilities ranging from neurological deficits and heart and lung damage to heightened risks for secondary cancers. The fear and uncertainty, and feelings of being out of step with or ostracized by peers, frequently have taken a heavy toll, too, in the form of depression and anxiety. A 2016 study of childhood survivors of brain cancer, to cite one example, found they not only had increased rates of stroke and hear-ing difficulties but also were at high risk of impaired academic skills and unemployment, and were less apt to live independently.

Doctors have worked hard to minimize these risks. "We had to figure out how to cure them without ruining their lives," says Jacqueline Casillas, director of the Pediatric, Adolescent and Young Adult Survivorship Program at UCLA's Jonsson Comprehensive Cancer Center and medical director of the cancer center at Miller Children's & Women's Hospital in Long Beach. Both hospitals provide comprehensive medical and psychosocial evaluations, and the staff works with young survivors to help them find the best support programs in their communities and reintegrate back into the world. There are now more than 150 pediatric survivorship programs across the U.S. and Canada, and many follow children into adulthood, addressing their unique issues such as dating, fertility and employment concerns. "Patients tell me all the time 'I look the same on the outside, but I feel different on the inside,'" says Casilla. "It's critical to connect them with different programs that can normalize their experiences."

The trend toward devising hospital-based programs for adults gained momentum after a 2005 Institute of Medicine report urged that all cancer patients get a formal ongoing care plan. But the real push came in 2012. That's when the Commission on Cancer, an initiative of the American College of Surgeons that recognizes programs providing high-quality patient-centered care, mandated a comprehensive after-treatment plan to gain the group's accreditation. The plans must include surveillance strategies, evaluations for health problems stemming from treatment, and recommendations for dealing with other issues. "Programs were slowly being implemented, but there was no real traction on this until the commission made this a standard," says Patricia Ganz, director of the Patients and Survivors Program at UCLA.

The Livestrong Foundation, a Texas-

life-altering events without Linda's consistent aid," Macy says.

The pioneering program at Penn, launched in 2001, now is one of dozens of hospital-based programs created across the country to provide long-term follow-up care – physical, emotional and even financial – to cancer survivors after treatment has ended. That's a growing group. "We're in a very different place than we were even in the 1990s," says Jacobs. "People are now living with cancer as a chronic illness." There are 15.5 million Americans now who are living as cancer survivors, and that number is expected to rise past 20 million by 2026 because of improvements in detection and treatment.

"There are 15.5 million Americans now living as cancer survivors.

based cancer charity, has designated several cancer centers as Survivorship Centers of Excellence: Memorial Sloan-Kettering in New York, Penn, UCLA, Ohio State University, Boston's Dana-Farber Cancer Institute, the Fred Hutchinson Cancer Research Center in Seattle and the University of North Carolina Lineberger Comprehensive Cancer Center. Such major centers that draw patients from all over may refer them to resources at the center or use a simple consultative model for those who don't live close by: Patients get a care plan and work with a nurse navigator to find resources that meet their needs in their own community.

At UNC, for example, patients fill out a distress screener to uncover their most pressing issues and can attend classes over a four-week period to help them transition. They get access to nutrition and exercise programs, along with personal trainers, on campus or in their local areas. "As an institution, we cover the whole state," says Deborah Mayer, director of cancer survivorship. "Our job is to figure out what is available where the patient lives."

Similarly, Ganz does extensive evaluations of UCLA patients' physical activity, nutrition and mental outlook and creates a plan that includes referral to a genetic counselor for input about the risk for secondary cancers and to local support groups. When they're at UCLA, they can be seen for counseling and consult a nutritionist. "We make both institutional and community referrals," says Ganz.

"This is a very difficult journey," says Dikla Benzeevi of Los Angeles, who has been battling advanced breast cancer for 15 years. Having a place where she can connect with other survivors provides "great comfort," she says. Diagnosed at 32, Benzeevi has undergone years of harrowing treatments at UCLA that included five months in a back brace after a spinal tumor had eaten away a vertebra. "That was a very scary time," recalls Benzeevi. Her support group at UCLA has helped her cope over the years with everything from weight gain and "emotional chaos" to dealing with stomach cramps and nausea and finding a great wig.

The survivorship clinic at Ohio State University's cancer center (known as

A FEW ONLINE RESOURCES

If your hospital doesn't provide you with an after-treatment plan, here are some other places to find help:

■ OncoLink (oncolink.org/oncolife) is a website sponsored by the University of Pennsylvania. Patients can use the OncoLife tool to answer questions about their cancer treatments and receive a care plan that they can use to navigate in their community.

■ Cancer Support Community (cancersupportcommunity.org) has over 150 locations worldwide, including Arizona, California, Pennsylvania, South Carolina, New York and New Mexico; dozens of on-site and online support groups; and a wealth of cancer survivorship information and other resources.

■ The Survivorship Center (cancer.org/survivorshipcenter), a collaboration between the American Cancer Society and George Washington University Cancer Institute, has a directory of post-treatment survivorship resources.

OSUCCC–James) offers a broad range of on- and off-site services geared to both survivors and their families, including financial, spiritual, genetic and nutritional counseling; yoga and tai chi; massage therapy; more than a dozen support groups; and vocational rehabilitation and employment assistance. The clinic even sponsors monthly lunch-and-learn workshops in which patients are educated about nutrition and go grocery shopping with a dietitian. "It's a real paradigm shift," says Maryam Lustberg, a medical oncologist at OSUCCC–James.

Smaller community hospitals are committing to serve survivors, too. "We have to be focused not just on medical treatment but on their recovery and on a holistic approach to their lives," says Randall Oyer, medical director of the oncology program at Lancaster General Hospital in Pennsylvania, which uses a combination of onsite nutritional counselors and support groups and such community resources as exercise programs at the local YMCA to customize care plans for patients and families.

For Rob Wood, 61, who has had surgery twice for colon cancer and thyroid cancer and is now in remission, the survivorship program at OSUCCC–James promises to be a huge help as he adjusts to being "a member of a club that I didn't ask to join." A professor and administrator at a small university in Columbus, Ohio, Wood has gained more than 60 pounds without a properly functioning thyroid, weight he hasn't been able to shed even though he now takes thyroid supplements. He hopes to get encouragement and lose a few pounds, and that peer counseling will eventually help him "feel better and be more positive." In fact, he thinks he might become a peer mentor himself. ●

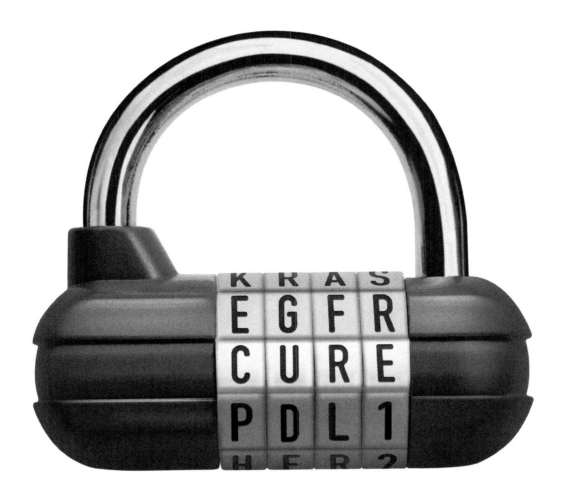

We're cracking the cancer code.

We're pursuing breakthroughs every day to help put an end to cancer. Exploring every idea and continually refining our approach to explore cancer genomes as never before. Identifying cancer mutations and mechanisms, like PD-1 interactions and EGFR, which has led to more targeted and effective cancer treatments. We are finding solutions to the toughest problems, because the more answers we find, the more lives we save.

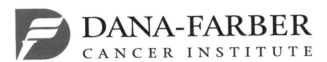

DANA-FARBER
CANCER INSTITUTE

Discover. Care. Believe.

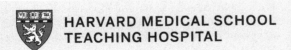

REBOOTING THE BRAIN

Transcranial magnetic stimulation may offer relief from all sorts of disorders

By Stacey Colino

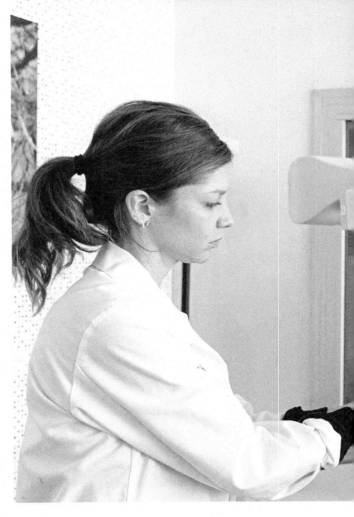

The idea of placing a special device against your head, flicking a switch, and resetting your mood or zapping away unpleasant symptoms may sound like the stuff of science fiction. But with the growing use of repetitive transcranial magnetic stimulation, a noninvasive technique that uses magnetic pulses to stimulate targeted areas of the brain, this scenario is becoming a reality. Approved by the Food and Drug Administration a decade ago to treat major depression that hasn't responded to antidepressants, TMS is now being used or studied for a host of other ills, from anxiety and obsessive-compulsive disorder to autism, dementia and chronic pain.

"Before I had the treatment, the pain was severe and walking was difficult," recalls a Los Angeles physician who was getting TMS therapy for depression in 2014 when she experienced a debilitating flare-up of nerve pain in her groin, a complication from an earlier surgery. Her doctor suggested TMS to treat her pain, aiming the pulses in such a way that they would inhibit pain signaling in her sensory cortex. "Scientifically, it made sense to me," the physician-patient says. "I felt remarkably better after each session – 80 percent of my pain was gone, just like that."

The common denominator behind the seemingly disparate disorders that may be treatable with TMS – which also include post-traumatic stress disorder, Parkinson's disease, stroke, attention deficit hyperactivity disorder, chronic migraines, traumatic brain injury, tinnitus (aka ringing in the ears) and multiple sclerosis – is that they're disorders of brain network function. "The brain is an electric organ," explains Joan Camprodon-Gimenez, director of the division of neuropsychiatry and neuromodulation at Massachusetts General Hospital and an assistant professor of psychiatry at Harvard Medical School. "With TMS, we are using electromagnetic pulses to change brain activities – to excite or inhibit activ-

ity in a particular brain region – in ways that will reverse or modulate the symptoms of a particular disorder."

During treatment, an electromagnetic coil is placed against the patient's skull near the forehead while pulses are delivered, stimulating neurons to fire and excite other neurons. "Every part of the brain is interconnected," notes Mehmet Dokucu, director of the neuromodulation program in psychiatry at Northwestern Memorial Hospital in Chicago. "So even if we target a particular part of the brain, other deeper areas get stimulated, too."

How this translates into specific gains isn't completely understood. But the theory is that the treatment is enhancing the brain's ability to change and "run circuits more efficiently, make new neural connections, and restore neural rhythms," says Linda Carpenter, a psychiatrist and research professor of psychiatry and human behavior at Brown University and director of the Butler Hospital TMS Clinic and Neuromodulation Research Facility in Providence, Rhode Island. There may be some other effects, too, she says, such as improving blood flow and the functioning of the cells' mitochondria – their energy producers.

Data on how effective TMS is for various conditions and how long the effects last is limited. The evidence that TMS makes a substantial difference for many cases of chronic pain "is not super compelling," Camprodon-Gimenez says, and it's only just beginning to be studied for autism, ADHD, OCD and other conditions. In Parkinson's and stroke patients, some

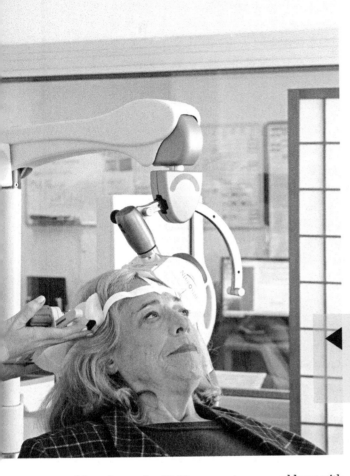

Nancy Lewis, Andrew Leuchter's patient at UCLA, has seen her depression symptoms ease by over 70 percent.

of clinical psychiatry and director of the Neuromodulation Service at Vanderbilt University Medical Center. For chronic pain, the sensory motor cortex, which receives physical sensations from the body, is being studied as the target. Generally, fast pulses at a high frequency enliven the targeted areas, while pulses at a low frequency can suppress activity, says Andrew Leuchter, a professor of psychiatry and director of the TMS Clinical and Research Service at the David Geffen School of Medicine at UCLA. While patients with depression typically benefit from having certain parts of their brain revved up, people with chronic pain, anxiety or PTSD often require a dialing down of activity in key areas of the brain. Patients often describe the sensation as feeling like a woodpecker is tapping on their head – not quite painful but not exactly comfortable, either. The magnetic pulses are similar to those generated by magnetic resonance imaging machines.

Compared with electroconvulsive therapy, which uses electrical stimulation in a more generalized fashion to treat severe treatment-resistant depression and other mental disorders, targeted TMS treatments involve a lower risk of side effects such as seizures, and there is no memory loss. While some people experience a mild headache or slight fatigue after sessions in the first week, most don't have any lingering side effects. The protocol typically involves five days a week for four to eight weeks. Each session generally lasts 20 to 40 or 60 minutes and is done on an outpatient basis. Many people begin to notice changes after about two weeks, though some people are early responders, some are late responders and others don't benefit at all.

TMS is not a cure, which means that supportive interventions such as medication, psychotherapy and exercise for depression may be needed to maintain improvements. "Just because a medication didn't get you well, that doesn't mean it can't keep you well," Becker says. Over the following year, depression symptoms typically return for about one-third of people who've had successful TMS. Those who have a relapse of depression can receive additional sessions of TMS. "There's no limit to the number of booster or maintenance sessions a person can have," Carpenter says.

The bad news: Most insurance plans cover TMS for major depression only. Leonore Gordon, 61, who had Parkinson's-induced challenges with mobility and motor skills, saw significant improvement when she participated in a study of TMS for Parkinson's at New York University. "I got married in 2014, and I was able to dance at my wedding," says Gordon, a retired therapist in Brooklyn. Some of the improvements have since faded, and Gordon would like to have TMS again. Since it would be outside of a clinical trial this time, though, she'll need to wait until TMS is approved for Parkinson's – and insurance coverage kicks in. ●

research has shown that TMS appears to ease problems with movement. On the other hand, there's strong research regarding depression. A 2012 study found that nearly 60 percent of people with treatment-resistant depression who underwent TMS were in remission at the three-month follow-up.

The severity of symptoms may influence the results. A 2015 study at the Walter Reed National Military Medical Center found that patients with mild to moderate depression had significantly better responses than those with severe depression did. Meanwhile, a 2016 study in the journal Neurology examined the effects of 10 daily sessions of repetitive TMS on the motor and mood symptoms of patients with Parkinson's: In people with both Parkinson's and depression, TMS led to improvements in motor function but not mood.

In other cases, motor skills and frame of mind improve in tandem, whether because of a neurological or a psychological ripple effect. Debbie Hall, of New Albany, Ohio, underwent TMS to stimulate the areas that control mobility and fine motor control in her left arm and hand after having a stroke in 2013. After six sessions, "I could pick up BBs – I was so excited!" says Hall, 52. Her mood also improved dramatically – as a result of the treatment, the physical improvement, or both. Since then, Hall has retained much of the functionality she gained.

To treat depression, magnetic pulses are directed at a brain region that is underactive in people with the condition, explains Jonathan Becker, an assistant professor

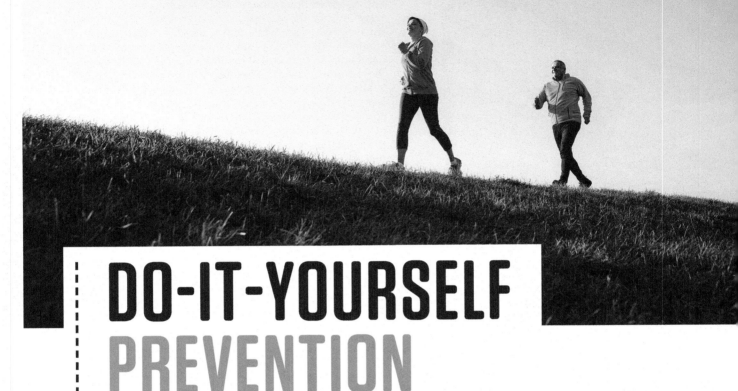

DO-IT-YOURSELF
PREVENTION

Your genes have a lot to say about whether you get cancer. But you have power to affect the story

By Courtney Rubin

There's been plenty of debate about whether developing cancer is simply a matter of genetic bad luck and how much, if anything, changing your habits can affect risk. The latest entry: Researchers at Johns Hopkins published a paper this spring in the journal Science suggesting that roughly two-thirds of cancers are due to DNA typos – essentially, random errors. That's a far cry from what a 2015 study found: that as many as 9 out of 10 cancers may be a result of environmental and lifestyle factors that could potentially be controlled. Still, the new findings are not an excuse to sit back and let fate take its course.

The Hopkins researchers said some 40 percent of cancers can be avoided.

There are a number of lifestyle changes you can make to affect your cancer risk – and, as an additional benefit, also reduce the odds of diabetes and heart disease. Below are eight suggestions on how to protect yourself that are supported by recent science. One not included: smoking, which pretty much everybody should know by now "is probably the single most important risk factor" for most types of cancer, never mind its effect on the respiratory system, says Edward Giovannucci, a professor of nutrition and epidemiology at Harvard's T.H. Chan

School of Public Health who has published several studies on risk.

Moderate your alcohol intake. According to the American Institute for Cancer Research, there's "convincing evidence" that alcohol increases the risk of several types of cancer, including mouth, liver, breast and – at least in men – colorectal. In 2016, a British expert advisory group examined data since 1995 and concluded that there was strong evidence that the risk of a range of cancers, including breast, increased directly in line with consumption of alcohol.

It's really excessive consumption that you need to worry about, experts say. Current recommendations call for no more than one drink a day for women and two for men. "If you want to make your risk zero, it should be zero intake," says Giovannucci. "But increased risk is pretty minimal with one to two drinks."

And of course, consider that a little bit of alcohol may have a cardioprotective effect – resveratrol, an antioxidant found in red wine, is particularly good at vacuuming up chemicals responsible for causing blood clots.

Limit sweets. "Sugar really has extreme adverse effects on human physiology," warns Patricia Thompson, the deputy director for research at Stony Brook University Cancer Center. For one, it contributes to obesity, which fosters widespread inflammation, and that puts various organ systems at risk of disease.

Unlike the inflammation of, say, a wound, the chronic or systemic kind has been linked to everything from bloating and acne to heart attacks, Alzheimer's and cancer. Excess sugar also is thought to negatively affect metabolism and the population of bacteria in your gut. Unbelievable as it may seem, what goes on in your "gut microbiome" is "really, really important" to the proper functioning of the body's primary defense against tumors, the immune system, says Thompson, whose own research fo-

cuses on cancers of the colorectum as well as the breast. And sugar increases insulin levels, a risk factor for diabetes and for colon cancer.

Add resistant starch. This type of starch – good sources include legumes, bananas (the less ripe, the better), rolled oats, and boiled potatoes that have cooled, as in potato salad – resists digestion, meaning it hasn't broken down by the time it passes through the small intestine and provides nutrition to those important bacteria.

Researchers are still trying to pinpoint how diet changes the microbiome, but they do know that when you feed certain bacteria, they release a variety of good-for-you compounds, including butyrate, which "knocks off cancer cells," says Michael Michael, a scientist at the Flinders Centre for Innovation in Cancer in Adelaide, Australia. In one of his studies, volunteers consumed 300 grams (roughly 10 ounces) of red meat a day, plus 40 grams of a powdered form of resistant starch mixed into orange juice. Normally the levels of a small group of microRNAs associated with cancer would go up with that kind of extreme meat-eating, but the starch brought almost all of the levels back to baseline. "That shows that at a molecular level this protects you against elevated cancer risk," says Michael. As a bonus, studies suggest resistant starch can also help lower blood sugar and boost gut health.

Scale back on red meat. And when you eat it, marinate it. Besides being a heart-healthy move, cutting back may offer protection against cancer. One of the links between red meat and cancer that researchers are investigating involves heme, an iron-containing compound that has been shown to damage the lining of the bowel.

Why should you marinate? Cooking meat at high temperatures produces compounds that cause potentially harmful changes in your DNA. Vari-

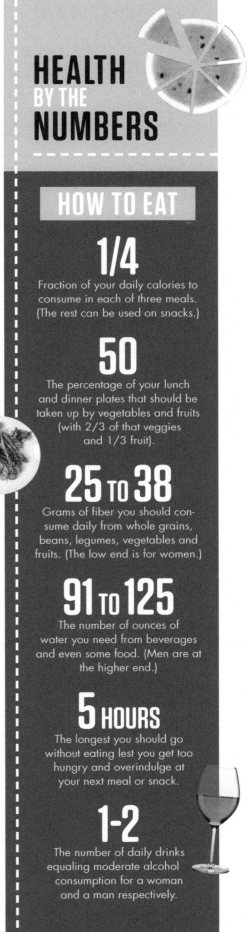

HEALTH BY THE NUMBERS

HOW TO EAT

1/4
Fraction of your daily calories to consume in each of three meals. (The rest can be used on snacks.)

50
The percentage of your lunch and dinner plates that should be taken up by vegetables and fruits (with 2/3 of that veggies and 1/3 fruit).

25 TO 38
Grams of fiber you should consume daily from whole grains, beans, legumes, vegetables and fruits. (The low end is for women.)

91 TO 125
The number of ounces of water you need from beverages and even some food. (Men are at the higher end.)

5 HOURS
The longest you should go without eating lest you get too hungry and overindulge at your next meal or snack.

1-2
The number of daily drinks equaling moderate alcohol consumption for a woman and a man respectively.

ous herbs, spices, and marinades have been shown to block the formation of cancer-causing compounds. A Kansas State University study, for example, found that rubbing rosemary onto uncooked meat reduced the compounds by 30 to 100 percent.

Limit processed meat.

Or better yet, cut it entirely. The International Agency for Research on Cancer, a group of international experts who scrutinize the evidence, has classified processed meat as carcinogenic to humans, putting it in the same category as tobacco smoking and asbestos. (This doesn't mean they're equally dangerous; classifications are based on the strength of evidence, not the risk level.) Researchers think substances used in the processing may create cancer-causing compounds. And nitrites, which are used as preservatives, may also form compounds that damage DNA.

One fringe benefit of cutting down on these types of meats is that it will help curb your salt intake, a step that could lessen your risk of heart disease, stroke and stomach cancer. Most peo-

ple eat more than the World Health Organization-recommended maximum of 5 grams per day. A 2017 Tufts University study found that a global drive to cut salt intake by 10 percent would save millions of lives currently lost to cardiovascular disease. In the U.S., a different study found, consuming too much salt was associated with 9.5 percent of deaths from heart disease, stroke and Type 2 diabetes.

Do more cardio.

Centers for Disease Control and Prevention guidelines call for 150 minutes of moderate exercise – or 75 minutes of vigorous exercise – per week. These are aimed at heart health, but also may have a protective effect against 13 types of cancer, according to a 2016 review of studies published in JAMA Internal Medicine. The review found that working out for just a couple of hours a week appeared to shrink the risk of breast, colon and lung cancer, among others. The more you exercise, the greater the benefit, the study suggested.

Activities that result in sustained

10
The maximum percentage of your total calories each day that should be comprised of sweet treats.

2
Minimum number of times per week you should eat fish (especially fatty fish like salmon, lake trout, mackerel or sardines) to protect your heart health.

HOW TO MOVE

150
Minimum minutes of moderate-intensity aerobic exercise you should get weekly. Or 75 minutes of vigorous aerobic exercise weekly gives you the same perks.

2
Times per week to do strength-training exercises to build muscle mass, which helps you burn calories faster.

48 HOURS
The longest you should go without a workout unless you're sick.

10
The maximum percentage you should increase the length of your workout each week to give your body ample time to adjust and avoid injury.

1
Workout-free day each week. What you should allow yourself to enable muscle recovery and repair.

increases in heart rate tend to burn the most calories and help people maintain their weight. One particularly efficient activity: high-intensity interval training (story, Page 89). Besides burning calories, it also burns fat and boosts metabolism.

In addition, physical activity is thought to lower levels of hormones such as estrogen that have been linked to different cancers. And people who work out have been shown to have lower levels of systemic inflammation, with some evidence suggesting that physical activity boosts the capacity of cells to repair damaged DNA. Exercise also has an effect on metabolism as well as the health and function of the gut microbiome.

Keep in mind that a brisk walk counts as exercise. In fact, a walk actually is as good as a run for cutting risk of heart disease, according to a 2013 study published in the journal Arteriosclerosis, Thrombosis and Vascular Biology.

Get at least seven hours of sleep. Sleep is the body's opportunity to do its repair work, but beyond that, disease researchers are particularly interested in the metabolic changes a sleep deficit creates. You've probably seen headlines to the effect that lack of sleep can make you fat – and your adipose tissue doesn't just sit there innocently. It contains hormones and vitamin D that are needed for energy balance. Loss of sleep can change some of the mechanisms underpinning a healthy hormone and energy balance, creating conditions that can lead to insulin resistance.
That state,

TURNING DOWN THE HEAT

The latest buzzword in diets these days seems to be "anti-inflammatory." Organizations from the Arthritis Foundation to Epicurious have featured the concept, and Andrew Weil, the alternative medicine guru, has created an anti-inflammatory food pyramid. Little wonder, since inflammation has developed such a bad reputation.

Stress, smoking and lack of sleep are some of the lifestyle choices that can cause chronic inflammation. Diet, too: What you eat can make matters worse – or better. Researchers don't recommend sticking with any particular anti-inflammatory diet, but if you abide by general healthy diet guidelines, you'll be on track, advises Edward Giovannucci, a professor of nutrition and epidemiology at Harvard's T.H. Chan School of Public Health and an author on a 2016 Journal of Nutrition Study on diet and inflammatory markers.

Red meat, processed meat and sugar-sweetened beverages all increase inflammation. Whole grains, leafy green and richly colored vegetables, and fruits such as berries, tart cherries (which are particularly powerful), pears and apples reduce inflammation. So do fatty fish such as salmon and tuna, and other sources of omega-3 fatty acids, like walnuts. One way to include a lot of anti-inflammatory foods without trying too hard is to follow the Mediterranean diet, which emphasizes fish, vegetables and olive oil. Giovannucci's study reveals just one surprise: People who ate more pizza had lower inflammation; tomato paste boasts bioavailable lycopene, a compound found in the tomatoes that mitigates inflammation. (That's not license to raise your pizza intake, though.)

"We don't want too much emphasis on a specific nutrient or food. More fruits and vegetables and less processed foods is something many people can attempt to do that will have a huge effect," Giovannucci says.

You can potentially gain some of the benefits by taking a fish oil supplement. But will that move overcome a bad diet? Nice idea, but it "doesn't seem to work," says Patricia Thompson, deputy director for research for the Stony Brook University Cancer Center. "It's been very difficult to identify something and just add it to a person's diet, and ask it to fix all the problems." –C.R.

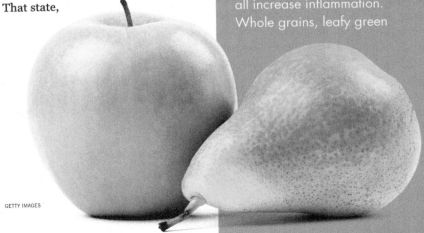

which impedes the body's ability to regulate glucose levels, may contribute to chronic inflammation and is a significant risk factor for developing Type 2 diabetes – itself a major risk factor for heart disease or stroke because excess glucose damages the arteries.

Moreover, chronic inflammation can put stress on the cells and interfere with normal cellular maintenance, so that "an event that would never have become a problem may move a line of healthy cells into a precancerous stage," says Linda Nebeling, the deputy associate director of the National Cancer Institute's Behavioral Research Program.

Keep an eye on your Vitamin D. You could say that Vitamin D, which is created when ultraviolet rays hit your skin, is having a moment in the sun. In 2016 alone, nearly 5,000 studies suggested its myriad health benefits. Aids the immune system! Maintains cognitive function! Reduces risk of cancer, heart attacks, MS and Type 2 diabetes! Helps you lose weight! Not bad for a vitamin whose earlier claim to fame was all about bone health: When D levels are too low, the body can't effectively absorb calcium. Vitamin D plays a role in cell growth, particularly in how cells divide and multiply. Giovannucci co-authored a 2014 study that found that cancer mortality decreased by up to 15 percent with Vitamin D supplementation. And Vitamin D receptors are widespread in brain tissue, suggesting that the vitamin may have a neuroprotective effect. Older adults with low levels of Vitamin D have four times the risk of cognitive impairment compared to those with adequate levels.

One problem: While there's strong observational data that Vitamin D is essential for good health and that people with low levels are at increased risk for several cancers, this is by association only – there could be another factor occurring with low vitamin D that explains the association, Thompson says. There's also little consensus about how much you need, how you should get it, and exactly how many diseases it can help prevent. In writing 2010 guidelines on Vitamin D, recommending 600 IUs (international units) for adults, the Institute of Medicine considered only the amount needed for bone health: 20 nanograms per milliliter. To find out if you're deficient, you'll need a blood test.

Under the right circumstances – tricky to nail down, because season, time of day, cloud cover, and even pollution affect the amount of UVB that reaches your skin – a fair-skinned person needs roughly 15 minutes in the sun three times a week to generate sufficient Vitamin D. It's tough to get Vitamin D from diet alone; a serving of fortified milk has just 100 IU.

That leaves supplements. If you go that route, look for Vitamin D3 instead of D2, because D3 is the compound you'd make from sun exposure, says Giovannucci. (He takes just one supplement himself: Vitamin D.) Most multivitamins contain 400 IU, a good start. ●

HOW TO LIVE

7 TO 9 HOURS
The amount of shut-eye adults need on a nightly basis; kids between ages 3 and 17 need 10 to 13 hours per night.

15
Minutes before going outside that you should apply sunscreen to allow your skin to absorb it. Reapply every two hours.

24.9
That's the upper threshold that distinguishes a healthy body mass index from being considered overweight (25 to 29.9) or obese (30 or higher).

5-10
Percentage of your total body weight you can aim to lose to achieve major health benefits, such as lower blood pressure and improved cholesterol numbers.

2
Number of times per day you should grab a soft-bristled toothbrush to keep your teeth healthy.

15 MINUTES
Roughly how long you can listen to your MP3 player cranked up to maximum volume before you harm your hearing.

20-20-20
The Rx for preventing or relieving eye strain from staring at a screen: Every 20 minutes, take a 20-second break to look at something 20 feet away.

By Stacey Colino

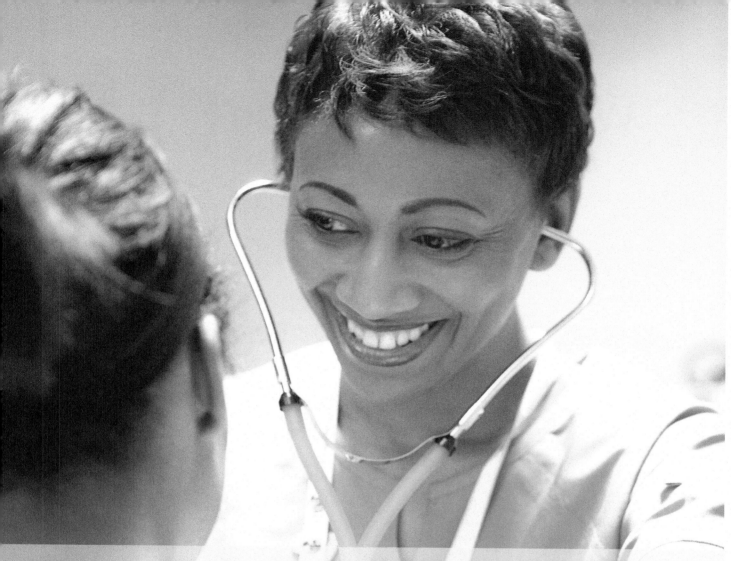

Quality Healthcare
Could Be Closer Than You Think.

Too often, we don't consider hospitals until life events make it necessary. But it's never too soon to research where to receive care. Find your best option from the **American Heart Association's** list of recognized hospitals, all of which are dedicated to providing up-to-date, scientific, guidelines-based treatment to the patients in their communities.

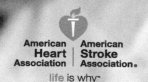

American
Heart
Association

American
Stroke
Association.

life is why™

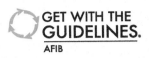 Brand*Fuse*

What Do the Awards Mean for You?

Everyone who has heart disease or a stroke should receive treatment at a hospital with the resources to correctly and consistently make time-critical decisions. Our awards recognize those that do, and chances are, one of these hospitals is near you.

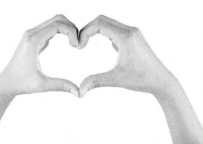

THE ISSUES

795,000
people in the United States have a stroke each year.

1 in 7
die from heart disease.

2,200
Americans die of cardiovascular disease each day.

Approximately
790,000
Americans have heart attacks each year.

The American Heart Association offers Get With The Guidelines®, an online tool, to assist hospitals in measuring and improving heart disease and stroke care through research-based guidelines.

This content is produced by or on behalf of our sponsor; it is not written by and does not necessarily reflect the view of U.S. News & World Report editorial staff. Learn more at mediakit.usnews.com.

THE IMPACT

✔ Nearly 1/2 of the nation's hospitals participate in at least one Get With The Guidelines quality improvement module.

✔ 80% of the U.S. population has access to a Get With The Guidelines-participating hospital.

✔ 6 million patients have been treated at Get With The Guidelines-participating hospitals.

✔ 4 million patient records have been entered into the Get With The Guidelines-Stroke program.

A Big Thanks to Our Sponsors

We appreciate these sponsors for supporting our healthcare quality programs and for respecting our clinical independence.

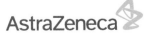

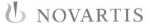 Cardiovascular

ᴕ NOVARTIS

THE AWARDS

Each year, the American Heart Association recognizes participating hospitals that demonstrate high commitment to following guidelines shown to improve patient outcomes.

Use the following guide to learn more about the award categories and locate award-winning hospitals near you. »

Key to the Awards

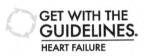 **GET WITH THE GUIDELINES.**
AFIB

Ⓖ **Gold Achievement.** These hospitals are recognized for two or more consecutive years of 85% or higher adherence on all achievement measures applicable to atrial fibrillation.

Ⓢ **Silver Achievement.** These hospitals are recognized for 1 calendar year of 85% or higher adherence on all achievement measures applicable to atrial fibrillation.

GET WITH THE GUIDELINES.
HEART FAILURE

Ⓖ⁺ **Gold Plus Achievement.** These hospitals are recognized for two or more consecutive years of 85% or higher adherence on all achievement measures applicable and 75% or higher adherence with four or more select quality measures in heart failure.

Ⓖ **Gold Achievement.** These hospitals are recognized for two or more consecutive years of 85% or higher adherence on all achievement measures applicable to heart failure.

Ⓢ⁺ **Silver Plus Achievement.** These hospitals are recognized for 1 calendar year of 85% or higher adherence on all achievement measures applicable and 75% or higher adherence with four or more select quality measures in heart failure.

Silver Achievement. These hospitals are recognized for 1 calendar year of 85% or higher adherence on all achievement measures applicable to heart failure.

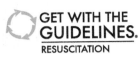

Gold Achievement. These hospitals are recognized for two or more consecutive years of 85% or higher adherence to designated achievement measures applicable to resuscitation.

Silver Achievement. These hospitals are recognized for one calendar year of 85% or higher adherence to designated achievement measures applicable to resuscitation.

*This hospital received Get With The Guidelines-Resuscitation awards for two or more patient populations.

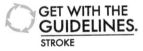

Gold Plus Achievement. These hospitals are recognized for two or more consecutive years of 85% or higher adherence on all achievement measures applicable and at least 75% or higher adherence with five or more select quality measures in stroke.

Gold Achievement. These hospitals are recognized for two or more consecutive years of 85% or higher adherence on all achievement measures applicable to stroke.

Silver Plus Achievement. These

---

hospitals are recognized for 1 calendar year of 85% or higher adherence on all achievement measures applicable and at least 75% or higher adherence with five or more select quality measures in stroke.

Silver Achievement. These hospitals are recognized for 1 calendar year of 85% or higher adherence on all achievement measures applicable to stroke.

TO BE RECOGNIZED IN 2018:

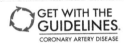

All 2018 Mission Lifeline awards will use 2017 GWTG-CAD data

Mission: Lifeline®
STEMI

Gold Receiving. These hospitals are recognized for consecutive 2 year intervals of 85% or higher composite adherence to all STEMI Receiving Center Performance Achievement indicators and 75% or higher compliance on each performance measure.

Gold Plus Receiving. These hospitals meet Gold Receiving Center criteria and in addition are recognized for 75% or higher achievement of First Door-to-Device time of 120 minutes or less for transferred STEMI patients.

Silver Receiving. These hospitals are recognized for 1 calendar year interval of 85% or higher composite adherence to all STEMI Receiving Center Performance Achievement indicators and 75% or

---

higher compliance on each performance measure.

Silver Plus Receiving. These hospitals meet Silver Receiving criteria and in addition are recognized for 75% or higher achievement of First Door-to-Device time of 120 minutes or less for transferred STEMI patients.

Gold Referring. These hospitals are recognized for consecutive 2 year intervals of 85% or higher composite adherence to all STEMI Receiving Center Performance Achievement indicators and 75% or higher compliance on each performance measure.

Silver Referring. These hospitals are recognized for 1 calendar year interval of 85% or higher composite adherence to all STEMI Referring Center Performance Achievement indicators and 75% or higher compliance on each performance measure.

Mission: Lifeline®
NSTEMI

Silver. These hospitals are recognized for 1 calendar year interval of achieving 65% adherence to Dual Antiplatelet prescription at discharge and 75% or higher compliance on each of the other 4 performance measures.

Bronze. These hospitals are recognized for at least one consecutive 90 day interval of achieving 65% adherence to Dual Antiplatelet prescription at discharge and 75% or higher compliance on each of the other 4 performance measures.

TARGET: HF™

Honor Roll. These hospitals are recognized for at least one calendar quarter of 50% or higher adherence to all relevant Target: Heart Failure measures in addition to current Bronze, Silver or Gold Get With The Guidelines-Heart Failure recognition status.

TARGET: STROKE™

Honor Roll - Elite Plus. These hospitals are recognized for at least four consecutive quarters of 75% or higher achievement of door-to-needle times within 60 minutes AND 50% achievement of door-to-needle times within 45 minutes in applicable stroke patients in addition to current Silver or Gold Get With The Guidelines-Stroke recognition status.

Honor Roll - Elite. These hospitals are recognized for at least four consecutive quarters of 75% or higher achievement of door-to-needle times within 60 minutes in applicable stroke patients in addition to current Silver or Gold Get With The Guidelines-Stroke recognition status.

Honor Roll. These hospitals are recognized for one calendar quarter or more of 50% or higher achievement of door-to-needle times within 60 minutes in applicable stroke patients in addition to current Bronze, Silver or Gold Get With The Guidelines-Stroke recognition status.

Find Your Hospital Listed Alphabetically By State

For a searchable map of hospitals within this region and across the U.S. visit heart.org/myhealthcare

ALABAMA

Baptist Medical Center South, Montgomery, AL .... G+
Brookwood Baptist Medical Center, Birmingham, AL .... G+ G+ HR
Coosa Valley Medical Center, Sylacauga, AL .... G+ E
Crestwood Medical Center, Huntsville, AL .... S G+
Eliza Coffee Memorial Hospital, Florence, AL .... G+ E
Flowers Hospital, Dothan, AL .... G+ B
Gadsden Regional Medical Center, Gadsden, AL .... G+ HR
Grandview Medical Center, Birmingham, AL .... G+ S G+
Huntsville Hospital, Huntsville, AL .... S G+ E
Mobile Infirmary, Mobile, AL .... G G G+ E
Princeton Baptist Medical Center, Birmingham, AL .... G+ E+
Providence Hospital, Mobile, AL .... G G+ HR
South Baldwin Regional Medical Center, Foley, AL .... G+ E
Southeast Alabama Medical Center, Dothan, AL .... G+ E
St. Vincent's Birmingham, Birmingham, AL .... S G+
Stringfellow Memorial Hospital, Anniston, AL .... G G+
UAB Hospital, Birmingham, AL .... G+ E+
University of South Alabama Medical Center, Mobile, AL .... G+ G+ E+
Walker Baptist Medical Center, Jasper, AL .... G

ALASKA

Alaska Regional Hospital, Anchorage, AK .... G+ HR
Providence Alaska Medical Center, Anchorage, AK .... G+ E+ S

ARIZONA

Abrazo Arrowhead Campus, Glendale, AZ .... G+ E S+
Abrazo Central Campus, Phoenix, AZ .... G+ HR
Abrazo Maryvale Campus, Phoenix, AZ ....
Abrazo Scottsdale Campus, Phoenix, AZ .... G+
Abrazo West Campus, Goodyear, AZ .... S+ HR
Banner Baywood Medical Center, Mesa, AZ .... G+ E
Banner Boswell Medical Center, Sun City, AZ .... G+ E
Banner Del E. Webb Medical Center, Sun City West, AZ .... G+ E+
Banner Desert Medical Center, Mesa, AZ .... G+ HR
Banner Estrella Medical Center, Phoenix, AZ .... G+ E
Banner Thunderbird Medical Center, Glendale, AZ .... G+ E
Banner University Medical Center Phoenix, Phoenix, AZ .... G+ E+
Banner University Medical Center Tucson, Tucson, AZ .... G+ HR
Carondelet St. Mary's Hospital, Tucson, AZ .... G+ E+
Dignity Health Mercy Gilbert Medical Center, Gilbert, AZ .... S G+ E
Dignity Health Chandler Regional Medical Center, Chandler, AZ ...... S G+ E+
Dignity Health St. Joseph's Hospital and Medical Center | Barrow
    Neurological Institute, Phoenix, AZ .... G+ E
HonorHealth Deer Valley Medical Center, Phoenix, AZ .... G+ E
HonorHealth John C. Lincoln Medical Center, Phoenix, AZ .... G+ E
HonorHealth Scottsdale Osborn Medical Center, Scottsdale, AZ ...... G+ E
Mayo Clinic Hospital Arizona, Phoenix, AZ .... G+ E+
Mountain Vista Medical Center, Mesa, AZ .... G+ HR
Southern Arizona VA Health Care System, Tucson, AZ .... S
The Carondelet Neurological Institute at St. Joseph's Hospital,
    Tucson, AZ .... G+ E+
Tucson Medical Center, Tucson, AZ .... G+ E

ARKANSAS

Baptist Health Medical Center, Little Rock, AR .... G+ HR
CHI St. Vincent Hot Springs, Hot Springs, AR .... G+
Medical Center of South Arkansas, El Dorado, AR .... S S
Mercy Hospital Rogers, Rogers, AR .... G+ HR
NEA Baptist Memorial Hospital, Jonesboro, AR .... B
Sparks Health System, Fort Smith, AR .... G+ HR
St. Bernards Medical Center, Jonesboro, AR .... G+ B
University of Arkansas for Medical Sciences, Little Rock, AR .... G+ E+
Washington Regional Medical Center, Fayetteville, AR .... G+ E
White County Medical Center, Searcy, AR .... S

CALIFORNIA

Alameda Hospital, Alameda, CA .... G+ G+ E+ B
Alta Bates Summit Medical Center-Alta Bates Campus,
    Berkeley, CA .... G+ E
Alta Bates Summit Medical Center-Summit Campus, Oakland, CA ...... G+ E
Arrowhead Regional Medical Center, Colton, CA .... G+ E
Bakersfield Heart and Surgical Hospital, Bakersfield, CA .... S+
California Pacific Medical Center, San Francisco, CA .... G+ HR S+ B
Cedars-Sinai Medical Center, Los Angeles, CA .... G+ E+
CHA Hollywood Presbyterian Medical Center, Los Angeles, CA ...... G+ E
Citrus Valley Medical Center, Inter-Community Campus,
    Covina, CA .... G HR
Citrus Valley Medical Center, Queen of the Valley Campus,
    West Covina, CA .... G HR G+ E
Community Hospital of the Monterey Peninsula, Monterey, CA .... G+ E+
Community Memorial Hospital, Ventura, CA .... G
Community Regional Medical Center, Fresno, CA .... S+ E
Corona Regional Medical Center, Corona, CA .... S+ E
Desert Regional Medical Center, Palm Springs, CA .... G G G+ E
Dignity Health California Hospital Medical Center, Los Angeles, CA ... G+ E
Dignity Health Dominican Hospital, Santa Cruz, CA .... G+ HR
Dignity Health French Hospital Medical Center, San Luis Obispo, CA ... S
Dignity Health Memorial Hospital, Bakersfield, CA .... G+ E E+
Dignity Health Mercy General Hospital, Sacramento, CA .... G+ E+
Dignity Health Mercy Hospital of Folsom, Folsom, CA .... G+ E
Dignity Health Mercy Hospitals of Bakersfield, Bakersfield, CA ...... G+ HR
Dignity Health Mercy Medical Center, Merced, CA .... G+ E
Dignity Health Mercy Medical Center Redding, Redding, CA .... G+ E
Dignity Health Mercy San Juan Medical Center, Carmichael, CA ..... G+ E+
Dignity Health Methodist Hospital of Sacramento, Sacramento, CA ... G+ E
Dignity Health Northridge Hospital Medical Center, Northridge, CA ... G+ E+
Dignity Health Saint Francis Memorial Hospital, San Francisco, CA ... G+ E+
Dignity Health Sequoia Hospital, Redwood City, CA .... G+ E
Dignity Health St. Bernardine Medical Center, San Bernardino, CA ... G+ E
Dignity Health St. John's Pleasant Valley Hospital, Camarillo, CA .... G+ E
Dignity Health St. John's Regional Medical Center, Oxnard, CA .... G+ E
Dignity Health St. Joseph's Medical Center, Stockton, CA .... S E S
Dignity Health St. Mary's Medical Center, San Francisco, CA .... G+ E
Dignity Health Woodland Memorial Hospital, Woodland, CA .... G+ E
Doctors Hospital of Manteca, Manteca, CA .... S+
Doctors Medical Center, Modesto, CA .... G+ G+ E G
El Camino Hospital - Mountain View and El Camino Hospital -
    Los Gatos, Mountain View and Los Gatos, CA .... G+ E
Emanuel Medical Center, Turlock, CA .... G
Encino Hospital Medical Center, Encino, CA .... G+ E+
Enloe Medical Center, Chico, CA .... G+ E
Fountain Valley Regional Hospital and Medical Center,
    Fountain Valley, CA .... G+ G+ E S B
Garfield Medical Center, Monterey Park, CA .... G+ E
Glendale Adventist Medical Center, Glendale, CA .... G+ E
Good Samaritan Hospital, San Jose, CA .... G+ E
Henry Mayo Newhall Hospital, Valencia, CA .... G+ HR
Hoag Memorial Hospital Presbyterian, Newport Beach, CA .... G G+ E
Huntington Hospital, Pasadena, CA .... G+ HR
John F. Kennedy Memorial Hospital, Indio, CA ....
John Muir Medical Center - Concord, Concord, CA .... G+ G+ E G
John Muir Medical Center - Walnut Creek, Walnut Creek, CA .... G+ G+ E S E
Kaiser Foundation Hospital - Antioch, Antioch, CA .... G+ G+ E
Kaiser Foundation Hospital - Fremont, Fremont, CA .... G+ E
Kaiser Foundation Hospital - Fresno, Fresno, CA .... G+ E
Kaiser Foundation Hospital - Manteca, Manteca, CA .... S S
Kaiser Foundation Hospital - Modesto, Modesto, CA .... G+ E
Kaiser Foundation Hospital - Oakland, Oakland, CA .... G+ E
Kaiser Foundation Hospital - Redwood City, Redwood City, CA ...... G+ E
Kaiser Foundation Hospital - Richmond, Richmond, CA .... S+ E

Kaiser Foundation Hospital - Roseville, Roseville, CA .... (G+) (E+)
Kaiser Foundation Hospital - Sacramento, Sacramento, CA .... (G+) (E+)
Kaiser Foundation Hospital - San Diego, San Diego, CA .... (G+) (E+)
Kaiser Foundation Hospital - San Francisco, San Francisco, CA .... (G+) (E+)
Kaiser Foundation Hospital - San Jose, San Jose, CA .... (G+) (E+)
Kaiser Foundation Hospital - San Leandro, San Leandro, CA .... (S) (S+)
Kaiser Foundation Hospital - San Rafael, San Rafael, CA .... (G+) (E+)
Kaiser Foundation Hospital - Santa Clara, Santa Clara, CA .... (G+) (E+)
Kaiser Foundation Hospital - Santa Rosa, Santa Rosa, CA .... (S) (G+)
Kaiser Foundation Hospital - South Sacramento, Sacramento, CA .... (G+) (E+)
Kaiser Foundation Hospital - South San Francisco,
    South San Francisco, CA .... (G+) (E+)
Kaiser Foundation Hospital - Vacaville, Vacaville, CA .... (G+) (E+)
Kaiser Foundation Hospital - Vallejo, Vallejo, CA .... (G+) (E+)
Kaiser Foundation Hospital - Walnut Creek, Walnut Creek, CA .... (G+) (G+) (E+)
Kaiser Foundation Hospital Orange County, Anaheim and Irvine, CA.... (S+) (E)
Kaiser Permanente Baldwin Park Medical Center,
    Baldwin Park, CA .... (G+) (G+) (E+)
Kaiser Permanente Downey Medical Center, Downey, CA .... (G+) (E)
Kaiser Permanente Fontana Medical Center, Fontana, CA .... (G+) (E+)
Kaiser Permanente Los Angeles Medical Center, Los Angeles, CA........ (G+) (E+)
Kaiser Permanente Moreno Valley Medical Center, Moreno Valley, CA. (G+) (E+)
Kaiser Permanente Ontario Medical Center, Ontario, CA........................ (G+) (E+)
Kaiser Permanente Panorama City Medical Center,
    Panorama City, CA .... (G+) (E+)
Kaiser Permanente Riverside Medical Center, Riverside, CA .... (G+) (E+)
Kaiser Permanente South Bay Medical Center, Harbor City, CA .... (G+) (E)
Kaiser Permanente Woodland Hills Medical Center,
    Woodland Hills, CA .... (G+) (E+)
Kaweah Delta Health Care District, Visalia, CA .... (G+)
Keck Hospital of USC, Los Angeles, CA........... (S)
Kern Medical, Bakersfield, CA........... (S)
Lakewood Regional Medical Center, Lakewood, CA........... (G+) (HR)
Loma Linda University Medical Center - Murrieta, Murrieta, CA .... (S+)
Long Beach Memorial, Long Beach, CA .... (G+) (HR) (G+) (E)
Los Alamitos Medical Center, Los Alamitos, CA .... (G+) (HR) (G+) (E+)
Los Angeles County + USC Medical Center, Los Angeles, CA................ (S+) (HR)
Los Robles Hospital & Medical Center, Thousand Oaks, CA .... (G+) (HR) (G+) (E+)
Marin General Hospital, Greenbrae, CA .... (G+) (HR)
Marshall Medical Center, Placerville, CA .... (G+) (E)
Methodist Hospital of Southern California, Arcadia, CA .... (G+) (HR)
Mills-Peninsula Health Services, Burlingame, CA........... (G+) (HR)
NorthBay Healthcare Group, Fairfield, CA .... (G+) (E) (S+)
O'Connor Hospital, San Jose, CA........... (G+) (E+)
Oroville Hospital, Oroville, CA........... (G+) (HR)
Palmdale Regional Medical Center, Palmdale, CA .... (S+)
PIH Health Hospital-Whittier, Whittier, CA .... (G+) (E)
Placentia-Linda Hospital, Placentia, CA .... (G+)
Pomona Valley Hospital Medical Center, Pomona, CA .... (G+) (G+) (E)
Providence Holy Cross Medical Center, Mission Hills, CA .... (G+) (HR)
Providence Little Company of Mary Medical Center San Pedro,
    San Pedro, CA .... (G+) (HR)
Providence Little Company of Mary Medical Center Torrance,
    Torrance, CA .... (S) (S+) (HR)
Providence Saint John's Health Center, Santa Monica, CA................... (S+) (E+)
Providence Saint Joseph Medical Center, Burbank, CA .... (G+) (HR)
Providence Tarzana Medical Center, Tarzana, CA........... (G+) (HR)
Redlands Community Hospital, Redlands, CA........... (G+) (HR)
Regional Medical Center of San Jose, San Jose, CA .... (G+) (HR)
Rideout Memorial Hospital, Marysville, CA .... (S+) (E+)
Riverside Community Hospital, Riverside, CA .... (G+) (E)
Riverside University Health System - Medical Center,
    Moreno Valley, CA .... (G+) (E)
Ronald Reagan UCLA Medical Center, Los Angeles, CA................... (G+) (HR) (G+) (E)
Saddleback Memorial Medical Center, Laguna Hills, CA................ (G+) (HR) (G+) (E)
Salinas Valley Memorial Hospital, Salinas, CA .... (G+) (HR) (G+) (HR) (B)
San Antonio Regional Hospital, Upland, CA........... (G+)
San Joaquin Community Hospital, Bakersfield, CA..................... (G+) (E) (G) (S)
San Joaquin General Hospital, French Camp, CA........... (G+) (E)
San Ramon Regional Medical Center LLC, San Ramon, CA................ (G+) (G+) (E+)

Santa Monica UCLA Medical Center and Orthopaedic Hospital,
    Santa Monica, CA .... (S+)
Scripps Green Hospital, La Jolla, CA........... (G+)
Scripps Memorial Hospital Encinitas, Encinitas, CA .... (G+) (E)
Scripps Memorial Hospital La Jolla, La Jolla, CA........... (G+) (E+)
Scripps Mercy Hospital, San Diego and Chula Vista, CA........... (G+) (E)
Seton Medical Center, Daly City, CA........... (G+) (E)
Sharp Chula Vista Medical Center, Chula Vista, CA........... (G+) (E+)
Sharp Grossmont Hospital, La Mesa, CA........... (G+) (E+)
Sharp Memorial Hospital, San Diego, CA........... (G+) (E)
Sherman Oaks Hospital, Sherman Oaks, CA........... (G+) (HR)
Sierra Nevada Memorial Hospital, Grass Valley, CA........... (G+) (E)
Sierra Vista Regional Medical Center, San Luis Obispo, CA .... (G+)
Simi Valley Hospital, Simi Valley, CA........... (G+) (HR)
Southwest Healthcare Systems Inland Valley Medical Center
    and Rancho Springs Medical Center, Wildomar and Murrieta, CA .... (G+) (HR)
St. Jude Medical Center, Fullerton, CA........... (G+) (E+)
St. Francis Medical Center, Lynwood, CA........... (G+) (E)
St. Louise Regional Hospital, Gilroy, CA........... (G+) (E+)
Stanford Health Care, Stanford, CA........... (S) (HR)
Sutter Health Eden Medical Center, Castro Valley, CA........... (G+) (E)
Sutter Health Memorial Medical Center, Modesto, CA........... (G+) (HR) (G) (B)
Sutter Medical Center Sacramento, Sacramento, CA........... (S+) (HR)
Sutter Santa Rosa Regional Hospital, Santa Rosa, CA........... (S+)
Temecula Valley Hospital, Temecula, CA........... (G+) (E)
Torrance Memorial Medical Center, Torrance, CA .... (G+) (HR) (G) (S+) (HR) (S)
Tri-City Medical Center, Oceanside, CA .... (G+) (HR) (S) (G+) (HR) (G)
Twin Cities Community Hospital, Templeton, CA........... (G+)
UC San Diego Health System, San Diego, CA........... (G+) (E+)
University of California Irvine Medical Center, Orange, CA........... (G+) (HR) (G+) (E)
University of California San Francisco (UCSF), San Francisco, CA .... (S+) (E+)
University of California, Davis Medical Center, Sacramento, CA........... (G+) (HR)
USC Verdugo Hills Hospital, Glendale, CA........... (G+)
VA Loma Linda Healthcare System, Loma Linda, CA .... (S+)
Ventura County Medical Center/Santa Paula Hospital, Ventura, CA........... (G+)
Washington Hospital Healthcare System, Fremont, CA........... (G+) (E+)
White Memorial Medical Center, Los Angeles, CA .... (G+) (E+)

COLORADO

Boulder Community Health Foothills Hospital, Boulder, CO........... (G+) (HR)
Good Samaritan Medical Center, Lafayette, CO .... (G+) (E+) (G+) (B)
Littleton Adventist Hospital, Littleton, CO........... (S) (G+) (E) (G+) (B)
Lutheran Medical Center, Wheat Ridge, CO........... (G+) (E+)
Medical Center of the Rockies, Loveland, CO .... (S+) (HR) (S+) (HR) (G+) (B)
Memorial Health System, Colorado Springs, CO .... (G+) (E) (G) (S)
North Colorado Medical Center, Greeley, CO .... (G+) (E) (G) (S)
North Suburban Medical Center, Thornton, CO .... (S+) (E+)
Parker Adventist Hospital, Parker, CO........... (G+) (E+) (G) (S)
Parkview Medical Center, Pueblo, CO........... (G+) (S)
Penrose-St. Francis Health Services, Colorado Springs, CO.... (G) (G+) (E+) (G) (S)
Platte Valley Medical Center, Brighton, CO........... (G+) (HR)
Porter Adventist Hospital- Centura Health, Denver, CO........... (G+) (HR) (G+) (E+)
Poudre Valley Hospital, Fort Collins, CO........... (S+) (HR) (S+) (E+)
Presbyterian/St. Luke's Medical Center, Denver, CO .... (G) (S)
Rose Medical Center, Denver, CO........... (G+) (E+) (G) (S)
Sky Ridge Medical Center, Lone Tree, CO........... (G+) (S)
St. Anthony Hospital, Lakewood, CO .... (G+) (E) (G+) (B)
St. Anthony North Hospital, Westminster, CO........... (B)
St. Francis Medical Center, Colorado Springs, CO .... (S+) (E+) (S) (S)
St. Mary - Corwin Medical Center, Pueblo, CO .... (G+) (HR)
St. Mary's Hospital and Medical Center, Grand Junction, CO........... (G+) (HR)
Swedish Medical Center, Englewood, CO .... (G+) (B)
The Medical Center of Aurora, Aurora, CO .... (G+) (E+) (G) (S)
University of Colorado Hospital, Aurora, CO........... (G) (HR) (G+) (E+) (G+) (B)

CONNECTICUT

Bridgeport Hospital, Bridgeport, CT........... (S) (HR)
Connecticut Children's Medical Center, Hartford, CT........... (G)
Eastern Connecticut Health Network, Manchester and Rockville,
    Manchester, CT........... (G)

Greenwich Hospital, Greenwich, CT .... (S) (G+)
Hartford Hospital, Hartford, CT .... (G+) (E+)
John Dempsey Hospital/UCONN Health Center,
    Farmington, CT .... (G+) (HR) (G) (E) (G+) (B)
Lawrence + Memorial Hospital, New London, CT .... (G) (HR) (S+)
Saint Francis Hospital and Medical Center, Hartford, CT .... (G+) (HR)
Saint Mary's Health System, Waterbury, CT .... (G)
St. Vincent's Medical Center, Bridgeport, CT .... (G+) (G+) (HR) (S) (B)
Stamford Hospital, Stamford, CT .... (G+) (E) (S) (B)
The Hospital of Central Connecticut, New Britain, CT .... (G+) (HR) (G+)
Waterbury Hospital, Waterbury, CT .... (G) (HR)
Yale - New Haven Hospital, New Haven, CT .... (G+) (E) (S)

DELAWARE

Bayhealth Medical Center - Kent General Hospital, Dover, DE ...... (S) (B)
Beebe Healthcare, Lewes, DE .... (HR) (G+) (HR) (B)
Christiana Care Health System, Newark, DE .... (G+) (E+) (G+) (S)
Nanticoke Memorial Hospital, Seaford, DE .... (S+) (HR) (G+) (E)
Saint Francis Hospital, Wilmington, DE .... (G+) (HR)

DISTRICT OF COLUMBIA

Howard University Hospital, Washington, DC .... (G+) (HR)
MedStar Washington Hospital Center, Washington, DC .... (G+) (E)
Providence Hospital, Washington, DC .... (G+)
Sibley Memorial Hospital, Washington, DC .... (G+) (HR)
The George Washington University Hospital, Washington, DC .... (G+) (E+)

FLORIDA

Arnold Palmer Hospital for Children, Orlando, FL .... (G)
Aventura Hospital and Medical Center, Aventura, FL .... (G+) (E+)
Baptist Hospital of Miami, Miami, FL .... (G+) (E+)
Baptist Medical Center - Beaches (Baptist Health),
    Jacksonville Beach, FL .... (S) (G+) (HR)
Baptist Medical Center - Jacksonville (Baptist Health),
    Jacksonville, FL .... (G+) (E)
Baptist Medical Center - South (Baptist Health), Jacksonville, FL .... (G) (S+)
Bayfront Health St. Petersburg, Saint Petersburg, FL .... (G+) (HR)
Boca Raton Regional Hospital, Boca Raton, FL .... (G+) (E)
Brandon Regional Hospital, Brandon, FL .... (G+) (HR) (G)
Broward Health Coral Springs, Coral Springs, FL .... (G+) (E+)
Broward Health Medical Center, Fort Lauderdale, FL .... (G+) (HR)
Broward Health North, Pompano Beach, FL .... (G+) (E+)
Cape Coral Hospital, Cape Coral, FL .... (G+) (E+)
Capital Regional Medical Center, Tallahassee, FL .... (G+)
Central Florida Regional Hospital, Sanford, FL .... (G+)
Citrus Memorial Hospital, also known as Citrus Memorial
    Health System, Inverness, FL .... (S)
Cleveland Clinic Florida, Weston, FL .... (G+) (E+)
Coral Gables Hospital, Miami, FL .... (S+)
Delray Medical Center, Delray Beach, FL .... (G+) (E+)
Doctors Hospital of Sarasota, Sarasota, FL .... (S+) (G+) (E+) (S+)
Englewood Community Hospital, Englewood, FL .... (G+) (S+)
Flagler Hospital, Inc., Saint Augustine, FL .... (G+) (S+)
Florida Hospital Altamonte, Altamonte Springs, FL .... (G+) (S+)
Florida Hospital Apopka, Apopka, FL .... (G+)
Florida Hospital Celebration Health, Celebration, FL .... (G+) (HR)
Florida Hospital DeLand, DeLand, FL .... (G+) (E+)
Florida Hospital East Orlando, Orlando, FL .... (G+)
Florida Hospital Fish Memorial, Orange City, FL .... (G+) (E+)
Florida Hospital Flagler, Palm Coast, FL .... (G+) (E+)
Florida Hospital Kissimmee, Kissimmee, FL .... (G+) (HR)
Florida Hospital Memorial Medical Center, Daytona Beach, FL .... (G+) (E+)
Florida Hospital New Smyrna, New Smyrna Beach, FL .... (G+) (E)
Florida Hospital North Pinellas, Tarpon Springs, FL .... (G+) (E+)
Florida Hospital Orlando, Orlando, FL .... (G+) (E) (G+) (B)
Florida Hospital Tampa/Florida Hospital Pepin Heart Institute,
    Tampa, FL .... (G+) (HR) (G+) (E+) (G)
Florida Hospital Wesley Chapel, Wesley Chapel, FL .... (G)
Florida Hospital Zephyrhills, Zephyrhills, FL .... (G+) (G+) (HR) (S+)
FLORIDA MEDICAL CENTER a campus of North Shore,
    Fort Lauderdale, FL .... (S+) (G+) (E+)

Fort Walton Beach Medical Center, Fort Walton Beach, FL .... (G+) (HR)
Good Samaritan Medical Center, West Palm Beach, FL .... (G+) (G+) (E)
Gulf Coast Medical Center, Fort Myers, FL .... (G+) (E+)
Halifax Health, Daytona Beach, FL .... (G+) (E)
Health Park Medical Center, Fort Myers, FL .... (G+)
Hialeah Hospital, Hialeah, FL .... (G+) (G+)
Holmes Regional Medical Center, Melbourne, FL .... (G+) (E)
Holy Cross Hospital, Fort Lauderdale, FL .... (HR) (G) (G+) (E+)
Indian River Medical Center, Vero Beach, FL .... (G+) (G) (B)
Jackson Memorial Hospital, Miami, FL .... (G+) (E+)
Jackson North Medical Center, North Miami Beach, FL .... (G+) (E+)
Jupiter Medical Center, Jupiter, FL .... (G+)
Lakeland Regional Health, Lakeland, FL .... (G+) (HR)
Lakewood Ranch Medical Center, Bradenton, FL .... (S+) (E+)
Largo Medical Center, Largo, FL .... (G) (G+) (G+)
Lee Memorial Hospital, Fort Myers, FL .... (G+) (HR)
Manatee Memorial Hospital, Bradenton, FL .... (G+) (E) (G)
Mease Countryside Hospital, Safety Harbor, FL .... (G+) (HR)
Mease Dunedin Hospital, Dunedin, FL .... (S+) (E)
Memorial Hospital, Jacksonville, FL .... (G+) (E+)
Memorial Hospital Pembroke, Pembroke Pines, FL .... (G+) (E+)
Memorial Hospital West, Pembroke Pines, FL .... (G+) (E+)
Memorial Regional Hospital, Hollywood, FL .... (G+) (E+)
Mercy Hospital, Miami, FL .... (G+)
Morton Plant Hospital, Clearwater, FL .... (G+) (E)
Morton Plant North Bay Hospital, New Port Richey, FL .... (G+) (HR)
Mount Sinai Medical Center, Miami Beach, FL .... (G+) (E+) (B)
NCH Healthcare System, Naples, FL .... (G) (S)
Nicklaus Children's Hospital, Miami, FL .... (G) (S)
North Florida Regional Medical Center, Gainesville, FL .... (S+) (E+)
North Shore Medical Center, Miami, FL .... (G+) (HR)
Northside Hospital and Tampa Bay Heart Institute,
    Saint Petersburg, FL .... (G+) (G+) (E+) (G+)
Ocala Health, Ocala, FL .... (G+) (HR)
Orange Park Medical Center, Orange Park, FL ...... (G) (G+) (HR) (G) (G+) (E+) (S+)
Orlando Regional Medical Center, Orlando, FL .... (S) (G+) (E)
Osceola Regional Medical Center, Kissimmee, FL .... (G+) (E+)
Palm Beach Gardens Medical Center,
    Palm Beach Gardens, FL .... (G+) (HR) (G+) (E+)
Palmetto General Hospital, Hialeah, FL .... (G+) (E+)
Palms of Pasadena Hospital, South Pasadena, FL .... (G+) (HR) (G)
Physicians Regional Healthcare System, Naples, FL .... (G+) (E+)
Sacred Heart Health System, Pensacola, FL .... (G+) (HR)
Sarasota Memorial Health Care System, Sarasota, FL .... (G+) (HR)
South Florida Baptist Hospital, Plant City, FL .... (G+)
St. Anthony's Hospital, Saint Petersburg, FL .... (S+) (E) (S)
St. Joseph's Hospital, Tampa, FL .... (G+) (HR)
St. Joseph's Hospital - South, Riverview, FL .... (S+)
St. Joseph's Hospital- North, Lutz, FL .... (G+) (E) (S)
St. Mary's Medical Center, West Palm Beach, FL .... (G+) (E+)
St. Vincent's Medical Center Riverside, Jacksonville, FL .... (G+) (HR)
St. Vincent's Medical Center Southside, Jacksonville, FL .... (HR) (E+)
Tallahassee Memorial HealthCare, Tallahassee, FL .... (G+) (E)
Tampa Community Hospital, Tampa, FL .... (S+)
Tampa General Hospital, Tampa, FL .... (G+) (E+)
The Villages Regional Hospital, The Villages, FL .... (S)
UF Health Jacksonville, Jacksonville, FL .... (S)
UF Health Shands Hospital, Gainesville, FL .... (G+) (E)
University of Miami Hospital, Miami, FL .... (G+) (E+)
Venice Regional Bayfront Health, Venice, FL .... (G+) (E+)
Wellington Regional Medical Center, Wellington, FL .... (G+) (HR)
West Boca Medical Center, Boca Raton, FL .... (G+) (E+)
West Florida Hospital, Pensacola, FL .... (G+) (E) (S)
West Kendall Baptist Hospital, Miami, FL .... (S+) (HR)
Winter Park Memorial Hospital, Winter Park, FL .... (G+) (E+)
Wuesthoff Medical Center Rockledge, Rockledge, FL .... (G+) (E+) (B)

GEORGIA

Appling Healthcare System, Baxley, GA .... (S+)
Athens Regional Medical Center, Athens, GA .... (S+) (E+)
AU Medical Center, Augusta, GA .... (S+) (E+)

Candler Hospital, Savannah, GA .... S+
Cartersville Medical Center, Cartersville, GA .... G+ E+
Coliseum Medical Centers, Macon, GA .... G+ HR
DeKalb Medical Center, Inc., Decatur, GA .... G+
DeKalb Medical Hillandale, Lithonia, GA .... S+
Doctors Hospital Augusta, Augusta, GA .... S+
Emory Johns Creek Hospital, Duluth, GA .... G S
Emory Saint Joseph's Hospital, Atlanta, GA .... S B
Emory University Hospital, Atlanta, GA .... G+ E+ G+ B
Emory University Hospital Midtown, Atlanta, GA .... G+ HR B
Fairview Park Hospital, Dublin, GA .... G
Floyd Medical Center, Rome, GA .... G+ E
Grady Health System, Atlanta, GA .... G+ G+ E+ G
Gwinnett Hospital System, Lawrenceville, GA .... G+ E G+
Hamilton Medical Center, Dalton, GA .... G+ E+
Meadows Regional Medical Center, Vidalia, GA .... S HR
Medical Center Navicent Health, Macon, GA .... G+ E+
Memorial Health University Medical Center, Savannah, GA .... G+ HR G+ E
Midtown Medical Center, Columbus, GA .... S
Northeast Georgia Medical Center, Gainesville, GA .... G+ E G B
Northside Hospital Atlanta, Atlanta, GA .... G+ G G E G B
Northside Hospital Cherokee, Canton, GA .... G+ G G E G B
Northside Hospital Forsyth, Cumming, GA .... G+ HR S G+ E G S
Phoebe Putney Memorial Hospital, Albany, GA .... G+
Piedmont Fayette Hospital, Fayetteville, GA .... G+ E S
Piedmont Henry Hospital, Stockbridge, GA .... G+ E+
Piedmont Hospital, Atlanta, GA .... G+ E+
Piedmont Newnan Hospital, Newnan, GA .... S+
Polk Medical Center, Cedartown, GA .... G+
Redmond Regional Medical Center, Rome, GA .... G+ HR G+ E+ S
Rockdale Medical Center, Conyers, GA .... S HR
South Georgia Medical Center, Valdosta, GA .... G G+ E+
St. Francis Hospital, Inc., Columbus, GA .... G+ E
St. Joseph's Hospital, Savannah, GA .... G+ E B
St. Mary's Health Care System, Athens, GA .... G+ G+ HR B
Tanner Medical Center/Villa Rica, Villa Rica, GA .... S
University Hospital, Augusta, GA .... G+
WellStar Atlanta Medical Center, Atlanta, GA .... G+ HR
WellStar Cobb Hospital, Austell, GA .... G+ E B
WellStar Douglas Hospital, Douglasville, GA .... G+
WellStar Kennestone Hospital, Marietta, GA .... G+ E+ S+
WellStar North Fulton Hospital, Roswell, GA .... G+ G+ E+ S
WellStar Paulding Hospital, Dallas, GA .... S
WellStar Spalding Regional Hospital, Griffin, GA .... G+ E
West Georgia Medical Center, LaGrange, GA .... B

HAWAII

Castle Medical Center, Kailua, HI .... G+
Kaiser Foundation Hospital - Moanalua Medical Center,
    Honolulu, HI .... G+ G+ E
Maui Memorial Medical Center, Wailuku, HI .... G+ HR G+ E
Pali Momi Medical Center, Aiea, HI .... G+ E
Straub Medical Center, Honolulu, HI .... G+ HR
The Queen's Medical Center Punchbowl, Honolulu, HI .... G+ E+
The Queen's Medical Center West Oahu, Ewa Beach, HI .... G+ HR
Wahiawa General Hospital, Wahiawa, HI .... G
Wilcox Memorial Hospital, Lihue, HI .... G G+ G+ E+

IDAHO

Eastern Idaho Regional Medical Center, Idaho Falls, ID ..... S+ G B
Kootenai Health, Coeur d'Alene, ID .... S
Portneuf Medical Center, Pocatello, ID .... S
Saint Alphonsus Regional Medical Center, Boise, ID .... S
St. Luke's Boise and Meridian Medical Centers, Boise, ID .. G+

ILLINOIS

Adventist Bolingbrook Hospital, Bolingbrook, IL .... B
Adventist Hinsdale Hospital, Hinsdale, IL .... S
Adventist LaGrange Memorial Hospital, La Grange, IL .... S S
Advocate BroMenn Medical Center, Normal, IL .... G+ HR G S
Advocate Christ Medical Center, Oak Lawn, IL .... G E G+

Advocate Condell Medical Center, Libertyville, IL .... G+ E
Advocate Good Samaritan Hospital, Downers Grove, IL ..... HR S
Advocate Good Shepherd Hospital, Barrington, IL .... G+ E S
Advocate Illinois Masonic Medical Center, Chicago, IL ...... G+ E S
Advocate Lutheran General Hospital, Park Ridge, IL .... G+ E+
Advocate Sherman Hospital, Elgin, IL .... G+ E S S
Advocate South Suburban Hospital, Hazel Crest, IL .... G+ E
Advocate Trinity Hospital, Chicago, IL .... G+ E
Amita Alexian Brothers Medical Center, Elk Grove Village, IL ..... G+
Amita St. Alexius Medical Center, Hoffman Estates, IL ...... G+ E+
Carle Foundation Hospital, Urbana, IL .... G+
Centegra Hospital -Woodstock, Woodstock, IL .... G+
Centegra Hospital- McHenry, McHenry, IL .... G+ E S+
Community First Medical Center, Chicago, IL .... S+ E
Decatur Memorial Hospital, Decatur, IL .... G+ E
Edward Hospital, Naperville, IL .... G+ HR G S+ E B
Elmhurst Hospital, Elmhurst, IL .... G+ HR
FHN Memorial Hospital, Freeport, IL .... G+ HR
Holy Cross Hospital, Chicago, IL .... G+ HR G+ E+ G S
HSHS St. John's Hospital, Springfield, IL .... S
Little Company of Mary Hospital , Evergreen Park, IL .... G+ E S+ S
Loyola University Medical Center, Maywood, IL .... G+ E
MacNeal Hospital, Berwyn, IL .... S G G+ E+ G+
Memorial Hospital of Carbondale, Carbondale, IL .... G+ S+ E+ S B
Memorial Medical Center, Springfield, IL .... S+ E
Mercy Hospital & Medical Center, Chicago, IL .... G+ HR B
MetroSouth Medical Center, Blue Island, IL .... G+ E
Mount Sinai Hospital, Chicago, IL .... G+ HR
Northwest Community Hospital, Arlington Heights, IL .... G+ HR
Northwestern Lake Forest Hospital, Lake Forest, IL .... S+ E G S
Northwestern Medicine Delnor Hospital, Geneva, IL .... G+ E+ S S
Northwestern Medicine- Central DuPage Hospital, Winfield, IL .. G+ E G
Northwestern Memorial Hospital, Chicago, IL .... S+ E+ G+ S
OSF Saint Anthony Medical Center, Rockford, IL .... G+ HR B
OSF Saint Francis Medical Center, Peoria, IL .... S+ E
OSF St. Joseph Medical Center, Bloomington, IL .... G+ E
Presence Resurrection Medical Center, Chicago, IL .... S+ B
Presence Saint Francis Hospital, Evanston, IL .... G
Presence Saint Joseph Hospital Chicago, Chicago, IL .... S B
Presence Saint Joseph Hospital-Elgin, Elgin, IL .... S+ HR
Presence Saint Joseph Medical Center, Joliet, IL .... S+ HR
Riverside Medical Center, Kankakee, IL .... G+ HR G+ HR S B
Rockford Memorial Hospital, Rockford, IL .... S+ HR
Rush Copley Medical Center, Aurora, IL .... G+ E+ S
Rush Oak Park Hospital, Oak Park, IL .... G+ HR G
Rush University Medical Center, Chicago, IL .... S G+ E
SIU Herrin Hospital, Herrin, IL .... S+ HR
Silver Cross Hospital, New Lenox, IL .... S G+ HR
SSM Health Good Samaritan, Mount Vernon, IL .... S G+ HR
Swedish American a Division of UW Health, Rockford, IL .. B
Swedish Covenant Hospital, Chicago, IL .... S S+
Trinity Medical Center, Rock Island, IL .... S G+ G+ E S
UnityPoint Health- Proctor, Peoria, IL ....
UnityPoint Methodist, Peoria, IL .... G+
University of Chicago Medical Center, Chicago, IL ....
University of Illinois Hospital and Health Sciences Systems,
    Chicago, IL .... S G+ E+
Vista Medical Center East, Waukegan, IL .... G+ HR G+ HR
West Suburban Medical Center, Oak Park, IL .... B

INDIANA

Baptist Health Floyd, New Albany, IN .... G+ E+
Columbus Regional Hospital, Columbus, IN .... G+
Community Hospital of Anderson, Anderson, IN .... G+ HR
Community Hospital of Munster, Munster, IN .... G+ G+ G+ S
Franciscan Health Indianapolis, Indianapolis, IN .... G+ HR
Franciscan St. Anthony Health – Michigan City, Michigan City, IN ...... G+ HR S+
Franciscan St. Ellizabeth Health – Lafayette East, Lafayette, IN ...... S
Indiana University Health, Fishers, IN .... S G+ E
Indiana University Health Ball Memorial Hospital, Muncie, IN ...... S G+ E S
Indiana University Health Methodist Hospital, Indianapolis, IN ...

IU Health Bloomington Hospital, Bloomington, IN .... G+ HR
IU Health West Hospital, Avon, IN .... G+
Lutheran Hospital, Fort Wayne, IN .... G+
Methodist Hospitals, Inc., Gary, IN .... G+
Parkview Health, Fort Wayne, IN .... G+ E+
Porter Regional Hospital, Valparaiso, IN .... G+
Riverview Hospital, Noblesville, IN .... S B
St. Catherine Hospital, Inc., East Chicago, IN .... G+ E
St. Mary Medical Center, Hobart, IN .... G+
St. Vincent Heart Center of Indiana, Indianapolis, IN .... G
St. Vincent Heart Center of Indiana on the St. Vincent Indianapolis
    Hospital Campus, Indianapolis, IN .... G+

IOWA

Genesis Medical Center, Davenport, IA .... S
Iowa City VA Health Care System, Iowa City, IA .... G
Mercy Iowa City, Iowa City, IA .... G+ S B
Mercy Medical Center - Des Moines, Des Moines, IA .... S+ HR S S
Mercy Medical Center - Dubuque, Dubuque, IA .... G+ HR
Mercy Medical Center - North Iowa, Mason City, IA .... S+
Mercy Medical Center - Sioux City, Sioux City, IA .... G+ G S
St. Luke's Hospital, Cedar Rapids, IA .... S B
St. Luke's Regional Medical Center, Sioux City, IA .... G S
Trinity Bettendorf, Bettendorf, IA .... B
UnityPoint Health- Iowa Methodist Medical Center, Des Moines, IA .... S
University of Iowa Hospitals and Clinics, Iowa City, IA .... G+ E+ B

KANSAS

Hays Med, Hays, KS .... G+ E
Hutchinson Regional Medical Center, Hutchinson, KS .... S HR
Lawrence Memorial Hospital, Lawrence, KS .... S S+ E+
Menorah Medical Center, Overland Park, KS .... G+ HR B
Olathe Medical Center, Olathe, KS .... G+
Overland Park Regional Medical Center, Overland Park, KS .... G+ E G
Saint Catherine Hospital, Garden City, KS .... G HR
Saint Francis Health Center, Topeka, KS .... G+ E S S
Saint Luke's South Hospital, Overland Park, KS .... G+ E+
Salina Regional Health Center, Salina, KS .... S+ E
Shawnee Mission Medical Center, Shawnee Mission, KS .... G+ S+ E G+
Stormont-Vail HealthCare, Topeka, KS .... G+ HR G+ E+ G
The University of Kansas Health System, Kansas City, KS . G+ HR G+ E+ G S
Via Christi Hospital St. Francis, Wichita, KS .... G+ E+
Wesley Medical Center, Wichita, KS .... G+ HR

KENTUCKY

Baptist Health LaGrange, LaGrange, KY .... G+
Baptist Health Lexington, Lexington, KY .... G+ HR G+ E+ G
Baptist Health Louisville, Louisville, KY .... G+ E+ G+
Baptist Health Paducah, Paducah, KY .... G+ HR B
Jewish Hospital, Louisville, KY .... G+ E+ G+
King's Daughters Medical Center, Ashland, KY .... G+ E+
Methodist Hospital, Henderson, KY, Henderson, KY .... S
Norton Audubon Hospital, Louisville, KY .... S
Norton Brownsboro Hospital, Louisville, KY .... G+ E+ G+
Norton Hospital, Louisville, KY .... G
Paul B. Hall Regional Medical Hospital, Paintsville, KY .... S
Pikeville Medical Center, Pikeville, KY .... G+ E B
Saint Joseph Hospital, Lexington, KY .... G+ E
Saint Joseph Hospital East, Lexington, KY .... S+
St. Elizabeth Edgewood, Edgewood, KY .... S S+ E B
St. Elizabeth Florence, Florence, KY .... S S+ S+ E
St. Elizabeth Ft. Thomas, Fort Thomas, KY .... S S+ HR S+ E
Sts. Mary and Elizabeth Hospital, Louisville, KY .... G+ E
University of Kentucky Hospital, Lexington, KY .... G G+ E+
University of Louisville Hospital, Louisville, KY .... G+ E+

LOUISIANA

Children's Hospital, New Orleans, LA .... S S
CHRISTUS St. Patrick Hospital, Lake Charles, LA .... G S B
East Jefferson General Hospital, Metairie, LA .... G+ HR G+ E

Lakeview Regional Medical Center, Covington, LA .... G+ E
Leonard J. Chabert Medical Center, Houma, LA .... S
Ochsner Medical Center - New Orleans, New Orleans, LA .... G+ HR
Our Lady of Lourdes Regional Medical Center, Lafayette, LA .... G+ E+
Our Lady of the Lake Regional Medical Center, Baton Rouge, LA .... G+ E
Rapides Regional Medical Center, Alexandria, LA .... S S G+ E
Slidell Memorial Hospital, Slidell, LA .... S+
St. Francis Medical Center, Monroe, LA .... S
St. Tammany Parish Hospital, Covington, LA .... S+ E
Terrebonne General Medical Center, Houma, LA .... G HR G+ S
Tulane University Hospital and Clinic, New Orleans, LA .... G S G+ E
University Medical Center New Orleans (UMCNO), New Orleans, LA .... S+ E
West Jefferson Medical Center, Marrero, LA .... G G+ E+ S B

MAINE

Central Maine Medical Center, Lewiston, ME .... G+
Eastern Maine Medical Center, Bangor, ME .... G+ E
Maine Medical Center, Portland, ME .... S
Mercy Hospital, Portland, ME .... B
Pen Bay Medical Center, Rockport, ME .... G+ E
St. Mary's Regional Medical Center, Lewiston, ME .... S
York Hospital, York, ME .... G

MARYLAND

Adventist HealthCare Shady Grove Medical Center, Rockville, MD ... G+ E+ G
Anne Arundel Medical Center, Annapolis, MD .... G+ E S+ B
Atlantic General Hospital, Berlin, MD .... G+ HF
Calvert Memorial Hospital, Prince Frederick, MD .... G+ HF
Doctor's Community Hospital, Lanham, MD .... G+ E
Frederick Memorial Hospital, Frederick, MD .... G+ HR S S
Greater Baltimore Medical Center, Baltimore, MD .... G+ E
Holy Cross Germantown Hospital, Germantown, MD .... S
Holy Cross Hospital, Silver Spring, MD .... G+ E S
Howard County General Hospital, Columbia, MD .... G
Johns Hopkins Bayview Medical Center, Baltimore, MD .... G+ E+ G
MedStar Franklin Square Medical Center, Baltimore, MD .... G+ E G
MedStar Good Samaritan Hospital, Baltimore, MD .... G+ HI
MedStar Montgomery Medical Center, Olney, MD .... G+ E
MedStar Southern Maryland Hospital Center, Clinton, MD .... G+ HI
MedStar Union Memorial Hospital, Baltimore, MD .... G+ HI
Mercy Medical Center, Baltimore, MD .... G
Meritus Medical Center, Hagerstown, MD .... G+ E S
Northwest Hospital, Randallstown, MD .... G+ E
Peninsula Regional Medical Center, Salisbury, MD .... G+ E
Prince George's Hospital Center, Cheverly, MD .... G+ HR
Saint Agnes Hospital, Baltimore, MD .... G+ E
Sinai Hospital, Baltimore, MD .... G+ HI
Suburban Hospital Johns Hopkins Medicine, Bethesda, MD .... G+ E
The Johns Hopkins Hospital, Baltimore, MD .... G+ E
Union Hospital of Cecil County, Elkton, MD .... G+ E
University of Maryland Baltimore Washington Medical Center,
    Glen Burnie, MD .... G E
University of Maryland Charles Regional Medical Center,
    La Plata, MD .... G+ E
University of Maryland Harford Memorial Hospital,
    Havre De Grace, MD .... S+ E
University of Maryland Medical Center, Baltimore, MD .... G+ E S
University of Maryland Medical Center Midtown Campus,
    Baltimore, MD .... S
University of Maryland Shore Medical Center at Easton, Easton, MD .... G+ E
University of Maryland St. Joseph Medical Center, Towson, MD .... G+ E
University of Maryland Upper Chesapeake Medical Center,
    Bel Air, MD .... G+ E
Washington Adventist Hospital, Takoma Park, MD .... G+ E+ E
Western Maryland Health System, Cumberland, MD .... G+ E

MASSACHUSETTS

Addison Gilbert Hospital, Gloucester, MA .... G
Baystate Franklin Medical Center, Greenfield, MA .... G+ E
Baystate Medical Center, Springfield, MA .... S+ E

Baystate Wing Hospital, Palmer, MA .... G+

Berkshire Medical Center, Pittsfield, MA .... G G+ HR G E+

Beth Israel Deaconess Hospital-Plymouth, Inc., Plymouth, MA ... G+

Beth Israel Deaconess Medical Center, Boston, MA .... HR G+ E

Beverly Hospital, Beverly, MA .... G+

Boston Medical Center, Boston, MA .... G+ E+

Brigham and Women's Faulkner Hospital, Boston, MA .... G G+

Brigham and Women's Hospital, Boston, MA .... G+ HR

Cape Cod Hospital, Hyannis, MA .... S+ HR

Carney Hospital, Dorchester Center, MA .... S+

Charlton Memorial Hospital, Southcoast Hospitals Group, Fall River, MA ... S+

Cooley Dickinson Hospital, Northampton, MA .... G+

Emerson Hospital, Concord, MA .... G+ HR

Fairview Hospital, Great Barrington, MA .... G

Falmouth Hospital/Cape Cod Healthcare, Falmouth, MA .... G+

Heywood Hospital, Gardner, MA .... G

Holyoke Medical Center, Holyoke, MA .... G+ E+

Lahey Hospital & Medical Center, Burlington, Burlington, MA .... G G+ E

Lowell General Hospital - Saints Campus, Lowell, MA .... G+ E

Massachusetts General Hospital, Boston, MA .... G+ E+

Melrose Wakefield Hospital, Melrose, MA .... G+

Mercy Medical Center, Springfield, MA .... G+ HR

MetroWest Medical Center - Framingham Union Hospital, Framingham, MA .... G+ G+ B

MetroWest Medical Center - Leonard Morse Hospital, Natick, MA .... G+

Milford Regional Medical Center, Milford, MA .... G+

Mount Auburn Hospital, Cambridge, MA .... G+ E+

Nashoba Valley Medical Center, Ayer, MA .... G+

Newton-Wellesley Hospital, Newton, MA .... G+ HR G+ E

North Shore Medical Center - Salem, Salem, MA .... G+ E

North Shore Medical Center - Union Hospital, Lynn, MA .... G+ HR

Norwood Hospital, Norwood, MA .... G+ HR

Saint Anne's Hospital, Fall River, MA .... G

Saint Vincent Hospital, Worcester, MA .... G+ HR

Signature Healthcare Brockton Hospital, Brockton, MA .... G

South Shore Hospital, South Weymouth, MA .... G

St. Elizabeth's Medical Center, Brighton, MA .... G+ HR

Sturdy Memorial Hospital, Attleboro, MA .... G+ E+ S

Tufts Medical Center, Boston, MA .... S G+ S

UMass Memorial Medical Center, Worcester, MA .... G G+ E+

MICHIGAN

Beaumont Hospital, Grosse Pointe, Grosse Pointe, MI .... G+

Beaumont Hospital, Troy, Troy, MI .... G HR

Borgess Medical Center, Kalamazoo, MI .... G+ HR G+

Bronson Methodist Hospital, Kalamazoo, MI .... S+ E+

Covenant HealthCare, Saginaw, MI .... G+ HR

DMC Detroit Receiving Hospital, Detroit, MI .... G+ E

DMC Harper University Hospital, Detroit, MI .... G+ E

DMC Sinai-Grace Hospital, Detroit, MI .... G+ E

Garden City Hospital, Garden City, MI .... G+ HR

Genesys Regional Medical Center, Grand Blanc, MI .... G+ HR

Henry Ford Hospital and Health Network, Detroit, MI .... G+ E

Henry Ford Macomb Hospital, Clinton Township, MI .... G+ E

Henry Ford West Bloomfield Hospital, West Bloomfield, MI .... S+

Holland Hospital, Holland, MI .... G S

Lakeland Healthcare, Saint Joseph, MI .... S E

McLaren Northern Michigan, Petoskey, MI .... S HR

Mercy Health Saint Mary's, Grand Rapids, MI .... G+ HR G+ E+

Metro Health – University of Michigan Health, Wyoming, MI .... G+ E B

Munson Medical Center, Traverse City, MI .... G+ HR

ProMedica Bixby Hospital, Adrian, MI .... G+ HR

Sparrow Hospital, Lansing, MI .... G+ E S

St. Joseph Mercy Ann Arbor, Ypsilanti, MI .... S G+ HR

St. Joseph Mercy Livingston Hospital, Ann Arbor, MI .... G+ E

St. Joseph Mercy Oakland, Pontiac, MI .... S G+ E

University of Michigan Health System, Ann Arbor, MI .... S G+ E

MINNESOTA

CentraCare Health St. Cloud Hospital, Saint Cloud, MN ...... G+ G S G+ HR G

Essentia Health East. St. Mary's Medical Center, Duluth, MN .... G+ E+ S

Fairview Northland Hospital, Princeton, MN .... S+

Fairview Range Hospital, Hibbing, MN .... S+

Fairview Southdale Hospital, Edina, MN .... G+ S+ E

Hennepin County Medical Center, Minneapolis, MN .... S S+ E+

Mayo Clinic Health System in Mankato, Mankato, MN .... G+ S

Mayo Clinic Hospital, Saint Marys Campus, Rochester, MN .... G+ S

Mercy Hospital, Coon Rapids, MN .... G

North Memorial Medical Center, Robbinsdale, MN .... G+ E+ S

Park Nicollet Methodist Hospital, Saint Louis Park, MN .... S+ S+ E+

Regions Hospital, Saint Paul, MN .... G+ E+

St. Joseph's Hospital, Saint Paul, MN .... S

St. Luke's, Duluth, MN .... G+ E G S

University of Minnesota Heart Care at Fairview Ridges Hospital, Burnsville, MN .... G+

University of Minnesota Medical Center, Minneapolis, MN .... S G+ HR

Woodwinds Health Campus, Woodbury, MN .... S

MISSISSIPPI

Baptist Memorial Hospital - DeSoto, Southaven, MS .... G+ E B

Baptist Memorial Hospital - Golden Triangle, Columbus, MS .... G+ S

Baptist Memorial Hospital - North Mississippi, Oxford, MS .... G B

Forrest General Hospital, Hattiesburg, MS .... G+ HR G+ S

Magnolia Regional Health Center, Corinth, MS .... G+ S

Merit Health Biloxi, Biloxi, MS .... S+

Merit Health Wesley, Hattiesburg, MS .... G+ HR S+

MS Baptist Medical Center, Jackson, MS .... S+ G+ E+

North Mississippi Medical Center, Tupelo, MS .... S+ HR B

Ocean Springs Hospital (Singing River Health System), Ocean Springs, MS .... G+ E G+

OCH Regional Medical Center, Starkville, MS .... S

River Oaks Hospital, Jackson, MS .... G+

Singing River Hospital (Singing River Health System), Pascagoula, MS .... G+ E

Southwest Mississippi Regional Medical Center, McComb, MS .... S+ B

St. Dominic Memorial Hospital, Jackson, MS .... G+ E S

University of Mississippi Health Care, Jackson, MS .... G+ HR G+ E+ G S

MISSOURI

Barnes-Jewish Hospital, Saint Louis, MO .... S G+ E+ S S

Barnes-Jewish St. Peters Hospital, Saint Peters, MO .... S+

Belton Regional Medical Center, Belton, MO .... S+

Boone Hospital, Columbia, MO .... G+ E+

Capital Region Medical Center, Jefferson City, MO .... S S

Centerpoint Medical Center, Independence, MO .... G+ HR HR

Christian Hospital, St. Louis, MO .... G+ HR S+

Citizens Memorial Hospital, Bolivar, MO .... G B

Cox Medical Center Branson, Branson, MO .... G+ E

CoxHealth, Springfield, MO .... S G+ E+

Des Peres Hospital, Saint Louis, MO .... G+ B

Freeman Health System, Joplin, MO .... S

Lake Regional Hospital, Osage Beach, MO .... G+ E

Lee's Summit Medical Center, Lees Summit, MO .... G+ E

Liberty Hospital, Liberty, MO .... S+ HR

Mercy Hospital Joplin, Joplin, MO .... S+ HR S

Mercy Hospital Springfield, Springfield, MO .... G+ E+ B

Mercy Hospital St. Louis, Saint Louis, MO .... S G+ E+ G+ S

Mercy Hospital Washington, Washington, MO .... S+ E

Mosaic Life Care, Saint Joseph, MO .... G S+ E

Phelps County Regional Medical Center, Rolla, MO .... S+ HR

Progress West Hospital, O'Fallon, MO .... G+ HR

Research Medical Center, Kansas City, MO .... G+ HR G+ E+ S+

Saint Francis Medical Center, Cape Girardeau, MO .... S

Saint Luke's East Hospital, Lees Summit, MO .... G+ E+

Saint Luke's Hospital of Kansas City, Kansas City, MO .... G+ HR G+ E+ G S

Saint Luke's North Hospital, Kansas City, MO .... G+ E G S

SSM Health DePaul Hospital, Bridgeton, MO .... S+

SSM Health Saint Louis University Hospital, Saint Louis, MO .... G+ E+ G B

SSM Health St. Joseph -St. Charles, Saint Charles, MO .... G+ E+

SSM St. Joseph Hospital Lake St. Louis, Lake St. Louis, MO .... G+ E

SSM Health St. Mary's Hospital, Richmond Heights, MO .... G+ E+ S+

St. Anthony's Medical Center, Saint Louis, MO .... S+ G+ E+ S+

American Heart Association | American Stroke Association.
life is why™

St. Joseph Medical Center, Kansas City, MO .... (G+) (S+)
St. Luke's Hospital, Chesterfield, MO .... (G) (B)
St. Mary's Medical Center, Blue Springs, MO .... (G+) (HR) (B)
Truman Medical Center, Kansas City, MO .... (S+)
University of Missouri Health Care, Columbia, MO .... (G+) (E+)

MONTANA

Benefis Health System, Great Falls, MT .... (G+) (HR)
Billings Clinic, Billings, MT .... (G) (B)
Bozeman Health Deaconess Hospital, Bozeman, MT .... (B)
Kalispell Regional Healthcare, Kalispell, MT .... (G+) (HR) (B)
Providence St. Patrick Hospital, Missoula, MT .... (S) (S+) (B)
St. Vincent Healthcare, Billings, MT .... (B)

NEBRASKA

Bryan Medical Center, Lincoln, NE .... (G)
CHI Health Good Samaritan Hospital, Kearney, NE .... (G+) (HR)
CHI Health St. Elizabeth, Lincoln, NE .... (G) (G+)
Faith Regional Health Services, Norfolk, NE .... (B)
Great Plains Health, North Platte, NE .... (G+) (E+)
Kearney Regional Medical Center, Kearney, NE .... (B)
Nebraska Medicine, Omaha, NE .... (G+) (E) (G)
Nebraska Medicine - Bellevue , Bellevue, NE .... (S+)
Nebraska Methodist Hospital, Omaha, NE .... (B)

NEVADA

Centennial Hills Hospital Medical Center, Las Vegas, NV .... (G+) (E)
Desert Springs Hospital Medical Center, Las Vegas, NV .... (G+) (E)
Dignity Health St. Rose Dominican Hospital - Rose de Lima,
    Henderson, NV .... (G+)
Dignity Health St. Rose Dominican Hospital - Siena,
    Henderson, NV .... (G+) (HR) (G+)
                                     (G+) (E) (S)
MountainView Hospital, Las Vegas, NV .... (G+) (E)
Northern Nevada Medical Center, Sparks, NV .... (G+) (E)
Renown Regional Medical Center, Reno, NV .... (G) (G+) (E) (G)
Saint Mary's Regional Medical Center, Reno, NV .... (G+) (E+) (G+)
Southern Hills Hospital, Las Vegas, NV .... (G+)
Spring Valley Hospital Medical Center, Las Vegas, NV .... (G+) (E) (S)
Summerlin Hospital Medical Center, Las Vegas, NV .... (G+) (E)
Sunrise Hospital & Medical Center, Las Vegas, NV .... (G+) (E+)
University Medical Center of Southern Nevada, Las Vegas, NV .... (G)
Valley Hospital Medical Center, Las Vegas, NV .... (G+) (E)

NEW HAMPSHIRE

Catholic Medical Center, Manchester, NH .... (G+) (HR)
Concord Hospital, Concord, NH .... (S+)
Dartmouth-Hitchcock Medical Center, Lebanon, NH .... (S) ✶ (S) (HR)
Portsmouth Regional Hospital, Portsmouth, NH .... (S+) (E)
Southern New Hampshire Medical Center, Nashua, NH .... (G+) (HR)
St. Joseph Hospital, Nashua, NH .... (G+) (E)

NEW JERSEY

Bayshore Community Hospital, Holmdel, NJ .... (G+) (E+) (G) (S)
Capital Health Regional Medical Center, Trenton, NJ .... (G+) (HR)
CarePoint Health - Bayonne Medical Center, Bayonne, NJ .... (S+) (G)
CarePoint Health - Christ Hospital, Jersey City, NJ .... (G+) (HR)
CarePoint Health - Hoboken University Medical Center, Hoboken, NJ .... (G+)
CentraState Medical Center, Freehold, NJ .... (G+) (E)
Chilton Medical Center, Pompton Plains, NJ .... (G+) (E) (S)
Deborah Heart and Lung Center, Browns Mills, NJ .... (G+)
Hackensack University Medical Center, Hackensack, NJ .... (G+) (E)
HackensackUMC Mountainside, Montclair, NJ .... (G+)
HackensackUMC Palisades, North Bergen, NJ .... (G+) (HR) (G+) (E)
Holy Name Medical Center, Teaneck, NJ .... (G+) (E+)
Inspira Medical Center Elmer, Elmer, NJ .... (G+)
Inspira Medical Center Vineland, Vineland, NJ .... (G+)
Inspira Medical Center Woodbury, Woodbury, NJ .... (G)
Jersey City Medical Center – Barnabas Health, Jersey City, NJ .... (G+)
Jersey Shore University Medical Center, Neptune, NJ .... (G+) (G+) (E) (S)

JFK Medical Center, Edison, NJ .... (G+) (E+)
Kennedy University Hospitals- Cherry Hill, Cherry Hill, NJ .... (G+) (E+)
Kennedy University Hospitals- Stratford, Stratford, NJ .... (G+) (HR)
Kennedy University Hospitals- Washington Township,
    Turnersville, NJ .... (G+) (HR)
Monmouth Medical Center, Long Branch, NJ .... (G+) (E)
Morristown Medical Center, Morristown, NJ .... (G+) (E+) (S)
Newark Beth Israel Medical Center, Newark, NJ .... (S) (S)
Newton Medical Center, Newton, NJ .... (G+) (E+)
Ocean Medical Center, Brick, NJ .... (G+) (G+) (E) (B)
Our Lady of Lourdes Medical Center, Camden, NJ .... (G+) (E+)
Overlook Medical Center, Summit, NJ .... (G+) (E+)
Riverview Medical Center, Red Bank, NJ .... (G+) (G+) (E) (G) (S)
Robert Wood Johnson University Hospital, New Brunswick, NJ .... (G+)
Robert Wood Johnson University Hospital Hamilton,
    Hamilton, NJ .... (G+) (G+) (HR)
Robert Wood Johnson University Hospital Somerset,
    Somerville, NJ .... (G+) (HR) (S) (S)
Saint Clare's Hospital, Denville, NJ, Dover, NJ .... (S+) (HR)
Saint Peter's University Hospital, New Brunswick, NJ .... (G+)
Southern Ocean Medical Center, Manahawkin, NJ .... (G+) (E+) (B)
St. Francis Medical Center, Trenton, NJ .... (G+)
St. Joseph's Regional Medical Center, Paterson, NJ .... (S+) (E) (G)
St. Luke's Warren Hospital, Phillipsburg, NJ .... (G+)
The Valley Hospital, Ridgewood, NJ .... (S) (G+) (E+)
University Hospital, Newark, NJ .... (HR) (G+) (E)
Virtua Memorial Hospital, Mt. Holly, NJ .... (S)

NEW MEXICO

Lea Regional Medical Center, Hobbs, NM .... (G+)
Lovelace Medical Center, Albuquerque, NM .... (G+) (E+) (G+)
Presbyterian Hospital, Albuquerque, NM .... (S+) (S)
San Juan Regional Medical Center, Farmington, NM .... (G)
University of New Mexico Hospitals, Albuquerque, NM .... (G) (HR) (G+) (E+) (G+)

NEW YORK

Albany Medical Center, Albany, NY .... (G+) (G+)
Arnot Ogden Medical Center, Elmira, NY .... (G+) (E)
Auburn Community Hospital, Auburn, NY .... (G+) (HR)
Bassett Medical Center, Cooperstown, NY .... (S) (G+)
Bronx-Lebanon Hospital Center, Bronx, NY .... (S) (G+) (HR) (G+) (E) (S) (S)
Brookdale University Hospital Medical Center, Brooklyn, NY .... (G+) (E)
Brookhaven Memorial Hospital Medical Center, Patchogue, NY .... (G+)
Catholic Health - Kenmore Mercy Hospital, Buffalo, NY .... (G+)
Catholic Health - Mercy Hospital of Buffalo, Buffalo, NY .... (G+) (E+) (S)
Catholic Health - Mount St. Mary's Hospital, Lewiston, NY .... (G+)
Catskill Regional Medical Center, Harris, NY .... (S+)
Cohen Children's Medical Center, New Hyde Park, NY .... (G)
Columbia Memorial Hospital, Hudson, NY .... (G)
Crouse Hospital, Syracuse, NY .... (G) (G+) (E) (G)
Ellis Hospital, Schenectady, NY .... (G+) (E)
Erie County Medical Center, Buffalo, NY .... (G+) (HR) (G+)
F.F. Thompson Hospital, Canandaigua, NY .... (G+)
Faxton St. Luke's Healthcare, an affiliation of Mohawk Valley Health
    System, Utica, NY .... (G+) (E)
Flushing Hospital Medical Center, Flushing, NY .... (G+) (E)
Gates Vascular Institute / Buffalo General Medical Center,
    Buffalo, NY .... (G+) (E+)
Geneva General Hospital, Geneva, NY .... (S+)
Glen Cove Hospital, Glen Cove, NY .... (G+)
Good Samaritan Hospital Medical Center, West Islip, NY .... (G+) (E)
Good Samaritan Hospital, a Member of WMC Health Network,
    Suffern, NY .... (S) (HR)
Guthrie Corning Hospital, Corning, NY .... (G+) (HR)
Health Alliance Broadway Campus, a Member of the WMC Health
    Network, Kingston, NY .... (G+) (HR)
Highland Hospital, Rochester, NY .... (G+) (G+)
Huntington Hospital, Huntington, NY .... (G+) (E)
Jamaica Hospital Medical Center, Richmond Hill, NY .... (G+) (E) (B)
John T. Mather Memorial Hospital, Port Jefferson, NY .... (G+) (HR)

*This hospital received Get With The Guidelines - Resuscitation awards for two or more patient populations.

Kingsbrook Jewish Medical Center, Brooklyn, NY .... G+ E
Lenox Hill Hospital, New York, NY .... G+ E
LIJ Medical Center at Forest Hills, Forest Hills, NY .... G+ E
LIJ Valley Stream, Valley Stream, NY .... G+ E
Long Island Jewish Medical Center, New Hyde Park, NY .... G+ E
Maimonides Medical Center, Brooklyn, NY .... G+ E+
Mercy Medical Center, Rockville Centre, NY .... G+
MidHudson Regional Hospital, a Member of the WMCHealth Network, Poughkeepsie, NY .... G+
Montefiore Mount Vernon Hospital, Mount Vernon, NY .... G+
Mount Sinai Beth Israel, New York, NY .... G+ HR G+ E+ G
Mount Sinai Brooklyn, Brooklyn, NY .... G+
Mount Sinai Queens, Astoria, NY .... G+ E
Mount Sinai St. Luke's & Mount Sinai West, New York, NY .... G+ HR
Nassau University Medical Center, East Meadow, NY .... G+ HR S G+ HR
New York Community Hospital, Brooklyn, NY .... G+ E
Newark–Wayne Community Hospital, Newark, NY .... G+ HR
NewYork-Presbyterian / Hudson Valley Hospital, Cortlandt Manor, NY .... G+ E
NewYork-Presbyterian Brooklyn Methodist Hospital, Brooklyn, NY .... G+ E+
NewYork-Presbyterian/Columbia University Medical Center, New York, NY .... G+ E+
NewYork-Presbyterian/Lawrence Hospital, Bronxville, NY .... G G+
NewYork-Presbyterian/Lower Manhattan Hospital, New York, NY .... G+ E+
NewYork-Presbyterian/Queens, Flushing, NY .... G+ E+ S
NewYork-Presbyterian/The Allen Hospital, New York, NY .... G+ E+
NewYork-Presbyterian/Weill Cornell Medical Center, New York, NY .... G+ E+
Niagara Falls Memorial Medical Center, Niagara Falls, NY .... G+
North Shore University Hospital, Manhasset, NY .... G+ E
Northern Westchester Hospital, Mount Kisco, NY .... G+ E+
Noyes Health, Dansville, NY .... G
Nyack Hospital, Nyack, NY .... G+ HR
NYC Health + Hospitals/Bellevue, New York, NY .... G+ HR G+ E+ S
NYC Health + Hospitals/Coney Island, Brooklyn, NY .... G+ E+
NYC Health + Hospitals/Elmhurst, Flushing, NY .... G+
NYC Health + Hospitals/Harlem, New York, NY .... G+
NYC Health + Hospitals/Jacobi, Bronx, NY .... G+ E
NYC Health + Hospitals/Kings County, Brooklyn, NY .... S G+ E
NYC Health + Hospitals/Lincoln, Bronx, NY .... G+
NYC Health + Hospitals/Metropolitan, New York, NY .... S+ E+
NYC Health + Hospitals/North Central Bronx, Bronx, NY .... HR
NYC Health + Hospitals/Woodhull, Brooklyn, NY .... HR
NYU Langone Medical Center, New York, NY .... G G+ E+ S
NYU Lutheran Medical Center, Brooklyn, NY .... G+ E+
Orange Regional Medical Center, Middletown, NY .... G+ E
Our Lady of Lourdes Memorial Hospital, Binghamton, NY .... G+
Peconic Bay Medical Center, Riverhead, NY .... G+ E
Phelps Hospital, Sleepy Hollow, NY .... G+ E
Plainview Hospital, Plainview, NY .... G+
Putnam Hospital Center, Carmel, NY .... S+
Richmond University Medical Center, Staten Island, NY .... S G+ E+
Rochester General Hospital, Rochester, NY .... G+ E+
Saint Joseph's Medical Center, Yonkers, NY .... G+
SBH Health System, Bronx, NY .... G+ E+
South Nassau Communities Hospital, Oceanside, NY .... G+ HR G+ E+
Southampton Hospital, Southampton, NY .... G+
Southside Hospital, Bay Shore, NY .... G+ E+ G
St. Catherine of Siena Medical Center, Smithtown, NY .... G+
St. Charles Hospital, Port Jefferson, NY .... G+
St. Francis Hospital, The Heart Center, Roslyn, NY .... G+
St. John's Episcopal Hospital, Far Rockaway, NY .... G+ E+
St. John's Riverside Hospital, Yonkers, NY .... G+ E
St. Joseph Hospital, Bethpage, NY .... G G+ E
St. Luke's Cornwall Hospital, Newburgh and Cornwall Campuses, Newburgh, NY .... G+ E
St. Peter's Hospital, Albany, NY .... G+ HR
Staten Island University Hospital, Staten Island, NY .... G+ E+
Stony Brook University Hospital, Stony Brook, NY .... S G+ E
Syosset Hospital, Syosset, NY .... G+ E
The Brooklyn Hospital Center, Brooklyn, NY .... G+ HR G+ E

The Mount Sinai Hospital, New York, NY .... G+ E+ B
UHS Wilson Medical Center, Johnson City, NY .... G+ S+
Unity Hospital, Rochester, NY .... G+ E
University Hospital of Brooklyn - SUNY Downstate Medical Center, Brooklyn, NY .... G+ HR
University of Rochester Medical Center, Strong Memorial Hospital, Rochester, NY .... G+ HR G G+ E+ B
Upstate University Hospital, Syracuse, NY .... G+ G+ E+
Vassar Brothers Medical Center, Poughkeepsie, NY .... G+ HR
Westchester Medical Center, Valhalla, NY .... G+ HR
White Plains Hospital, White Plains, NY .... G+ E
Winthrop University Hospital, Mineola, NY .... G+ E
Wyckoff Heights Medical Center, Brooklyn, NY .... G+ E

NORTH CAROLINA

Angel Medical Center, Franklin, NC .... S+ HR
Cape Fear Valley Medical Center, Fayetteville, NC .... S G G G+ E G+
Carolinas HealthCare System Cleveland, Shelby, NC .... S G+
Carolinas HealthCare System Kings Mountain, Kings Mountain, NC .... S
Carolinas HealthCare System Lincoln, Lincolnton, NC .... S+
Carolinas HealthCare System NorthEast, Concord, NC .... G+ E G+ S
Carolinas HealthCare System Pineville, Charlotte, NC .... G+ HR G+ S
Carolinas HealthCare System Stanly, Albemarle, NC .... G+ E
Carolinas HealthCare System Union, Monroe, NC .... G+ HR
Carolinas HealthCare System University, Charlotte, NC .... S+ HR
Carolinas Medical Center, Charlotte, NC .... G+ E G+ S
CaroMont Regional Medical Center, Gastonia, NC .... HR G+ E S
Carteret Health Care Medical Center, Morehead City, NC .... G G HR G+ G+ HR
Central Carolina Hospital, Sanford, NC .... HR G+ HR
Columbus Regional Healthcare, Whiteville, NC .... S HR
Cone Health, Greensboro, NC .... S G+ E+ B
Duke Raleigh Hospital, Raleigh, NC .... G+ E
Duke Regional Hospital, Durham, NC .... G+ E S+ E+
Duke University Hospital, Durham, NC .... G+ HR G+ E+ G S
FirstHealth of the Carolinas Moore Regional Hospital, Pinehurst, NC .... S+ E+
Frye Regional Medical Center, Hickory, NC .... G+ G+ E G+ B
Hugh Chatham Memorial Hospital, Elkin, NC .... G+ E+
Iredell Memorial Hospital, Statesville, NC .... G+
Mission Hospitals, Inc., Asheville, NC .... G+ E+
Nash Hospitals Inc., Rocky Mount, NC .... S+ E S S
New Hanover Regional Medical Center, Wilmington, NC .... G+ E+ G S
Novant Health Brunswick Medical Center, Bolivia, NC .... HR G+ E+ G+
Novant Health Forsyth Medical Center, Winston-Salem, NC .... HR G+ E+ G+
Novant Health Huntersville Medical Center, Huntersville, NC .... G E G B
Novant Health Matthews Medical Center, Matthews, NC .... G+ HR G E B
Novant Health Presbyterian Medical Center, Charlotte, NC .... G+ HR G+ E+ G+ S
Novant Health Rowan Medical Center, Salisbury, NC .... G+ G+ HR S+
Novant Health Thomasville Medical Center, Thomasville, NC .... G
Onslow Memorial Hospital, Jacksonville, NC .... S
Pardee Hospital, Hendersonville, NC .... S
UNC Hospitals, Chapel Hill, NC .... G+ E+ G S
UNC Lenoir Health Care, Kinston, NC .... S
UNC REX Healthcare, Raleigh, NC .... G+ HR G
Vidant Medical Center, Greenville, NC .... G+ HR S S S
Wake Forest Baptist Medical Center, Winston-Salem, NC .... G+ E
WakeMed Cary Hospital, Cary, NC .... G
WakeMed Health & Hospitals - Raleigh Campus, Raleigh, NC .... S G+ E+ S+
Wayne UNC Health Care, Goldsboro, NC .... S+ HR
Wesley Long Hospital, Greensboro, NC .... S

NORTH DAKOTA

Altru Health System, Grand Forks, ND .... G+ E S+
CHI St. Alexius Health Bismarck, Bismarck, ND .... G+ HR S B
Essentia Health, Fargo, ND .... G+ E B
Sanford Medical Center Bismarck, Bismarck, ND .... S+ HR S
Sanford Medical Center Fargo, Fargo, ND .... S B
Trinity Health, Minot, ND .... G+ E S

OHIO

Adena Health System, Chillicothe, OH .... (S)
Affinity Medical Center, Massillon, OH .... (G)(S)
Ashtabula County Medical Center, Ashtabula, OH .... (G+)(S)
Atrium Medical Center, Franklin, OH .... (G+)(HR)(G+)(S)
Aultman Hospital, Canton, OH .... (HR)(S)(G+)(E)
Cleveland Clinic, Cleveland, OH .... (G+)(S)(G+)(E)
Cleveland Clinic Akron General, Akron, OH .... (S+)(HR)(S+)
Fairfield Medical Center, Lancaster, OH .... (S+)(HR)(G+)(S)
Fairview Hospital - A Cleveland Clinic Hospital, Cleveland, OH .... (G+)(E)
Firelands Regional Medical Center, Sandusky, OH .... (S+)(HR)
Genesis Healthcare System, Zanesville, OH .... (G)(G+)(HR)
Good Samaritan Hospital, Dayton, OH .... (G+)(E)
Hillcrest Hospital - A Cleveland Clinic Hospital, Mayfield Heights, OH .... (G+)(E)(B)
Kettering Medical Center, Dayton, OH .... (G+)(E)
Knox Community Hospital, Mount Vernon, OH .... (G)(S)
Licking Memorial Hospital, Newark, OH .... (G)(S)
Lima Memorial Health System, Lima, OH .... (G+)(B)
Louis Stokes Cleveland VA Medical Center, Cleveland, OH .... (G+)(HR)
Marymount Hospital, Garfield Heights, OH .... (G+)(E)
Medina Hospital, Medina, OH .... (G+)(S)
Mercy Health - Anderson Hospital, Cincinnati, OH .... (S)
Mercy Health - Fairfield Hospital, Fairfield, OH .... (S+)
Mercy Health - St. Elizabeth Youngstown Hospital, Youngstown, OH .... (G+)(HR)(G)(HR)
Mercy Medical Center, Canton, OH .... (G+)(HR)(G+)(HR)(G+)
Miami Valley Hospital, Dayton, OH .... (G+)(E)
Mount Carmel East, Columbus, OH .... (G+)
Mount Carmel Health System, Columbus, OH .... (G+)(E+)
Mount Carmel St. Ann's, Westerville, OH .... (G+)(E+)
Mount Carmel West, Columbus, OH .... (S+)
OhioHealth Doctors Hospital, Columbus, OH .... (G)
OhioHealth Grant Medical Center, Columbus, OH .... (G+)
OhioHealth Marion General Hospital, Marion, OH .... (G+)(HR)(G+)(B)
OhioHealth Riverside Methodist Hospital, Columbus, OH .... (G+)(E+)(G)
ProMedica Flower Hospital, Sylvania, OH .... (G+)(E)
ProMedica Toledo Hospital, Toledo, OH .... (G+)(E+)
Salem Regional Medical Center, Salem, OH ....
South Pointe Hospital, Warrensville Heights, OH .... (G+)(E)
Southwest General Health Center, Middleburg Heights, OH .... (G)(G+)(S)
St. Rita's Medical Center, Lima, OH .... (G)(S)
St. Vincent Charity Medical Center, Cleveland, OH .... (G+)
Summa Akron City Hospital, Akron, OH .... (G+)(E+)(G+)
Sycamore Medical Center, Miamisburg, OH .... (G+)(B)
The Christ Hospital, Cincinnati, OH .... (G+)(E+)(G)(S)
The MetroHealth System, Cleveland, OH .... (G)(G+)(G+)(E+)(G)(S)
The Ohio State University Wexner Medical Center, Columbus, OH .... (G+)(E)(G+)(S)
The University of Toledo Medical Center, Toledo, OH .... (G+)(G+)(E)
UH Regional Hospitals, Bedford Medical Center and Richmond Medical Center, Richmond Heights, OH .... (G+)(E)
Union Hospital, Dover, OH .... (G+)
University Hospitals Ahuja Medical Center, Beachwood, OH .... (G+)(E)
University Hospitals Cleveland Medical Center, Cleveland, OH .... (G+)(E)(G+)(S)
University Hospitals Elyria Medical Center, Elyria, OH .... (G+)(E)(G+)(S)
University Hospitals Geauga Medical Center, Chardon, OH .... (G+)(E+)
University Hospitals St. John Medical Center, Cleveland, OH .... (G)(B)
University of Cincinnati Medical Center, Cincinnati, OH .... (G+)(HR)(G+)(E+)(S+)
West Chester Hospital, West Chester, OH .... (S)(HR)(S)
West Hospital, Cincinnati, OH .... (B)(HR)
Western Reserve Hospital, Cuyahoga Falls, OH .... (G+)(HR)(S+)

OKLAHOMA

INTEGRIS Baptist Medical Center, Oklahoma City, OK .... (G+)(E+)(B)
INTEGRIS Southwest Medical Center, Oklahoma City, OK .... (G+)(E+)
Jane Phillips Medical Center, Bartlesville, OK .... (G+)(B)
Mercy Hospital Oklahoma City Comprehensive Stroke Center, Oklahoma City, OK .... (G+)(E+)

Norman Regional HealthPlex Heart Hospital, Norman, OK .... (B)
Oklahoma Heart Institute at Hillcrest Medical Center, Tulsa, OK .... (G+)(HR)(S+)(E+)(G)
Saint Francis Hospital, Tulsa, OK .... (S)(S+)(E+)
St. Anthony Hospital, Oklahoma City, OK .... (G+)(B)
St. John Medical Center, Tulsa, OK .... (G+)(E+)

OREGON

Adventist Medical Center - Portland, Portland, OR .... (S+)
Asante Rogue Regional Medical Center, Medford, OR .... (G+)
Good Samaritan Regional Medical Center, Corvallis, OR .... (G+)(E)
Kaiser Foundation Hospital - Westside, Hillsboro, OR .... (G+)
Kaiser Sunnyside Medical Center, Clackamas, OR .... (G+)(HF)
Legacy Emanuel Medical Center, Portland, OR .... (G+)(G+)(E+)(S+)(G)
Legacy Good Samaritan Medical Center, Portland, OR .... (S+)(G+)(G)
Legacy Meridian Park Medical Center, Tualatin, OR .... (G+)(E)(G)(G)
Legacy Mount Hood Medical Center, Gresham, OR .... (G+)(E)
Oregon Health & Science University, Portland, OR .... (G+)(HR)(G)(S)(G+)(G)(S)
PeaceHealth Sacred Heart Medical Center RiverBend, Springfield, OR .... (G+)
Providence Medford Medical Center, Medford, OR .... (G+)(E)(S)
Providence Newberg Medical Center, Newberg, OR .... (S)
Providence Portland Medical Center, Portland, OR .... (G+)(E)
Providence St. Vincent Medical Center, Portland, OR .... (G+)(E)(G)
Providence Willamette Falls Medical Center, Oregon City, OR .... (G+)(E)
Salem Hospital, Salem, OR .... (G+)(E)
Sky Lakes Medical Center, Klamath Falls, OR .... (G+)(E)
St. Charles Health System, Bend, OR .... (G)(G+)(B)
Tuality Healthcare, Hillsboro, OR .... (G)

PENNSYLVANIA

Abington Health - Abington Memorial Hospital, Abington, PA .... (G+)(G+)(E)(G+)
Allegheny General Hospital, Pittsburgh, PA .... (S)(G+)(HR)(G+)(E)
Allegheny Valley Hospital, Natrona Heights, PA .... (G+)(HR)
Aria Health, Philadelphia, PA .... (G+)(HR)(S)
Aria Jefferson Health Systems Bucks, Langhorne, PA .... (B)
Brandywine Hospital, Coatesville, PA .... (S)
Bryn Mawr Hospital, Bryn Mawr, PA .... (G+)(E)
Butler Memorial Hospital, Butler, PA .... (G+)(E)
Carlisle Regional Medical Center, Carlisle, PA .... (S)
Chambersburg Hospital, Chambersburg, PA .... (G+)(HR)(G+)(E)(G)
Chestnut Hill Hospital, Philadelphia, PA .... (G+)(E)
Conemaugh Valley Memorial Hospital, Johnstown, PA .... (S)(G+)(E)
Crozer-Chester Medical Center, Upland, PA .... (G+)(E)
Delaware County Memorial Hospital, Drexel Hill, PA .... (G)(S)
Doylestown Hospital, Doylestown, PA .... (G+)(HR)(G)(G+)(E+)(G)(S)
Einstein Medical Center - Philadelphia, Philadelphia, PA .... (S)(G+)(H)
Einstein Medical Center Montgomery, East Norriton, PA .... (G+)(H)
Evangelical Community Hospital, Lewisburg, PA .... (G+)(E)
Excela Health Westmoreland, Greensburg, PA .... (S)
Forbes Hospital, Monroeville, PA .... (G+)(E)
Geisinger Community Medical Center, Scranton, PA .... (G+)(E+)(G)
Geisinger Medical Center, Danville, PA .... (G+)(HR)(G)
Geisinger Wyoming Valley Medical Center, Wilkes Barre, PA .... (G+)(HR)(G)
Grand View Health, Sellersville, PA .... (H)
Hahnemann University Hospital, Philadelphia, PA .... (G+)(G)(G+)(H)
Hanover Hospital, Hanover, PA .... (G+)(G)(E)
Heritage Valley Beaver, Beaver, PA .... (G+)(E)
Holy Redeemer Hospital, Meadowbrook, PA .... (G+)(E+)(S)
Holy Spirit Hospital: A Geisinger Affiliate, Camp Hill, PA .... (G)(G+)(HR)(S)(G+)(E)(S)
Jeanes Hospital - Temple University Health System, Philadelphia, PA .... (G+)(E)
Jefferson Hospital, Clairton, PA .... (G+)(HR)(G+)(E)(G)
Lancaster General Hospital, Lancaster, PA .... (G+)(E)
Lancaster Regional Medical Center, Lancaster, PA .... (S)
Lancaster Regional Medical Center & Heart of Lancaster Regional Medical Center, Lititz, PA .... (S)
Lankenau Medical Center, Wynnewood, PA .... (G+)(E)(G)
Lansdale Hospital, Lansdale, PA .... (G+)(E)

Lehigh Valley Health Network Cedar Crest, Allentown, PA .... (G+) (E) (S)
Lehigh Valley Health Network Muhlenberg, Bethlehem, PA .... (G+) (E) (S)
Lehigh Valley Hospital- Hazleton, Hazleton, PA .... (G+) (HR) (G+) (E)
Memorial Hospital, York, PA .... (S)
Mercy Fitzgerald Hospital, Darby, PA .... (G) (G)
Mercy Philadelphia Hospital, Philadelphia, PA .... (G) (G)
Mercy Suburban Hospital, Norristown, PA .... (G+) (HR) (G+) (E+)
Monongahela Valley Hospital, Monongahela, PA .... (S+) (G+) (E) (B)
Moses Taylor Hospital, Scranton, PA .... (G+) (E)
Mount Nittany Medical Center, State College, PA .... (G+) (E+)
Nazareth Hospital, Philadelphia, PA .... (G+) (HR) (G+)
Paoli Hospital, Paoli, PA .... (S+) (S)
Penn Highlands DuBois, Du Bois, PA .... (S)
Penn Medicine Chester County Hospital, West Chester, PA .... (G+) (HR) (S)
Penn Presbyterian Medical Center, Philadelphia, PA .... (G+) (E+)
Penn State Hershey Medical Center, Hershey, PA .... (G+) (HR) (G+) (E+)
Pennsylvania Hospital, Philadelphia, PA .... (S+) (G+) (E+)
Phoenixville Hospital, Phoenixville, PA .... (G+) (HR)
Pinnacle Health System - Harrisburg Hospital,
   Harrisburg, PA .... (G+) (HR) (G+) (E) (S)
Pinnacle Health System - West Shore Hospital,
   Mechanicsburg, PA .... (G+) (S)
Pocono Medical Center, East Stroudsburg, PA .... (G+) (E)
Pottstown Memorial Medical Center, Pottstown, PA .... (G+) (HR)
Reading Hospital, West Reading, PA .... (G+) (HR) (G+) (HR) (G) (B)
Regional Hospital of Scranton, Scranton, PA .... (S) (HR)
Riddle Memorial Hospital, Media, PA .... (G+) (E)
Roxborough Memorial Hospital, Philadelphia, PA .... (G+) (HR)
Sacred Heart Hospital, Allentown, PA .... (G+)
Saint Vincent Health System, Erie, PA .... (G+) (HR) (S)
Schuylkill Medical Center East Norwegian Street, Pottsville, PA .... (G+) (HR)
Schuylkill Medical Center South Jackson, Pottsville, PA .... (G+) (HR)
Sharon Regional Health System, Sharon, PA .... (S)
St. Clair Hospital, Pittsburgh, PA .... (S+) (E)
St. Joseph Regional Health Network, Reading, PA .... (G+) (G+) (E)
St. Luke's Hospital - Anderson Campus, Easton, PA .... (S+) (HR)
St. Luke's Hospital Quakertown Campus, Quakertown, PA,
   Quakertown, PA .... (S+)
St. Luke's Hospital-Miners Campus, Coaldale, PA .... (G+) (HR)
St. Luke's University Hospital, Bethlehem, PA .... (G+) (E+)
St. Mary Medical Center, Langhorne, PA .... (G) (G) (G+) (E+) (G+)
Temple University Hospital, Philadelphia, PA .... (G+) (E+) (S+)
The Children's Hospital of Philadelphia, Philadelphia, PA .... (G) (S)
The Good Samaritan Health System, Lebanon, PA .... (G+) (HR) (G+) (HR)
The Hospital of the University of Pennsylvania,
   Philadelphia, PA .... (G+) (HR) (G+) (E)
Uniontown Hospital, Uniontown, PA .... (G+) (HR)
UPMC Altoona, Altoona, PA .... (G+) (E)
UPMC East, Monroeville, PA .... (S+)
UPMC Hamot, Erie, PA .... (G+) (HR) (G+) (E+)
UPMC Horizon, Greenville, PA .... (G+)
UPMC McKeesport, McKeesport, PA .... (G+) (HR)
UPMC Mercy Pittsburgh, Pittsburgh, PA .... (G+) (E)
UPMC Northwest, Seneca, PA .... (G+)
UPMC Passavant, Pittsburgh, PA .... (S+) (E+) (B)
UPMC Presbyterian, Pittsburgh, PA .... (G+) (E+)
UPMC Shadyside, Pittsburgh, PA .... (G+)
UPMC St. Margaret, Pittsburgh, PA .... (G+) (E)
Washington Health System, Washington, PA .... (G+) (E)
Wellspan Ephrata Community Hospital, Stevens, PA .... (G+) (G+) (E+)
WellSpan Gettysburg Hospital , Gettysburg, PA .... (G+)
WellSpan Health - York Hospital, York, PA .... (S) (S+) (G+) (HR)
Williamsport Regional Medical Center - Susquehanna Health,
   Williamsport, PA .... (S)

Administración De Servicios Médicos, San Juan, PR .... (G+) (E)
Hospital HIMA - San Pablo - Caguas, Caguas, PR .... (G+) (HR) (G+) (E)
Hospital HIMA San Pablo Bayamón, Bayamón, PR .... (G+) (HR) (S+) (HR)

Kent Hospital, Warwick, RI .... (G+) (HR)
Memorial Hospital of Rhode Island, Pawtucket, RI .... (G+)
Rhode Island Hospital, Providence, RI .... (G+) (E+)
South County Hospital Health Care System, Wakefield, RI .... (G+) (HR)
The Miriam Hospital, Providence, RI .... (S+) (E)

AnMed Health, Anderson, SC .... (G) (G+) (E) (G+)
Beaufort Memorial Hospital, Beaufort, SC .... (G+) (E+) (S) (B)
Bon Secours Saint Francis Health System, Greenville, SC . (G+) (HR) (G+) (HR) (G+) (B)
Bon Secours St. Francis Hospital, Charleston, SC .... (G+) (HR)
Coastal Carolina Hospital, Hardeeville, SC .... (G+) (HR)
Conway Medical Center, Conway, SC .... (S+) (E+)
Grand Strand Medical Center, Myrtle Beach, SC .... (G+) (E+)
Greenville Memorial Hospital, Greenville, SC .... (G+) (E+) (G+)
Greer Memorial Hospital, Greer, SC .... (G) (HR)
Hilton Head Hospital, Hilton Head, SC .... (G+) (G+)
Lexington Medical Center, West Columbia, SC .... (G+) (HR) (G+)
Mary Black Health System, Spartanburg, SC .... (G+) (E+)
McLeod Regional Medical Center, Florence, SC .... (G+) (E+)
Medical University of South Carolina Medical Center, Charleston, SC .. (G+) (E+)
Palmetto Health Richland, Columbia, SC .... (G+) (G+) (E+) (S+)
Piedmont Medical Center, Rock Hill, SC .... (G+) (G) (G+) (E+)
Regional Medical Center of Orangeburg & Calhoun Counties,
   Orangeburg, SC .... (G+) (HR) (S) (G+) (E)
Roper St. Francis Hospital, Charleston, SC .... (G+) (HR)
Self Regional Healthcare, Greenwood, SC .... (G+) (HR) (G+) (HR)
Spartanburg Regional Healthcare System, Spartanburg, SC .... (G+)
Summerville Medical Center, Summerville, SC .... (G+)
Tidelands Georgetown Memorial Hospital, Georgetown, SC .... (S+) (E)
Tidelands Waccamaw Community Hospital, Murrells Inlet, SC .... (G+) (E+)
Trident Medical Center, Charleston, SC .... (G+) (G+) (HR) (S+) (S)

Avera Heart Hospital of South Dakota, Sioux Falls, SD .... (S)
Rapid City Regional Hospital, Rapid City, SD .... (G+) (HR) (B)
Sanford USD Medical Center, Sioux Falls, SD .... (G) (G+) (S)

Baptist Memorial Hospital Memphis, Memphis, TN .... (G+) (E+) (S)
Blount Memorial, Maryville, TN .... (G)
Bristol Regional Medical Center, Bristol, TN .... (S) (G) (S)
Erlanger Health System, Chattanooga, TN .... (G+) (E+) (B)
Fort Sanders Regional Medical Center, Knoxville, TN .... (G+) (E+) (G+) (S)
Holston Valley Medical Center, Kingsport, TN .... (G) (S)
Jackson-Madison County General Hospital, Jackson, TN .... (S)
Johnson City Medical Center, Johnson City, TN .... (G+) (S+)
Maury Regional Medical Center, Columbia, TN .... (G+)
Methodist Healthcare University Hospital, Memphis, TN .... (S+) (E+)
NorthCrest Medical Center, Springfield, TN .... (B)
Parkridge Medical Center, Chattanooga, TN .... (G) (G) (S+)
Saint Francis Hospital - Memphis, Memphis, TN .... (G+) (G+) (E+)
St. Francis Hospital - Bartlett, Bartlett, TN .... (S+) (E)
Sumner Regional Medical Center, Gallatin, TN .... (S+) (E)
Tennova Healthcare Harton, Tullahoma, TN .... (B)
The University of Tennessee Medical Center, Knoxville, TN .... (G+) (G+) (E+)
TriStar Centennial Medical Center, Brentwood, TN .... (G+) (E+)
TriStar Skyline Medical Center, Nashville, TN .... (S+) (E)
TriStar Southern Hills Medical Center, Nashville, TN .... (S+)
TriStar Summit Medical Center, Hermitage, TN .... (S+) (E)
Vanderbilt University Medical Center, Nashville, TN .... (G+) (E+)

Baptist Health System, San Antonio, TX .... (G) (G+) (E)
Baylor Jack and Jane Hamilton Heart and Vascular Hospital,
   Dallas, TX .... (G+) (S)

Baylor Medical Center at Irving, Irving, TX .... (G+) (B)
Baylor Regional Medical Center at Plano, Plano, TX .... (S+)
Baylor Scott & White Hillcrest Medical Center, Waco, TX .... (G+) (E) (S)
Baylor Scott & White Medical Center - Centennial, Frisco, TX .... (G+) (G+)
Baylor Scott & White Medical Center - Garland, Garland, TX........... (G+) (S+)
Baylor Scott & White Medical Center - Grapevine, Grapevine, TX...... (G+) (E+) (G+)
Baylor Scott & White Medical Center - Lake Pointe, Rowlett, TX .... (G+) (G+) (HR)
Baylor Scott & White Medical Center - Lakeway, Lakeway, TX........... (S+) (E+)
Baylor Scott & White Medical Center - McKinney, McKinney, TX....... (G+) (HR) (S+)
Baylor Scott & White Medical Center - Round Rock,
      Round Rock, TX .... (S) (G+) (E+) (G+) (S)
Baylor Scott & White Medical Center - Temple , Temple, TX........... (G+) (E+) (G+) (B)
Baylor Scott & White Medical Center - White Rock, Dallas, TX .... (G+)
Baylor University Medical Center at Dallas, Dallas, TX................ (G+) (B)
Bayshore Medical Center, Pasadena, TX .... (G+) (E)
Ben Taub Hospital, Houston, TX .... (G+) (E+) (G+) (S)
Central Texas Medical Center, San Marcos, TX .... (S+) (HR)
CHI St. Joseph Health Regional Hospital, Bryan, TX....................... (G+) (E) (B)
CHI St. Luke's Health – Baylor St. Luke's Medical Center,
      Houston, TX.. (G+) (E+) (G)
CHI St. Luke's Health–The Woodlands Hospital, The Woodlands, TX.... (G+) (E)
CHRISTUS Hospital - St. Elizabeth & St. Mary, Beaumont, TX........... (S+) (S) (HR)
CHRISTUS Santa Rosa Health, New Braunfels, TX........................ (S+)
CHRISTUS Santa Rosa Health, San Antonio, TX......................... (S+)
CHRISTUS Spohn Hospital Corpus Christi - Shoreline,
      Corpus Christi, TX.. (G+) (HR) (S)
CHRISTUS St. Michael Health System, Texarkana, TX................... (G+) (E)
Citizens Medical Center, Victoria, TX.............................. (G+) (E) (B)
Clear Lake Regional Medical Center, Webster, TX.................... (S+) (E+)
Conroe Regional Medical Center, Conroe, TX....................... (G+) (E)
Corpus Christi Medical Center, Corpus Christi, TX .... (G+) (E)
Cypress Fairbanks Medical Center, Houston, TX.................... (G+) (G+) (HR)
Del Sol Medical Center, El Paso, TX............................... (G+) (HR) (G+) (E)
DeTar Healthcare System, Victoria, TX............................ (G+)
Doctors Hospital at Renaissance, Edinburg, TX................ (G+) (HR) (G+) (E) (G)
East Texas Medical Center, Tyler, TX............................. (G+) (HR)
Good Shepherd Medical Center, Longview, TX.................... (G+) (E+) (G+) (S)
Good Shepherd Medical Center - Marshall, Marshall, TX........... (G+)
HCA- West Houston Medical Center, Houston, TX.................. (B)
Heart Hospital of Austin, Austin, TX.............................. (G+) (E+)
Hendrick Medical Center, Abilene, TX............................. (G+) (E+)
Houston Methodist Hospital, Houston, TX......................... (G+) (E+)
Houston Methodist San Jacinto Hospital, Baytown, TX............ (S) (G+) (HR)
Houston Methodist St. John Hospital, Nassau Bay, TX............ (S+) (E+)
Houston Methodist Sugar Land Hospital, Sugar Land, TX............. (G+) (E) (S)
Houston Methodist West Hospital, Houston, TX .... (G+) (E)
Houston Methodist Willowbrook Hospital, Houston, TX........... (G+) (E) (S)
Houston Northwest Medical Center, Houston, TX................. (G+) (G) (G+) (E)
Huntsville Memorial Hospital, Huntsville, TX...................... (S+) (E+)
JPS Health Network, Fort Worth, TX............................... (S+)
Kingwood Medical Center Hospital, an HCA Affiliated Hospital,
      Kingwood, TX... (G+) (E)
Knapp Medical Center, Weslaco, TX............................... (S+) (HR)
Las Palmas Medical Center, El Paso, TX .... (G+) (G+) (HR)
Matagorda Regional Medical Center, Bay City, TX................. (S)
McAllen Heart Hospital, McAllen, TX.............................. (S+)
Medical Center Hospital, Odessa, TX............................. (G+) (HR) (S)
Medical City Arlington, Arlington, TX............................. (S)
Medical City Dallas Hospital, Dallas, TX.......................... (G)
Memorial Hermann - Texas Medical Center, Houston, TX............ (G+) (E+) (G) (B)
Memorial Hermann Greater Heights Hospital, Houston, TX .... (G+) (E+)
Memorial Hermann Katy Hospital, Katy, TX....................... (G+) (E) (S)
Memorial Hermann Memorial City Medical Center, Houston, TX......... (G+) (E+)
Memorial Hermann Northeast Hospital, Humble, TX .... (S)
Memorial Hermann Pearland Hospital, Pearland, TX............... (S)
Memorial Hermann Southeast Hospital, Houston, TX............. (G+) (E) (S+)
Memorial Hermann Southwest Hospital, Houston, TX............. (G+) (E+)
Memorial Hermann Sugar Land Hospital, Sugar Land, TX .... (B)
Memorial Hermann The Woodlands, The Woodlands, TX.............. (G+) (HR) (S)

Methodist Charlton Medical Center, Dallas, TX .... (S+)
Methodist Dallas Medical Center, Dallas, TX........................ (G+) (E)
Methodist Hospital, San Antonio, TX................................ (G+) (E) (G+) (B)
Methodist Mansfield Medical Center, Mansfield, TX.................. (G+)
Methodist Stone Oak Hospital, San Antonio, TX.................... (G+) (E)
Metroplex Hospital, Killeen, TX................................... (S+) (G+) (B)
Metropolitan Methodist Hospital, San Antonio, TX................ (S+) (S) (B)
Midland Memorial Hospital, Midland, TX.......................... (B)
North Central Baptist Hospital, San Antonio, TX.................. (G+)
North Cypress Medical Center, Cypress, TX .... (G+) (E) (S) (B)
North Hills Hospital, North Richland Hills, TX.................... (S) (S)
Northeast Baptist Hospital, San Antonio, TX..................... (S)
Northeast Methodist Hospital, San Antonio, TX.................. (S+) (S)
OakBend Medical Center, Richmond, TX......................... (G+) (HR)
OakBend Medical Center Williams Way Campus, Richmond, TX...... (S+)
Parkland Health & Hospital System, Dallas, TX .... (G+) (G+) (E) (S) (S)
Providence Health Center, Waco, TX............................ (G+) (HR) (B)
Resolute Health Hospital , New Braunfels, TX.................. (S+) (HR)
Seton Medical Center Austin, Austin, TX....................... (S+) (E+) (G+)
Seton Medical Center Hays, Kyle, TX .... (G+) (E) (S+)
Seton Medical Center Williamson, Round Rock, TX.............. (G+) (E) (S+)
Shannon Medical Center, San Angelo, TX...................... (G) (S+) (G) (S)
Southwest General Hospital, San Antonio, TX................. (G+) (HR)
St. David's Georgetown, Georgetown, TX .... (G+) (HR) (S)
St. David's Medical Center, Austin, TX........................ (G+) (E+) (S) (S)
St. David's North Austin Medical Center, Austin, TX........... (G+)
St. David's Round Rock Medical Center, Round Rock, TX....... (G+) (E) (G+) (B)
St. David's South Austin Medical Center, Austin, TX.......... (S+) (HR) (S+) (S)
St. Joseph Medical Center, Houston, TX....................... (G)
Texas Health Arlington Memorial Hospital, Arlington, TX ...... (G+) (G+) (HR)
Texas Health Denton, Denton, TX............................. (G+)
Texas Health Harris Methodist Hospital Azle, Azle, TX........ (S+) (HR)
Texas Health Heart and Vascular Hospital, Arlington, TX...... (G+)
Texas Health Huguley Hospital, Burleson, TX................. (S+)
Texas Health Hurst Euless Bedford, Bedford, TX.............. (G)
Texas Health Plano, Plano, TX............................... (S+) (HR) (S+)
Texas Health Presbyterian Hospital Dallas, Dallas, TX......... (G+) (E+) (G)
The Heart Hospital Baylor Plano, Plano, TX................. (G+) (G+) (B)
The Hospitals of Providence East Campus, El Paso, TX......... (G+) (E)
The Hospitals of Providence Memorial Campus, El Paso, TX .....
The Hospitals of Providence Sierra Campus, El Paso, TX........ (G+) (G+) (HR) (S+)
The Medical Center of Plano, Plano, TX...................... (HR)
The University of Texas Medical Branch - Galveston Campus,
      Galveston, TX.. (G) (S+) (E+)
Titus Regional Medical Center, MT Pleasant, TX............. (S+) (E+)
University Health System, San Antonio, TX................. (G+) (E+) (S)
University Medical Center, Lubbock, TX.................... (S+)
University Medical Center Brackenridge, Austin, TX......... (G+) (E)
University Medical Center of El Paso, El Paso, TX........... (G+) (E)
UT Southwestern Medical Center, Dallas, TX................ (G+) (E)
Valley Baptist Medical Center-Brownsville, Brownsville, TX ... (G+) (E)
Valley Baptist Medical Center-Harlingen, Harlingen, TX....... (G+) (E)
Valley Regional Medical Center, Brownsville, TX............. (G+) (E)
Wadley Regional Medical Center, Texarkana, TX .... (G+) (E)
Wise Health System, Decatur, TX........................... (G+)

UTAH

American Fork Hospital, American Fork, UT......................... (G+)
Davis Hospital and Medical Center, Layton, UT .... (G+) (HR)
Dixie Regional Medical Center, St. George, UT................. (G+) (E)
Intermountain Medical Center, Murray, UT..................... (G+)
Jordan Valley Medical Center/JVMC-West Valley Campus/Mountain Point
      Medical Center, a Campus of JVMC, West Jordan, UT......... (G+) (E)
Lakeview Hospital, Bountiful, UT............................. (G+) (HR)
McKay-Dee Hospital, Ogden, UT.............................. (G+) (HR)
Mountain View Hospital - Payson, Payson, UT................ (G+)
Ogden Regional Medical Center, Ogden, UT................... (G+)
St. Marks Hospital, Salt Lake City, UT...................... (G+) (E) (G+)

Timpanogos Regional Hospital, Orem, UT .... (G+)
University of Utah Health, Salt Lake City, UT .... (G+)(E+)(B)
Utah Valley Hospital - Intermountain Healthcare System, Provo, UT..... (G+)(HR)

VERMONT

The University of Vermont Medical Center, Burlington, VT .... (G+)(HR)

VIRGINIA

Augusta Health, Fishersville, VA.................................... (G+)(E+)(S+)
Bon Secours DePaul Medical Center, Norfolk, VA .... (G+)(E+)
Bon Secours Maryview Medical Center, Portsmouth, VA .... (G+)(E+)(G)
Bon Secours Memorial Regional Medical Center,
    Mechanicsville, VA.. (G)(S+)(E)
Bon Secours Rappahannock General Hospital, Kilmarnock, VA .... (G+)
Bon Secours St. Mary's Hospital, Richmond, VA.................... (G)(G+)(HR)(B)
Carilion Roanoke Memorial Hospital, Roanoke, VA .... (G+)(HR)
Centra Lynchburg General Hospital, Lynchburg, VA .... (HR)(G+)(E)(G)
Chesapeake Regional Medical Center, Chesapeake, VA.......... (G+)(E)
Chippenham Medical Center, Richmond, VA......................... (S+)
Inova Alexandria Hospital, Alexandria, VA .... (G+)(E+)(S+)(S)
Inova Fair Oaks Hospital, Fairfax, VA .... (G+)(E)
Inova Fairfax Hospital, Falls Church, VA...................... (G+)(E+)(G+)(B)
Inova Loudoun Hospital, Leesburg, VA.......................... (G+)(E+)(B)
Inova Mount Vernon Hospital, Alexandria, VA .... (G+)(E+)
John Randolph Medical Center, Hopewell, VA.................... (S)
Lewis Gale Medical Center, Salem, VA.......................... (S)
Martha Jefferson Hospital, Charlottesville, VA.................. (S+)
Novant Health UVA Health System Culpeper Medical Center,
    Culpeper, VA .... (S)
Novant Health UVA Health System Prince William Medical Center,
    Manassas, VA .... (HR)(S+)
Reston Hospital Center, Reston, VA............................. (G+)(E)
Riverside Regional Medical Center, Newport News, VA .... (G+)(E+)
Sentara CarePlex Hospital, Hampton, VA .... (G)(B)
Sentara Leigh Hospital, Norfolk, VA........................... (G)(B)
Sentara Louise Obici Memorial Hospital, Suffolk, VA........... (S)
Sentara Norfolk General Hospital/Sentara Heart Hospital, Norfolk, VA .... (B)
Sentara Northern Virginia Medical Center, Woodbridge, VA....... (G)(B)
Sentara Princess Anne Hospital, Virginia Beach, VA............ (B)
Sentara Virginia Beach General Hospital, Virginia Beach, VA.... (G+)(B)
Sentara Williamsburg Regional Medical Center, Williamsburg, VA .... (G)(B)
Stafford Hospital, Stafford, VA............................... (S+)
StoneSprings Hospital Center, Dulles, VA...................... (S+)
Twin County Regional Healthcare, Galax, VA.................... (G+)(HR)
University of Virginia Health System, Charlottesville, VA......... (HR)(G+)(E+)(S)
VCU Community Memorial Hospital, South Hill, VA .... (G+)(E)
Virginia Commonwealth University Medical Center,
    Richmond, VA... (G+)(E+)(G)(B)
Winchester Medical Center, Winchester, VA..................... (G)(S)(B)

WASHINGTON

Confluence Health-Central Washington Hospital, Wenatchee, WA..(G+)(HR)(G+)
Deaconess Hospital, Spokane, WA .... (G+)(E+)
EvergreenHealth, Kirkland, WA................................. (G+)(E+)
Harborview Medical Center, Seattle, WA........................ (G+)(E)(S)
Harrison Medical Center, Bremerton, WA .... (G+)(E)(S+)(S)
Highline Medical Center, Burien, WA........................... (S+)(HR)
Jefferson Healthcare, Port Townsend, WA....................... (G+)
Kittitas Valley Healthcare, Ellensburg, WA.................... (G+)(E)
MultiCare Auburn Medical Center, Auburn, WA .... (S)
MultiCare Good Samaritan Hospital, Puyallup, WA .... (S)(G+)(E)
MultiCare Tacoma General Allenmore Hospital,
    Tacoma, WA .... (G)(S)(G+)(E)(S+)
Northwest Hospital & Medical Center, Seattle, WA.............. (G+)(E+)(S)(S)
Overlake Medical Center, Bellevue, WA......................... (G+)(HR)
PeaceHealth St. Joseph Medical Center, Bellingham, WA......... (G+)(E+)(S)
Providence Regional Medical Center Everett, Everett, WA .... (G+)(E+)
Providence Sacred Heart Medical Center & Children's Hospital,
    Spokane, WA .... (G+)(E+)(B)

Skagit Valley Hospital, Mount Vernon, WA...................... (G+)(E)
St. Francis Hospital, Federal Way, WA .... (S+)(B)
St. Joseph Medical Center, Tacoma, WA .... (G+)(HR)(S+)(S)
Swedish Edmonds, Edmonds, WA................................. (G+)(E+)
Swedish Medical Center - Cherry Hill, Seattle, WA .... (G+)(E+)
Swedish Medical Center, Issaquah and Redmond Ambulatory Care,
    Issaquah, WA .... (G+)(E)
Trios Health, Kennewick, WA .... (G+)(HR)(S)
UW Medicine | Valley Medical Center, Renton, WA .... (G+)(E+)(S)
Virginia Mason Medical Center, Seattle, WA................... (G+)(HR)(G+)(HR)(B)
Virginia Mason Memorial, Yakima, WA.......................... (G)(G+)(E+)
Yakima Regional Medical and Cardiac Center, Yakima, WA........ (B)

WEST VIRGINIA

Cabell Huntington Hospital, Huntington, WV .... (G+)(E)
Camden Clark Medical Center, Parkersburg, WV .... (G)(G+)
Davis Medical Center, Elkins, WV............................. (G)
Monongalia General Hospital, Morgantown, WV .... (G)
St. Mary's Medical Center, Huntington, WV.................... (G+)(S)(G+)(S)
United Hospital Center, Bridgeport, WV .... (S)(S+)
West Virginia University Hospital, Inc., Morgantown, WV ...... (G+)(HR)(E+)(E)
Wheeling Hospital, Wheeling, WV.............................. (G)(G+)

WISCONSIN

Ascension- All Saints, Racine, WI............................ (G+)(S+)(E)
Aspirus Wausau Hospital, Wausau, WI.......................... (G+)(S)
Aurora BayCare Medical Center, Green Bay, WI................. (G)(G+)(G+)(E+)(G+)(B)
Aurora Lakeland Medical Center, Elkhorn, WI.................. (G+)(HR)(G+)
Aurora Medical Center - Grafton, Grafton, WI................. (G+)(G+)(E)(G+)(B)
Aurora Medical Center - Kenosha, Kenosha, WI................. (G+)(HR)(G+)
Aurora Medical Center- Oshkosh, Oshkosh, WI.................. (G+)
Aurora Medical Center Summit, Oconomowoc, WI................. (G+)(G+)(E+)(B)
Aurora Memorial Hospital Burlington, Burlington, WI.......... (G+)(HR)(G+)
Aurora Sheboygan Memorial Medical Center, Sheboygan, WI...... (G+)(E)
Aurora Sinai Medical Center, Milwaukee, WI.................. (G+)(HR)(G+)(HR)
Aurora St. Luke's Medical Center, Milwaukee, WI.............. (G+)(HR)(G+)(G+)(S)
Aurora St. Luke's South Shore, Cudahy, WI................... (G+)(HR)(G+)
Aurora West Allis Medical Center, West Allis, WI .... (G+)(G+)
Bellin Memorial Hospital, Green Bay, WI .... (G+)(E+)
Beloit Memorial Hospital, Beloit, WI .... (G+)(S)
Columbia - St. Mary's Hospital, Milwaukee, WI............... (G+)(HR)(B)
Columbia-St. Mary's Hospital - Ozaukee, Mequon, WI.......... (G)
Froedtert Hospital, Milwaukee, WI........................... (G+)
Gundersen Lutheran Medical Center, La Crosse, WI .... (G+)(E+)
Holy Family Memorial Medical Center, Manitowoc, WI .... (S+)(S)
HSHS St. Vincent Hospital, Green Bay, WI .... (G+)(S)
Mayo Clinic Health System in Eau Claire, Eau Claire, WI ..... (G+)(HR)
Mayo Clinic Health System LaCrosse, La Crosse, WI .... (G+)(E)
Mercy Hospital and Trauma Center, Janesville, WI .... (G+)(HR)(G+)(HR)
Meriter-UnityPoint Health, Madison, WI .... (G+)(HR)
Ministry Saint Joseph's Hospital, Marshfield, WI .... (G+)(E)
Oconomowoc Memorial Hospital, Oconomowoc, WI................ (G+)
Sacred Heart Hospital, Eau Claire, WI .... (G+)
SSM Health St. Mary's Hospital - Madison, Madison, WI ...... (G+)(E+)(G+)(B)
St. Agnes Hospital, Fond Du Lac, WI .... (G+)(HR)
St. Clare Hospital and Health Services, Baraboo, WI .... (G+)
St. Mary's Hospital Medical Center, Green Bay, WI .... (S+)(G)(B)
Theda Clark Medical Center, Neenah, WI .... (G+)(HR)
University of Wisconsin Hospital and Clinics, Madison, WI ... (G+)(E+)(S)
Waukesha Memorial Hospital, Waukesha, WI .... (G+)(E+)
Wheaton Franciscan Healthcare - Elmbrook, Brookfield, WI.... (G+)(HR)
Wheaton Franciscan Healthcare - St. Joseph, Milwaukee, WI ... (G+)(HR)

WYOMING

Cheyenne Regional Medical Center, Cheyenne, WY .... (S)(G)(S)
Wyoming Medical Center, Casper, WY .... (G+)(E+)(G+)(S)

American Heart Association American Stroke Association.
life is why™

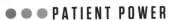
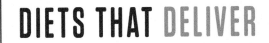

DIETS THAT DELIVER

U.S. News looks at how well 38 eating plans live up to the hype

AS FRUSTRATED DIETERS KNOW, losing weight is hard, and most diets don't work. This is why U.S. News has produced its Best Diets rankings, based on the views of a panel of nationally recognized experts (Page 85) on how effective some of the best-known eating plans are, whether the aim is to lose weight, improve heart health, or manage diabetes. Our panelists reviewed the research, added their own fact-finding, and rated the diets from 1 to 5 (the top score) in a number of areas: short-term weight loss (the likelihood of losing significant weight dur-ing the first 12 months); long-term weight loss (the likelihood of maintaining significant weight loss for two years or more); diabetes prevention and man-agement; heart health (effectiveness at preventing cardiovascular disease and reducing risk for heart patients); ease of compliance; nutritional complete-ness (how well a plan meets federal dietary guide-lines); and safety (whether, for example, it omits key nutrients). Which plan can help you achieve your goals? Check out the results in these pages. For more on the plans, visit usnews.com/bestdiets.

HOW THE PLANS COMPARE OVERALL

Thirty-eight diets were rated from 1 to 5 on multiple measures. Rank is based on a score compiled from panelists' average scores for each measure. The results:

Rank	Diet	Overall score	Short-term weight loss	Long-term weight loss	For diabetes	For heart health	Nutrition	Safety	Ease of complying
1	DASH	4.2	3.4	3.2	4.0	4.6	4.9	4.8	3.6
2	Mediterranean	4.1	3.4	3.2	3.8	4.3	4.7	4.7	3.7
3	Mind	4.0	3.2	3.1	3.7	4.2	4.6	4.6	3.7
4	Flexitarian	3.9	3.6	3.4	3.7	3.9	4.3	4.4	3.6
4	Mayo Clinic	3.9	3.5	3.0	3.7	3.9	4.5	4.6	3.4
4	TLC	3.9	3.4	2.9	3.5	4.5	4.5	4.6	3.3
4	Weight Watchers	3.9	4.3	3.7	3.6	3.5	4.4	4.5	3.7
8	Fertility	3.8	3.1	2.9	3.7	3.8	4.4	4.3	3.7
8	Volumetrics	3.8	3.9	3.5	3.5	3.6	4.3	4.5	3.5
10	Jenny Craig	3.7	4.1	3.3	3.3	3.3	3.9	4.2	3.6
10	Ornish	3.7	3.6	3.1	3.7	4.6	4.2	4.1	2.3
10	Vegetarian	3.7	3.2	3.2	3.7	3.9	4.1	4.1	3.1
13	Traditional Asian	3.6	3.2	3.0	3.4	3.6	4.1	4.2	3.1
14	Anti-Inflammatory	3.5	2.9	2.8	3.6	3.9	4.0	4.1	3.0
15	Biggest Loser	3.4	4.2	2.8	3.5	3.4	3.8	3.6	2.8
16	Flat Belly	3.3	3.4	2.7	3.2	3.4	3.8	3.9	2.9
16	Nutrisystem	3.3	3.6	2.7	3.0	2.9	3.6	3.7	3.2
16	Spark Solution	3.3	3.8	2.9	3.1	3.1	3.7	3.9	2.6
16	Vegan	3.3	3.7	3.4	3.8	4.1	3.3	3.1	2.1
20	Eco-Atkins	3.2	4.0	2.8	3.1	3.6	3.2	3.4	2.4
20	Engine 2	3.2	3.6	3.0	3.7	4.0	3.2	3.4	2.0
20	HMR	3.2	4.3	2.8	3.2	3.1	3.4	3.2	2.9
20	SlimFast	3.2	3.8	3.1	3.1	2.9	3.3	3.3	2.9
24	South Beach	3.1	3.8	2.6	2.9	3.1	3.3	3.4	2.8
25	Abs	3.0	3.2	2.1	2.7	2.9	3.4	3.6	2.6
25	Glycemic-Index	3.0	3.2	2.5	3.0	2.6	3.3	3.7	2.2
25	Zone	3.0	3.4	2.6	2.6	3.0	3.4	3.6	2.4
28	Macrobiotic	2.9	3.3	2.7	3.3	3.4	3.0	3.1	2.0
29	Medifast	2.8	3.9	2.3	2.8	2.9	3.0	2.9	2.5
29	Supercharged Hormone	2.8	3.3	2.5	2.8	2.9	2.9	3.1	2.3
31	Acid Alkaline	2.7	2.8	2.2	2.5	2.6	2.9	3.3	2.1
32	Body Reset	2.5	3.2	1.9	2.1	2.3	2.8	3.0	2.1
32	Fast	2.5	3.3	2.3	2.3	2.6	2.4	2.6	2.5
32	Raw Food	2.5	3.8	3.2	2.8	2.9	2.3	2.2	1.2
35	Atkins	2.4	4.0	2.5	2.6	2.2	2.0	2.4	2.2
36	Paleo	2.3	2.7	2.1	2.6	2.3	2.3	2.5	1.9
37	Dukan	2.1	3.3	2.1	2.1	2.0	2.1	2.5	1.7
38	Whole30	2.0	3.2	1.8	2.1	2.0	1.9	2.4	1.5

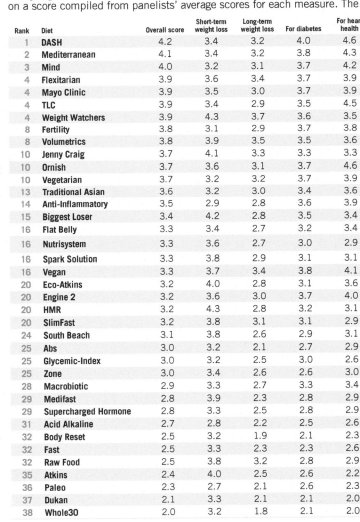

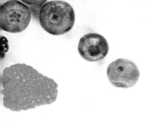

BEST WEIGHT-LOSS DIETS

Diets are ranked by the average of the scores experts assigned them for producing short- and long-term results.

Rank	Diet	Avg. score
1	Weight Watchers	4.1
2	Jenny Craig	3.7
2	Volumetrics	3.7
4	HMR	3.6
5	Biggest Loser	3.5
5	Flexitarian	3.5
5	Raw Food	3.5
5	SlimFast	3.5
5	Vegan	3.5
10	Ornish	3.4
10	Spark Solution	3.4

BEST DIABETES DIETS

These plans scored highest for both managing and preventing the condition.

Rank	Diet	Avg. score
1	DASH	4.0
2	Mediterranean	3.8
2	Vegan	3.8
4	Engine 2	3.7
4	Fertility	3.7
4	Flexitarian	3.7
4	Mayo Clinic	3.7
4	Mind	3.7
4	Ornish	3.7
4	Vegetarian	3.7
11	Anti-Inflammatory	3.6
11	Weight Watchers	3.6

BEST COMMERCIAL DIETS

Nutritional value, ease of use and safety are counted, as well as weight-loss effectiveness.

Rank	Diet	Avg. score
1	Mayo Clinic	3.9
1	Weight Watchers	3.9
3	Jenny Craig	3.7
4	Biggest Loser	3.4
5	Flat Belly	3.3
5	Nutrisystem	3.3
5	Spark Solution	3.3
8	HMR	3.2
8	SlimFast	3.2
10	South Beach	3.1

BEST DIETS FOR THE HEART

With these plans, you can take aim at cholesterol, blood pressure or triglycerides as well as weight.

Rank	Diet	Avg. score
1	DASH	4.6
1	Ornish	4.6
3	TLC	4.5
4	Mediterranean	4.3
5	Mind	4.2
6	Vegan	4.1
7	Engine 2	4.0
8	Anti-Inflammatory	3.9
8	Flexitarian	3.9
8	Mayo Clinic	3.9
8	Vegetarian	3.9
12	Fertility	3.8

BEST PLANT-BASED DIETS

These diets emphasize minimally processed foods from plants and are good bets for weight loss.

Rank	Diet	Avg. score
1	Mediterranean	4.1
2	Flexitarian	3.9
3	Ornish	3.7
3	Vegetarian	3.7
5	Traditional Asian	3.6
6	Anti-Inflammatory	3.5
7	Vegan	3.3
8	Eco-Atkins	3.2
8	Engine 2	3.2
10	Macrobiotic	2.9
11	Raw Food	2.5

EASIEST-TO-FOLLOW DIETS

The ranking is based on ease of use and a diet's ability to deliver weight loss and good nutrition.

Rank	Diet	Avg. score
1	Fertility	3.7
1	Mediterranean	3.7
1	Mind	3.7
1	Weight Watchers	3.7
5	DASH	3.6
5	Flexitarian	3.6
5	Jenny Craig	3.6
8	Volumetrics	3.5
9	Mayo Clinic	3.4
10	TLC	3.3

THE EXPERT PANEL

Twenty people reviewed detailed assessments of the U.S. News list of 38 diets and rated them on a number of key measures, described on Page 84.

Kathie Beals
Associate professor (clinical), division of nutrition, University of Utah

Amy Campbell
Nutrition and wellness consultant and writer

Lawrence Cheskin
Founder and director, Johns Hopkins Weight Management Center

Michael Davidson
Director of preventive cardiology, University of Chicago Medical Center

Teresa Fung
Professor of nutrition, Simmons College

Andrea Giancoli
Nutrition communications consultant

Carole V. Harris
Senior fellow, public health division, ICF International

David Katz
Director, Yale-Griffin Prevention Research Center

Penny Kris-Etherton
Distinguished professor of nutrition, Pennsylvania State University

Robert Kushner
Clinical director, Northwestern Comprehensive Center on Obesity

JoAnn Manson
Professor of women's health, Harvard Medical School

Lori Mosca
Director of preventive cardiology, New York-Presbyterian Hospital

Yasmin Mossavar-Rahmani
Associate professor of clinical epidemiology and population health, Albert Einstein College of Medicine

Elisabetta Politi
Nutrition director, Duke Diet and Fitness Center

Rebecca Reeves
Adjunct assistant professor, University of Texas School of Public Health

Michael Rosenbaum
Professor of clinical pediatrics and clinical medicine; associate director of the Clinical Research Resource at Columbia University Medical Center

Lisa Sasson
Clinical associate professor of nutrition, food studies and public health, New York University

Laurence Sperling
Founder and director of the Emory Heart Disease Prevention Center

Sachiko St. Jeor
Professor emeritus of internal medicine, University of Nevada School of Medicine

Brian Wansink
Director, Food and Brand Lab, Cornell University

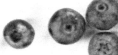

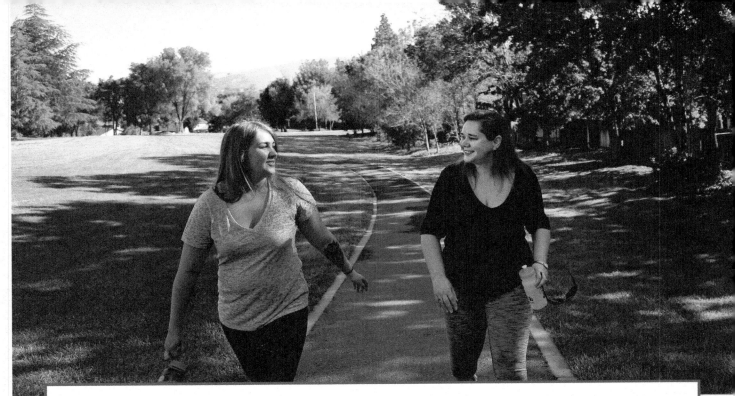

AN ANSWER IN YOUR GENES?

Some people swear by weight-loss plans tailored to their DNA

By Arlene Weintraub

If you've had the same experience as Donna Ridolfino, a clinical nurse supervisor for insurer Aetna who has been struggling to control her weight for more than 30 years, you might be both daunted and relieved by some of the latest obesity research. Daunted by news that the winds against you may be programmed into your genes; relieved that blaming yourself for faulty willpower may be the wrong response.

Ridolfino, 60, has tried everything from the Atkins diet to Weight Watchers, and every time she lost weight, she gained it back – and more. Then, when the scale registered 354 pounds in 2015, Aetna offered what she considers a "life-changing" breakthrough: a program that would use her genetic code to determine the best weight-loss plan for her. Testing revealed a variant of a gene called MC4R, often referred to as the "appetite" gene, which normally triggers signals in the brain that it's time to stop eating. "I started looking at how other people eat and suddenly I realized this was the key – my brain didn't know I was full," says Ridolfino, who lives in Myrtle Beach, South Carolina. Working with a weight-loss coach, she has adjusted her portion sizes and learned to pay close attention to signals of fullness coming from her stomach instead of her brain. Encouraged, she also started doing aerobics and strength training three times a week.

"I now have the tools to overcome what was defeating me," says Ridolfino, who has lost 25 pounds so far. "It's not a diet. This is now my lifestyle for the rest of my life."

MC4R is one of hundreds of genes believed to play a role in how people gain weight – their eating behaviors, how they metabolize fat – and how effectively they lose it. And even though researchers still have much to learn about how these genes can be employed in battling obesity, there's little doubt that at least some of the propensity to gain weight is predetermined.

Despite ongoing debate about the value now of using genetic data to guide weight loss, several companies have started marketing gene tests to insurers and employer groups, and sometimes to consumers. Ridolfino's plan was created by Newtopia, a company that works with groups to develop personalized wellness programs based on each participant's genetic makeup and behavioral profile. Newtopia counts 10,000 participants so far – a number it expects to triple by 2018. For consumers, 23andme sells a $199 kit online that promises to help people make the best diet and exercise choices. Dallas-based Genetic Direction sells a $349 test, GxSlim, that offers diet and exercise plans based on 16 genetic traits.

The tests look for mutations in genes that scientists have linked to body mass index, fat metabolism, addictive behavior, and other factors underlying a predisposition for weight gain. In addition to checking MC4R, Newtopia's test screens for variations in the gene FTO, which governs how efficiently fat is converted to energy rather than simply stored, and DRD2, a gene believed to be associated with addictive behaviors such as overeating. Aetna found that over 75 percent of employees who pilot-tested the plan lost an average of 10 pounds over a year by focusing on genetically driven recommendations – cutting fat instead of just calories if their FTO gene was the culprit, for instance, and finding pleasurable nonfattening habits to sub for eating if DRD2 was to blame. Someone who uses GxSlim and has a variant of a gene called GNPDA2 that has been tied to an increased body mass index might be prescribed strength training as a good way to burn fat. Someone who is shown to have certain variants of other genes governing how fat is stored might be told that simple cardio won't work off the excess pounds – high-intensity interval training is called for.

Brian Rudman, a doctor in Dallas who specializes in weight loss and uses GxSlim in his practice, says the test results often come as a revelation to patients. "I have people who will say they work out three hours on the treadmill and don't see any weight loss," says Rudman (who is also an investor in Genetic Direction). If the test shows that "a patient is going to have a poor response to cardio," he advises a switch to a regimen of intense bursts of activity. Anyone can lose weight eventually by modifying their diet and trying different exercise programs until they hit on the right one, he says. But without the genetic data "we're working with incomplete information."

Maybe so, but some scientists who specialize in genetics argue that the link between genes and weight loss isn't strong enough to justify testing for most people. About 175 genetic variants have been associated with body weight to date, and most of them are still not well understood, says Ruth Loos, a professor of environmental medicine and public health at Mount Sinai in New York. What's more, studies of twins and families have suggested that body weight is determined half by genetics and half by lifestyle factors. "Even people who carry genetic variants that make them prone to gain weight are able to overcome them" with extra effort, she says.

Moreover, it's too early to be sure that the purported links between particular genetic variants and weight-loss strategies are solid. For example, a study published a few years ago in the journal Obesity reported no link between GNPDA2 and favorable changes in body weight in young women who underwent 12 weeks of strength training.

Still, some experts counter, simply knowing you have a genetic predisposition to struggle can be empowering. Blaming oneself for being overweight "actually makes the weight loss much harder," says Gary Foster, chief scientific officer of Weight Watchers International, whereas people who have their genes tested "can say, 'I know the deck is stacked against me. Now I feel resolved that I can do something about it.'" Most people know it's possible to lose weight by eating less and exercising more, says Jeff Ruby, Newtopia's founder and CEO. But "something is missing to spark that behavioral change." The genetic information, he argues, "makes it real – it taps into their intrinsic motivation to change."

That's the case with Trish Brown, a genetic counselor in San Francisco who has learned from testing her genes that she has a rare genetic variant linked to a buildup of fat in the abdomen and a high risk of metabolic diseases like diabetes, as well as a gene that interferes with her ability to shed pounds in response to exercise. She took her results to a personal trainer, who developed a high-intensity workout designed to be performed three to five times a week. Though she temporarily is sticking to yoga and walking because of surgery, the combination of exercise and a low-fat diet has helped her shed 20 pounds so far.

Brown, 50, is well aware that many questions remain unanswered, and that determined people can lose weight without testing. But knowing her makeup has made all the difference for her, she says. "I spent tens of thousands of dollars at medical weight-loss clinics. I went to Weight Watchers. And I was not progressing on those programs," she says. "When I got my genetic information, I knew it would just take me a lot longer to lose weight. It was very validating." ●

> **It's not a diet. This is now my lifestyle.**

FITNESS
IN A FLASH

Interval training can bring
great results in minutes

By Beth Howard

Fitness fads come and go. Remember the Hula-Hoop workout? How about Jazzercise and pole dancing? But the latest trend – workouts that take mere minutes to complete – should have more staying power. Accumulating research shows that 10-, seven-, and even one-minute workouts of high-intensity interval training, or HIIT, can be as effective as the traditional variety, if not more so, in a fraction of the time. "A small time commitment can get you some pretty potent benefits," says Jonathan Little, assistant professor of health and exercise sciences at the University of British Columbia and an investigator funded by the Canadian Institutes of Health Research, which has been at the forefront of the HIIT research.

These routines, which are taught at many fitness facilities in boot camp-style programs, are characterized by quick bursts of intense activity interspersed with periods of mild activity. "You increase the intensity of your workout out of your comfort zone for a few seconds up to a few minutes and then you take a break and rest," Little explains. "You then repeat that two to 10 times throughout a workout."

The benefits of this approach can be striking. In landmark research, Martin Gibala, chair of the department of kinesiology at McMaster University in Ontario and author of "The One-Minute Workout" showed with his research team that the fitness gains from a somewhat more intensive version of HIIT, known as sprint interval training, or SIT (three 20-second exer-

cise spurts with two-minute recovery periods of light activity between them, performed three times a week) equaled those resulting from the recommended activity guidelines: 150 minutes of moderate exercise a week, or about 30 minutes, five times a week.

How does it work? Interval workouts force the heart and lungs to work harder in the "sprint" mode than they would in a typical workout, which leads to faster gains in aerobic capacity, helping the heart and lungs. "There are improvements in vascular function," says Little, so your blood vessels are "able to dilate better, and they're more elastic." In fact, two sessions a week of a high-intensity regimen lowered blood pressure by 9 percent, according to a study from Ab-

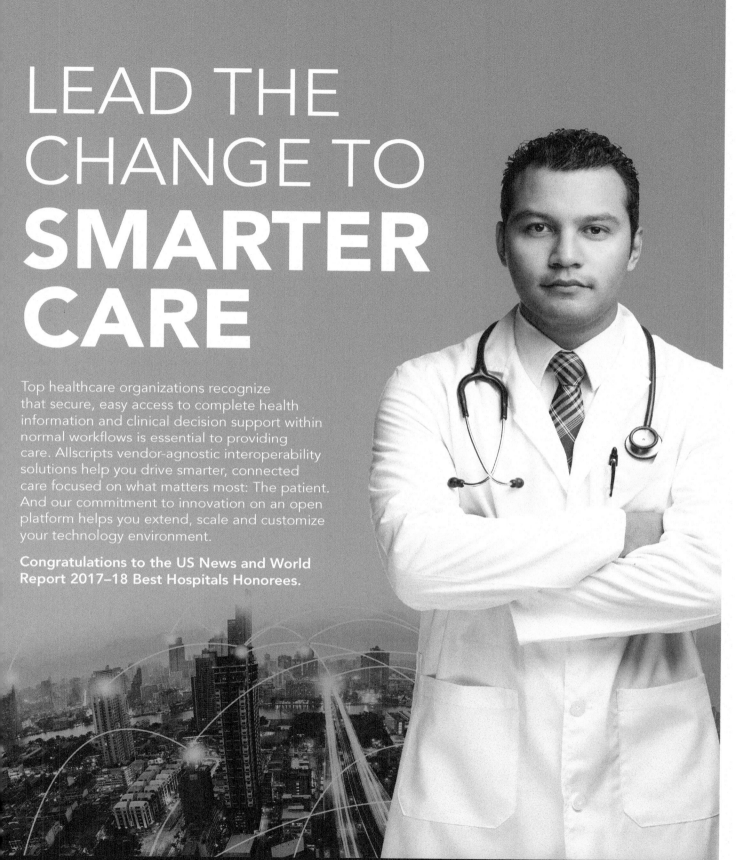

ertay University in Dundee, Scotland. Participants, each over age 60, pedaled all-out for a mere six seconds, followed by about a minute of rest, working up to 10 sprint-rest cycles per workout.

Muscles also seem to get an extra boost from HIIT-style exercise, which could be significant as people age and begin to lose muscle mass. "When you go out for a walk, only about 60 percent of the muscle fibers in your legs get any benefit," Little says. "The other 40 percent don't because you aren't working hard enough. Even if you're walking steadily every day you're going to lose some conditioning in muscle fibers that don't get called upon."

This is particularly important with the body's so-called fast-twitch muscle fibers, which help maintain the strength needed to carry out the tasks of daily living like climbing stairs. "If we're sedentary all the time or just do very light activity, we never call upon these fibers and they atrophy and shrink,"

Gibala says. "But when we challenge them, pushing the system a little bit in intervals, we recruit more fast-twitch fibers." By the way, you can turn an ordinary walk into one that activates more muscle fibers by incorporating HIIT principles: When you're walking, just speed walk (or even break into a run) for 30 seconds, then resume your normal pace for two minutes, repeating the cycle several times.

A new study from researchers at the Mayo Clinic in Rochester, Minnesota, revealed surprising changes at the cellular level from these workouts, according to senior author K. Sreekumaran Nair, a professor of medicine and endocrinology. Researchers assigned a group of people ages 18 to 30 and another group ages 65 to 80 to interval training, weight training, or a combination of the two for three months.

Muscle biopsies taken at the start of the study and 72 hours after the final exercise session showed that doing high-intensity interval training

improved the ability of mitochondria – the powerhouse of cells – to generate energy by an average of 49 percent in younger people and 69 percent in older individuals, effectively reversing many of the age-related changes in these proteins. HIIT also improved participants' insulin sensitivity.

Several studies have also shown that HIIT workouts may do a better job boosting glucose control than regular training. In new research from the University College of Southeast Norway, exercise scientists compared a group of people with Type 2 diabetes participating in HIIT workouts to another group that did a steady, moderate workout. Exercise led to lower body fat, blood pressure, and waist and hip circumference in both groups. But only those doing intervals significantly lowered their A1C levels, a measure of glucose control over time, says lead study author Eva Maria Støa. Meanwhile, new research from California State Uni-

PLAYGROUNDS FOR GROWN-UPS

Since Andrea Saunders began exercising at the outdoor "fitness zone" in Gwen Cherry Park in Miami about a year ago, she's lost 28 lbs., something she hadn't been able to accomplish before. "I love being outside," she explains. "And it's free."

The outdoor play space is just one of hundreds that have sprung up around the country in recent years as parks and municipalities take on two major population trends: aging and obesity. Two nonprofits – The Trust for Public Lands and KaBOOM!, which serves underprivileged communities – are key driving forces. Nationwide, KaBOOM!

has installed 65 multigenerational playgrounds, which include equipment for both children and adults, while the Trust for Public Lands has built 205 outdoor fitness zones for adults in 42 city parks, from Portland, Oregon, to Portland, Maine.

Such facilities often boast joint-friendly equipment and are

designed to help older people stay fit and independent. Research has shown that regular use of an adult playground improves balance, speed and coordination, capabilities that can boost seniors' ability to live on their own. Those that feature equipment for both kids and adults also allow the generations to bond, a plus versity at San Marcos indicates that HIIT workouts are more enjoyable than moderate continuous activity, which should make these regimens easier to stick with.

Still, Gibala notes, "There's no free lunch. There is an intensity duration trade-off. The more intense the exercise, the more uncomfortable it is." That means you might huff and puff more than you're used to during the high-intensity portion of the workout. Skeptics have also suggested that people doing interval training may be at a greater risk for injury. (Always get your doctor's OK before starting an exercise program if you have been sedentary.) "It makes sense to be a bit cautious with high-intensity interval training, because it is more vigorous," Little says, but "ultimately the risk of being sedentary and not doing anything at all is much greater."

Exercise scientists are just glad to

> ## " HIIT workouts may do a better job boosting glucose control than regular training.

have another effective fitness option. Currently only about half of Americans 18 and over manage to meet the recommended physical activity guidelines. Experts hope that these time-crunch-ing workouts will nudge more people off the couch, helping to turn the tide against rising rates of obesity, diabetes and heart disease. Says Gibala, "The more options we have, the better." ●

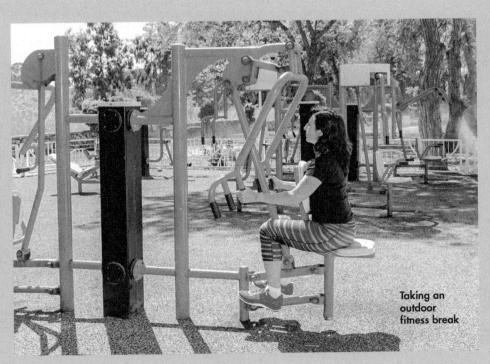

for older people who experience loneliness, which is linked to poorer heart and brain health. Just being in the open air offers an important benefit. Says Kellie May, director of health and wellness for the National Recreation and Park Association, "Exercising outdoors, surrounded by nature, makes it easier to stick with." –B.H.

Taking an outdoor fitness break

PHARMACIST FAVORITES

The experts share their top picks for your over-the-counter choices

#1 PHARMACIST RECOMMENDED BRAND 2017-2018 — U.S.News & WORLD REPORT — Pharmacy Times

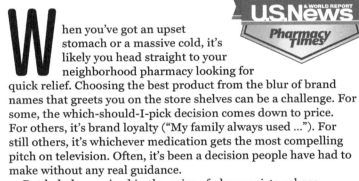

When you've got an upset stomach or a massive cold, it's likely you head straight to your neighborhood pharmacy looking for quick relief. Choosing the best product from the blur of brand names that greets you on the store shelves can be a challenge. For some, the which-should-I-pick decision comes down to price. For others, it's brand loyalty ("My family always used ..."). For still others, it's whichever medication gets the most compelling pitch on television. Often, it's been a decision people have had to make without any real guidance.

But help has arrived in the guise of pharmacists, whose mission includes educating patients on how and when to take a prescribed medicine, advising them on possible side effects, and warning about potential drug interactions. For over 20 years, the industry trade publication Pharmacy Times has surveyed thousands of pharmacists nationwide to pinpoint their top recommendations on a range of over-the-counter products. The results, published each year in its OTC Guide, are then shared widely among pharmacists throughout the nation to help them guide consumers' buying decisions. And now this inside intel is available to you, too.

U.S. News and Pharmacy Times have combed through the survey responses to show how different brands stack up in more than 150 over-the-counter product categories. The tables that follow here reveal the top brand-name picks for a number of popular product types, including decongestants, sunscreen, diaper rash and remedies for upset stomachs. Percentages have been rounded.

Though you should always read package labels for ingredients, directions and warnings, don't hesitate to consult with your pharmacist as you navigate the drugstore aisles. For the full results in all 150-plus categories, visit **usnews.com/tophealthproducts**.

ACID REDUCERS

Product	% Pharmacists recommending
Prilosec OTC	31%
Nexium 24HR	22%
Pepcid	21%
Zantac	20%
Prevacid 24HR	5%

ACNE PRODUCTS

Product	% Pharmacists recommending
Neutrogena	26%
Clearasil	21%
PanOxyl	17%
Oxy	10%
Differin Gel	10%
Clean & Clear Persa-Gel 10	7%

ADHESIVE BANDAGES

Product	% Pharmacists recommending
Band-Aid	73%
Nexcare	20%
Curad	7%

ANTIBIOTICS/ ANTISEPTICS (TOPICAL)

Product	% Pharmacists recommending
Neosporin	71%
Polysporin	13%
Bacitraycin Plus	6%
Hibiclens	6%
Betadine	2%

ANTIHISTAMINES (ORAL)

Product	% Pharmacists recommending
Claritin	39%
Zyrtec	38%
Allegra Allergy	11%
Benadryl	7%
Chlor-Trimeton	4%

ARTHRITIS TREATMENT (ORAL)

Product	% Pharmacists recommending
Aleve	30%
Tylenol Arthritis Pain	27%
Advil	26%
Motrin	16%

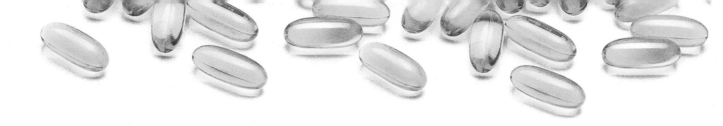

ARTIFICIAL TEARS

Product	% Pharmacists recommending
Refresh	32%
Systane	30%
Tears Naturale	13%
GenTeal	10%
Blink Tears	3%
Clear Eyes	3%
Hypo Tears	3%
Visine Tears	3%

ATHLETE'S FOOT/ ANTIFUNGAL PRODUCTS

Product	% Pharmacists recommending
Lotrimin	45%
Lamisil	40%
Tinactin	5%
Zeasorb	4%
Micatin	1%

BLOOD PRESSURE MONITORS

Product	% Pharmacists recommending
Omron	82%
LifeSource	11%
HoMedics	6%

BURN TREATMENTS

Product	% Pharmacists recommending
Neosporin	36%
Dermoplast	20%
Lanacane Spray	13%
Curad Silver Solution	8%
Bacitraycin Plus	7%
Polysporin	7%
A+D Ointment	5%

CHOLESTEROL MANAGEMENT

Product	% Pharmacists recommending
Nature Made Fish Oil	32%
Metamucil	19%
Nature's Bounty Fish Oil	17%
Slo-Niacin	14%
Nature Made CholestOff	6%
Schiff MegaRed	6%

COLD REMEDIES

Product	% Pharmacists recommending
Cepacol	32%
Zicam	21%
Cold-EEZE	16%
Halls Defense	16%
Sucrets	8%

CONTACT LENS SOLUTIONS

Product	% Pharmacists recommending
Opti-Free	43%
Renu multi-purpose solution	28%
Biotrue	12%
Clear Care Cleaning & Disinfecting Solution	8%
Boston Advance	5%

COUGH SUPPRESSANTS

Product	% Pharmacists recommending
Delsym	48%
Mucinex DM	26%
Robitussin	23%
NyQuil	1%
Tylenol Cold & Cough	1%

DANDRUFF SHAMPOO

Product	% Pharmacists recommending
Selsun Blue	32%
Head & Shoulders	26%
Nizoral	23%
T/Gel	18%
Denorex	2%

DECONGESTANTS (ORAL)

Product	% Pharmacists recommending
Sudafed (pseudoephedrine)	51%
Claritin-D	13%
Mucinex D	10%
Sudafed PE (phenylephrine)	8%
Zyrtec-D	7%

DIAPER RASH PRODUCTS

Product	% Pharmacists recommending
Desitin Diaper Rash	27%
A+D Diaper Rash Ointment	22%
Boudreaux's Butt Paste	17%
Calmoseptine	8%
Triple Paste	7%
Balmex	5%

DIGITAL THERMOMETERS

Product	% Pharmacists recommending
Braun ThermoScan	27%
Omron	26%
Vicks	20%
Nexcare	12%
Exergen Temporal Artery Thermometer	8%
3M Nexcare	7%

FIBER SUPPLEMENTS

Product	% Pharmacists recommending
Metamucil	44%
Benefiber	26%
Citrucel	14%
FiberCon	9%
Konsyl	3%

FLU TREATMENT PRODUCTS

Product	% Pharmacists recommending
Tylenol Cold & Flu Severe	22%
TheraFlu	21%
Coricidin HBP Cold & Flu	15%
DayQuil Cold & Flu	14%
NyQuil Cold & Flu	12%
Alka-Seltzer Plus Cold + Flu	9%

HAND SANITIZERS

Product	% Pharmacists recommending
Purell	87%
Germ-X	13%

INFANT FORMULAS

Product	% Pharmacists recommending
Enfamil	46%
Similac	32%
Gerber Good Start	3%
Earth's Best	3%
Isomil	2%

MIGRAINE RELIEVERS

Product	% Pharmacists recommending
Excedrin Migraine	72%
Advil Migraine	13%
Aleve	8%
Tylenol	3%

MULTIVITAMINS

Product	% Pharmacists recommending
Centrum	50%
One A Day	22%
Nature Made	13%
Nature's Bounty	9%
21st Century	3%

PRENATAL VITAMINS

Product	% Pharmacists recommending
One A Day Prenatal	40%
Nature Made Multi Prenatal	22%
Centrum Specialist Prenatal	13%
Nature's Bounty Prenatal	9%
Vitafusion PreNatal	6%
Similac Prenatal	5%

SLEEP AIDS

Product	% Pharmacists recommending
Unisom	38%
Tylenol PM	23%
Advil PM	9%
Vicks ZzzQuil	8%
Simply Sleep	7%
Sominex	5%

SUNSCREEN

Product	% Pharmacists recommending
Neutrogena	41%
Coppertone	20%
Banana Boat	10%
CeraVe	7%
Blue Lizard	6%
Bullfrog	6%

TOOTHPASTE

Product	% Pharmacists recommending
Crest	38%
Colgate	27%
Sensodyne	20%
Aquafresh	5%
Tom's of Maine	4%

UPSET STOMACH REMEDIES

Product	% Pharmacists recommending
Pepto-Bismol	56%
Emetrol	29%
Alka-Seltzer	9%
Kaopectate	6%

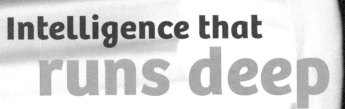

Intelligence that runs deep

usa.siemens.com/intelligence

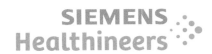

SIEMENS
Healthineers

BEST HOSPITALS

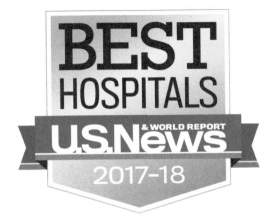

THE
HONOR ROLL

The 20 medical centers below excel in treating patients with complex diagnoses and those with relatively routine needs. Each hospital is nationally ranked in 10 or more of the 16 Best Hospitals specialties and is rated "high performing" in most or all of nine common procedures and conditions (full ratings at usnews.com/best-hospitals). Honor Roll standing is based on points. A hospital that was ranked No. 1 in all 16 specialties and rated high performing in all nine procedures and conditions would have received 448 points. The 20 highest scorers qualified for the Honor Roll.

BEST HOSPITALS
U.S.News & WORLD REPORT
HONOR ROLL 2017–18

1 Mayo Clinic
Rochester, Minn., 415 points

2 Cleveland Clinic
365 points

3 Johns Hopkins Hospital
Baltimore, 363 points

4 Massachusetts General Hospital
Boston, 358 points

5 UCSF Medical Center
San Francisco, 303 points

6 University of Michigan Hospitals and Health Centers
Ann Arbor, 294 points

7 Ronald Reagan UCLA Medical Center
Los Angeles, 292 points

8 New York-Presbyterian Hospital
New York, 267 points

9 Stanford Health Care-Stanford Hospital
Stanford, Calif., 251 points

10 Hospitals of the University of Pennsylvania-Penn Presbyterian
Philadelphia, 244 points

11 Cedars-Sinai Medical Center
Los Angeles, 239 points

12 Barnes-Jewish Hospital
St. Louis, 236 points

13 Northwestern Memorial Hospital
Chicago, 228 points

14 UPMC Presbyterian Shadyside
Pittsburgh, 218 points

15 University of Colorado Hospital
Aurora, 204 points

16 Thomas Jefferson University Hospitals
Philadelphia, 202 points

17 Duke University Hospital
Durham, N.C., 199 points

18 Mount Sinai Hospital
New York, 196 points

19 NYU Langone Medical Center
New York, 194 points

20 Mayo Clinic Phoenix
186 points

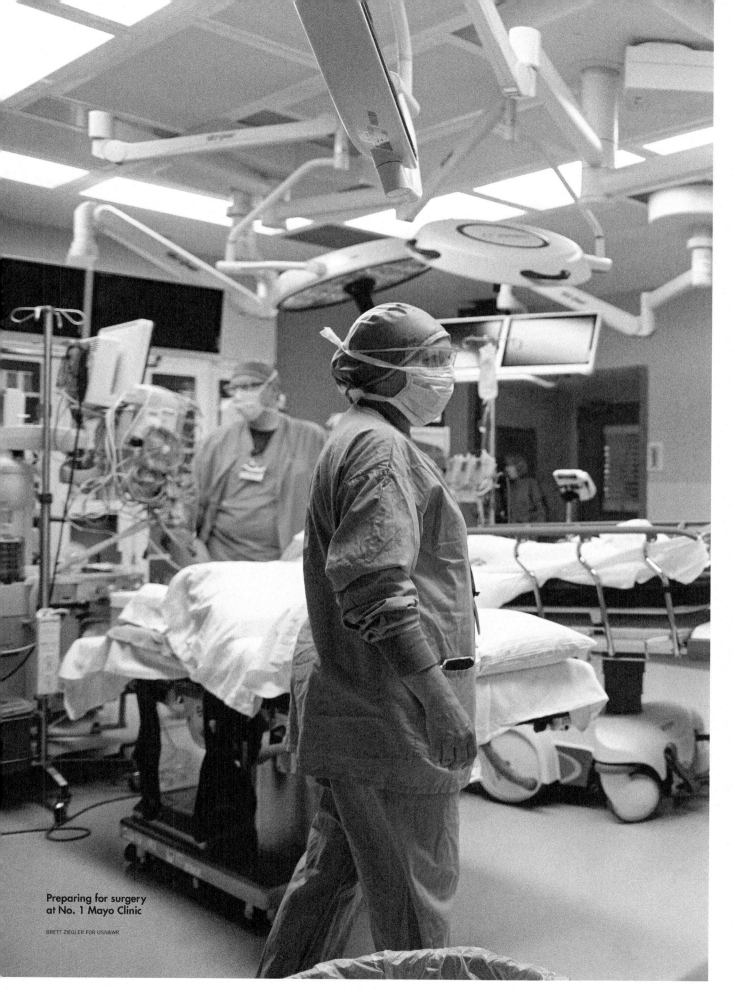

Preparing for surgery
at No. 1 Mayo Clinic

BRETT ZIEGLER FOR USN&WR

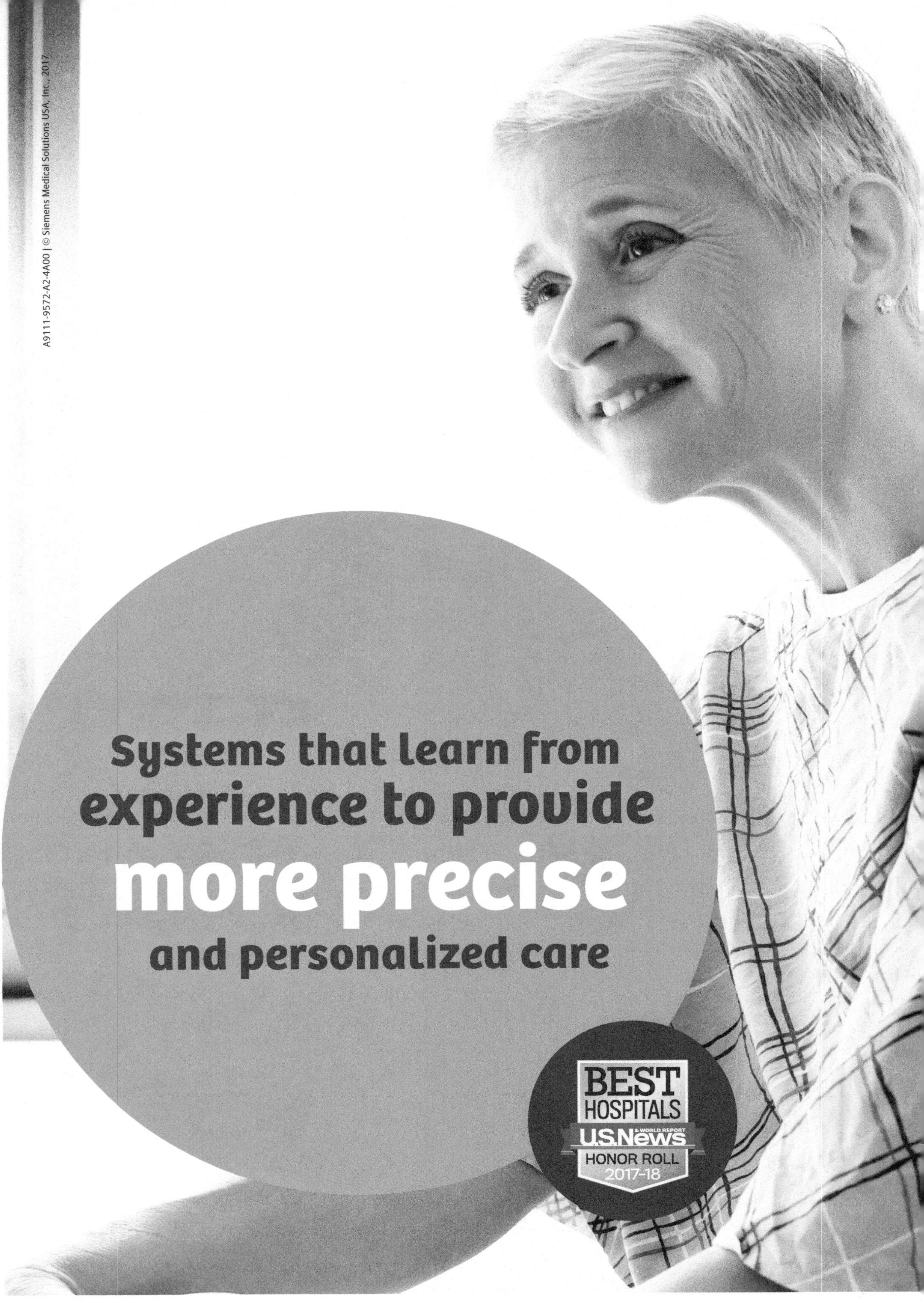

A9111-9572-A2-4A00 | © Siemens Medical Solutions USA, Inc., 2017
Systems that learn from
experience to provide
more precise
and personalized care
BEST
HOSPITALS
U.S.News & WORLD REPORT
HONOR ROLL
2017-18

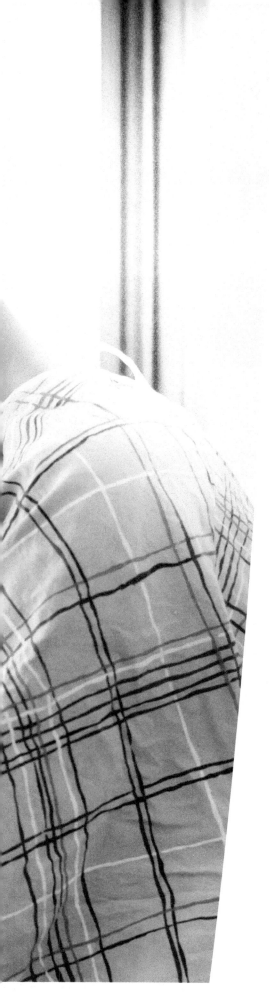

That's the power of Artificial Intelligence, and that's just the beginning.

We're developing more intelligent systems, with the goal of continuously learning from experience and improving their performance as they absorb more and more data. What does that mean for healthcare?

More personalized exams enabled by systems that adapt to every patient to satisfy individual patient needs and create a more efficient workflow for providers.

More accurate, reproducible, and predictable diagnostic results made possible by intelligent systems.

More precise disease classification that guides more personalized therapy and follow-up.

That means providers can spend more time with patients and less time analyzing and repeating exams.

Siemens Healthineers is proud to work with the top 20 Honor Roll hospitals, where we are pioneering more precise, more personalized, and more patient-centric healthcare.

Find out more at usa.siemens.com/intelligence

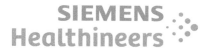

SIEMENS
Healthineers

Need help finding the right school for you?

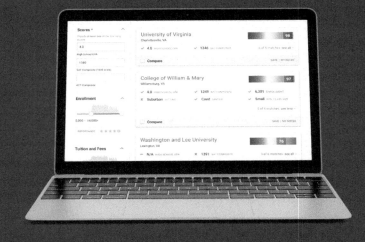
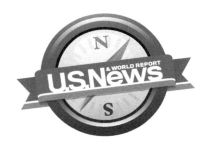

A GUIDE TO THE RANKINGS

How we identified 152 outstanding hospitals in 16 specialties

By Avery Comarow and Ben Harder

The mission of the Best Hospitals annual rankings, now in their 28th year, remains the same as always: to help guide patients who need an especially high level of care to the right place. These are patients whose surgery or condition is complex or difficult. Or whose advanced age, physical infirmity or existing medical condition puts them at heightened risk.

Such patients account for a small fraction of hospital patients, but they add up to millions of individuals, and most hospitals simply are not good enough for them. A hospital ranked by U.S. News in cardiology and heart surgery, say, is likely to have the experience and expertise to operate safely on a patient 85 or 90 years old with a leaky heart valve. The typical community hospital cannot supply the special techniques and precautions needed, and should instead send such a patient to a hospital that can. Many community hospitals do that. But not all.

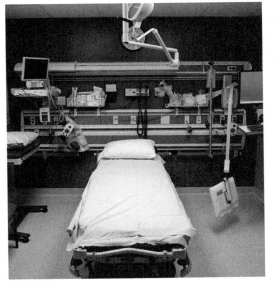

The following pages offer hospital rankings in 16 specialties, from cancer to urology. Of 4,658 hospitals evaluated this year, only 152 performed well enough to be ranked in any specialty. Based on input from experts and the professional literature, we implemented several significant methodology changes, described below, to improve the rankings' usefulness to consumers.

In 12 of 16 specialties, hard data, much of it from the federal government, mostly determined whether a hospital was ranked. Some kinds of data, such as death rates, are intimately related to quality. Numbers of patients and the balance of nurses to patients are examples of data that are also important, although the quality connection may seem less evident. We also factored in, as a form of peer review, results from annual surveys of physicians who were asked to name hospitals they consider tops in their specialty for difficult cases.

Hospitals in the other four specialties (ophthalmology, psychiatry, rehabilitation and rheumatology) were ranked solely on the basis of the annual physician surveys. That's because so few patients die in these specialties that mortality data, which carry heavy weight in the 12 other specialties, mean little.

To be considered for ranking in the 12 data-driven specialties, a hospital had to meet any of four criteria: It had to be a teaching hospital, or be affiliated with a medical school, or have at least 200 beds, or have at least 100 beds and offer at least four out of eight advanced medical technologies. This year 2,255 hospitals met that test.

The hospitals next had to meet a volume requirement in each specialty – a minimum number of Medicare inpatients from 2013 to 2015 who received certain procedures and treatment for specific conditions. The minimum number of patients for cardiology and heart surgery, for example, was 1,382, of which 500 had to be surgical. A hospital that fell short was still eligible if it was nominated in the specialty by at least 1 percent of the physicians responding to the 2015, 2016 and 2017 reputational surveys.

At the end of the process, 1,896 hospitals were candidates for ranking in at least one specialty. Each received a U.S. News score of 0 to 100 based on four elements: patient survival; patient safety; care-related factors such as nursing, volume, technology, and special accreditations and recognitions; and reputation. The 50 top performers in each of the 12 specialties were ranked. Scores and data for the rest, as well as more detail on the methodology, are available at usnews.com/best-hospitals. The four elements and their weights in brief:

Survival score (37.5 percent). Success at keeping patients alive was judged by comparing the number of Medicare inpatients with certain conditions who died within 30 days of admission in 2013, 2014 and 2015 with the number expected given the severity of their illness, the complexity of their care and risk-elevating factors such as advanced age, obesity and high blood pressure. New this year: Using dual eligibility for Medicare and Medicaid as a proxy, we adjusted scores to account for poverty, which is known to affect patient outcomes. We also tapped additional data to more completely exclude patients transferred into the hospital, so as not to penalize institutions taking on the sickest people. A score of 10 indicates the best chance of survival (and 1 the worst) relative to other hospitals. Industry-standard software (3M Health Information Systems' Medicare Severity Grouper) was used to adjust each patient's risk in calculating survival odds.

Patient safety score (5 percent). Every hospital harms patients unnecessarily. This score reflects efforts to prevent the four kinds of harm listed in the box below. The measure was changed this year to omit two types of harm too rare to be meaningful for most hospitals.

Other care-related indicators (30 percent). Trauma center status, arthritis center certification, and availability of intensive care specialists are examples.

Reputation (27.5 percent). This part of a hospital's total score was drawn from the last three years of annual physician surveys. Specialists were asked to name up to five hospitals, setting aside location and cost, that they consider best in their area of expertise for patients with the most difficult medical problems. In the lat-

est three-year period, responses were tallied from some 33,000 physicians.

The figures shown under "% of specialists recommending hospital" in the ranking tables are the average percentages of specialists in 2015, 2016 and 2017 who recommended a hospital. Adjustments are made to keep a relatively small number of hospitals with high reputational scores from monopolizing the final rankings. Hospitals with low reputational scores but strong clinical numbers can outrank centers with higher reputations.

In the four reputation-based specialties, a hospital had to be cited by at least 5 percent of responding physicians in the latest three years of U.S. News surveys to be ranked. That created lists of 12 hospitals in psychiatry, 13 in ophthalmology, and 14 in rehabilitation and rheumatology.

Be sure to monitor usnews.com over the year for new Best Hospitals content. You'll want to add your own fact-gathering to ours and consult with your doctor or other health professional. No hospital, no matter how excellent, is best for every patient. ●

A GLOSSARY OF TERMS

FACT accreditation level: hospital meets Foundation for the Accreditation of Cellular Therapy standards as of March 1, 2017, for harvesting and transplanting stem cells from a patient's own bone marrow and tissue (level 1) and from a donor (level 2) to treat cancer.

Intensivists: at least one critical-care specialist manages patients in intensive care units.

NAEC epilepsy center: designated by the National Association of Epilepsy Centers as of March 1, 2017, as a regional or national referral facility (level 4) for staffing, technology and training in epilepsy care.

NCI cancer center: designated by the National Cancer Institute as of March 1, 2017, as a clinical or comprehensive cancer hospital.

NIA Alzheimer's center: designated by the National Institute

on Aging as of March 1, 2017, as an Alzheimer's Disease Center, indicating high quality of research and clinical care.

Number of patients: estimated number of Medicare inpatients in 2013, 2014 and 2015 who received certain high-level care as defined by U.S. News. Based on an adjustment to the number of such patients with traditional Medicare insurance. In geriatrics, only patients age 75 and older are included.

A Nurse Magnet hospital: certified by the American Nurses Credentialing Center as of March 17, 2017, for nursing excellence.

Nurse staffing score: relative balance of nonsupervisory registered nurses (inpatient and outpatient) to average daily number of all patients. Inpatient staffing receives greater weight. Agency and temporary nurses are not counted.

Patient safety score: indicates ability to protect patients from four types of preventable harm: death from preventable postsurgical complications, major postsurgical bleeding and bruising, postsurgical respiratory failure, and injury during surgery.

Patient services score: number of services offered out of the number considered important to quality (such as genetic testing in cancer and an Alzheimer's center in geriatrics).

% of specialists recommending hospital: percentage of physicians responding to U.S. News surveys in 2015, 2016 and 2017 who named the hospital as among the best in their specialty for especially challenging cases and procedures, setting aside location and cost.

Rank: based on U.S. News score except in ophthalmology, psychiatry, rehabilitation and rheumatology, where specialist recommendations determine rank.

Survival score: reflects patient deaths in the specialty within 30 days of admission.

Technology score: reflects availability of technologies considered important to a high quality of care, such as PET/CT scanner in pulmonology and diagnostic radioisotope services in urology.

Transparency score: indicates whether hospital publicly reports heart outcomes through the American College of Cardiology and the Society of Thoracic Surgeons.

Trauma center: indicates Level 1 or 2 trauma center certification. Such a center can care properly for the most severe injuries.

U.S. News score: summary of quality of hospital inpatient care. In most specialties, survival is worth 37.5 percent, operational quality data such as nurse staffing and patient volume 30 percent, specialists' recommendations 27.5 percent, and patient safety 5 percent.

#1 HOSPITAL IN CALIFORNIA

ONE OF THE NATION'S TOP 5 HOSPITALS

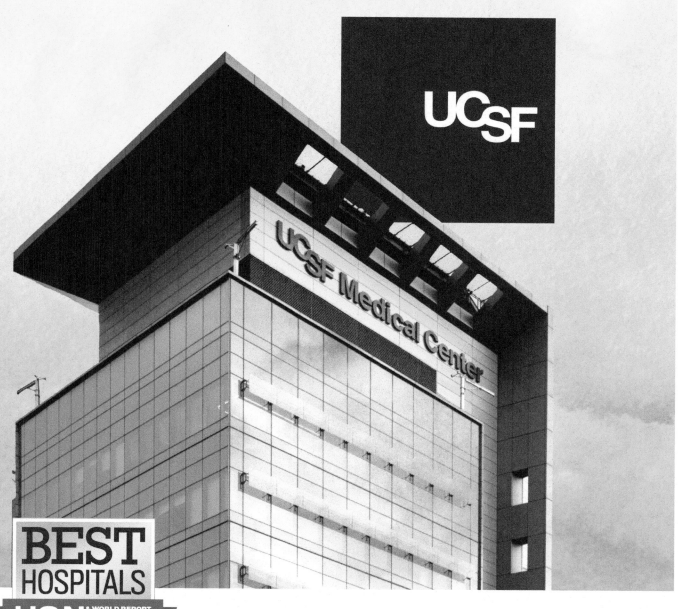

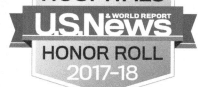

UCSF Health

CANCER

Rank	Hospital	U.S. News score	Survival score (10=best)	Patient safety score (9=best)	Number of patients	Nurse staffing score (higher is better)	A Nurse Magnet hospital	NCI cancer center	FACT accreditation level (2=best)	Patient services score (8=best)	% of specialists recommending hospital
1	University of Texas MD Anderson Cancer Center, Houston	100.0	10	5	7,488	1.9	Yes	Yes	2	8	56.9%
2	Memorial Sloan Kettering Cancer Center, New York	97.4	9	6	5,603	2.1	Yes	Yes	2	8	53.6%
3	Mayo Clinic, Rochester, Minn.	91.8	10	5	3,688	2.7	Yes	Yes	2	8	24.3%
4	Dana-Farber/Brigham and Women's Cancer Center, Boston	84.4	9	5	2,983	2.4	Yes	Yes	2	8	30.8%
5	Seattle Cancer Care Alliance/U. of Washington Medical Center	76.5	10	5	1,382	2.1	Yes	Yes	2	8	8.9%
6	Johns Hopkins Hospital, Baltimore	75.9	8	5	1,793	2.2	Yes	Yes	2	8	18.8%
7	Cleveland Clinic	75.0	9	6	2,619	2.1	Yes	Yes	2	8	9.1%
7	Hosps. of the Univ. of Pennsylvania-Penn Presby., Philadelphia	75.0	9	5	2,792	2.3	Yes	Yes	2	8	7.4%
9	Moffitt Cancer Center and Research Institute, Tampa	74.9	10	4	3,156	1.2	Yes	Yes	2	8	5.4%
10	UCSF Medical Center, San Francisco	73.3	9	6	1,944	2.4	Yes	Yes	2	8	6.9%
11	Stanford Health Care-Stanford Hospital, Stanford, Calif.	73.2	9	6	1,986	2.5	Yes	Yes	2	8	6.7%
12	Massachusetts General Hospital, Boston	71.4	8	5	2,617	2.4	Yes	Yes	2	8	10.4%
12	Ronald Reagan UCLA Medical Center, Los Angeles	71.4	9	5	2,005	3.0	Yes	Yes	2	8	6.1%
12	Univ. of Michigan Hospitals and Health Centers, Ann Arbor	71.4	9	6	2,060	2.8	Yes	Yes	2	8	3.7%
15	USC Norris Cancer Hosp.-Keck Medical Cen. of USC, Los Angeles	70.5	10	6	1,283	3.0	No	Yes	2	8	1.5%
16	Northwestern Memorial Hospital, Chicago	69.9	10	6	1,630	1.6	Yes	Yes	2	8	2.0%
17	Mayo Clinic Phoenix	69.6	10	6	1,647	2.9	No	Yes	2	8	2.6%
18	Mayo Clinic Jacksonville, Fla.	69.5	9	6	968	2.1	Yes	Yes	2	8	2.8%
19	Barnes-Jewish Hospital, St. Louis, Mo.	69.3	9	5	3,362	2.4	Yes	Yes	2	8	3.9%
20	Thomas Jefferson University Hospitals, Philadelphia	69.1	9	6	2,131	2.2	Yes	Yes	2	8	2.0%
21	City of Hope, Duarte, Calif.	68.8	10	5	1,758	2.2	No	Yes	2	8	5.1%
22	New York-Presbyterian Hospital	68.1	9	4	4,335	2.8	No	Yes	2	8	3.1%
23	Ohio State University James Cancer Hospital, Columbus	67.4	9	5	3,045	2.0	Yes	Yes	2	8	4.0%
24	University of North Carolina Hospitals, Chapel Hill	67.3	9	5	1,259	2.0	Yes	Yes	2	8	2.5%
25	University of Kansas Hospital, Kansas City	67.1	10	5	1,506	2.0	Yes	Yes	2	8	0.7%
26	OHSU Hospital, Portland, Ore.	66.1	9	5	1,659	2.0	Yes	Yes	2	8	1.2%
27	Wake Forest Baptist Medical Center, Winston-Salem, N.C.	65.8	9	5	2,463	1.6	Yes	Yes	2	8	1.8%
28	Fox Chase Cancer Center, Philadelphia	65.7	9	5	1,542	1.8	Yes	Yes	2	8	3.0%
29	University of Colorado Hospital, Aurora	65.6	9	5	1,611	2.3	Yes	Yes	2	8	1.1%
30	University of Virginia Medical Center, Charlottesville	65.5	10	5	984	2.0	Yes	Yes	2	8	0.8%
31	University of Chicago Medical Center	65.3	9	6	1,745	2.4	No	Yes	2	8	3.2%
32	University of California, Davis Medical Center, Sacramento	64.6	9	5	1,381	2.7	Yes	Yes	2	8	0.8%
33	Roswell Park Cancer Institute, Buffalo	64.4	9	5	1,310	2.1	No	Yes	2	8	2.8%
34	University Hospitals Seidman Cancer Center, Cleveland	64.1	9	5	1,467	2.4	Yes	Yes	2	8	1.2%
35	UPMC Presbyterian Shadyside, Pittsburgh	63.9	8	5	3,810	1.9	Yes	Yes	2	8	2.5%
36	University of Wisconsin Hospitals, Madison	63.7	9	5	1,325	2.5	Yes	Yes	2	8	0.6%
37	University of Minnesota Medical Center, Fairview	63.4	10	4	1,529	1.9	No	Yes	2	8	0.4%
38	Duke University Hospital, Durham, N.C.	63.1	7	5	1,915	2.1	Yes	Yes	2	8	5.6%
38	Huntsman Cancer Institute at the U. of Utah, Salt Lake City	63.1	10	5	1,098	2.2	No	Yes	2	8	0.6%
40	UC San Diego Health-Moores Cancer Center	62.9	8	5	1,270	2.1	Yes	Yes	2	8	1.4%
40	University of Iowa Hospitals and Clinics, Iowa City	62.9	9	5	1,234	1.8	Yes	Yes	2	8	1.1%
42	MUSC Health-University Medical Center, Charleston, S.C.	62.6	9	5	1,013	2.0	Yes	Yes	2	8	0.2%
43	Rush University Medical Center, Chicago	62.5	9	5	1,473	2.3	Yes	No	2	8	1.8%
44	Mount Sinai Hospital, New York	62.4	8	7	1,919	2.0	Yes	Yes	2	8	0.9%
44	NYU Langone Medical Center, New York	62.4	9	5	1,592	2.6	Yes	Yes	1	8	1.2%
44	Vanderbilt University Medical Center, Nashville	62.4	8	5	1,728	1.9	Yes	Yes	2	8	2.5%
47	Cedars-Sinai Medical Center, Los Angeles	62.0	8	5	2,627	2.6	Yes	No	2	8	1.9%
48	Banner University Medical Center Tucson, Ariz.	61.4	9	4	1,000	1.8	Yes	Yes	2	7	0.1%
48	University of Maryland Medical Center, Baltimore	61.4	10	2	1,127	2.1	Yes	Yes	2	7	0.7%
50	University of Kentucky Albert B. Chandler Hospital, Lexington	60.9	9	6	1,003	1.9	Yes	Yes	2	8	0.9%

Terms are explained on Page 102.

▶ **More** @ usnews.com/besthospitals

WE DON'T BELIEVE

THE FUTURE CAN WAIT

FOR THE FUTURE

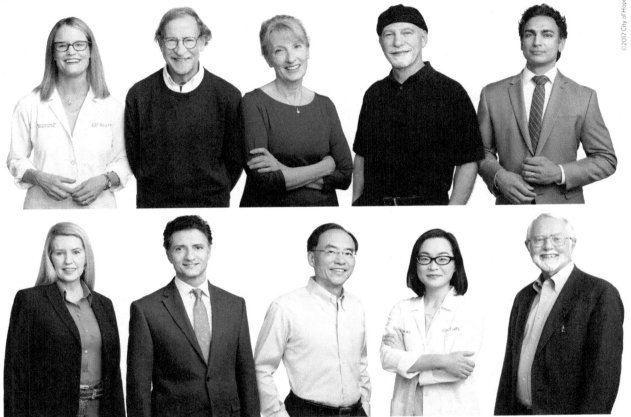

We are City of Hope doctors, advancing science that saves lives. We have performed more than 13,000 bone marrow and stem cell transplants to treat cancer, with a 12-year record of unparalleled survival rates. Our research has led to developing synthetic insulin and four of the most widely used cancer-fighting drugs. We are maximizing the potential of immunology and making precision medicine a reality. Bottom line, it's not enough to promise future cures. We have to find them sooner. This is the passion that drives us every day. Find out more at **CityofHope.org**

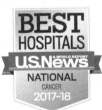

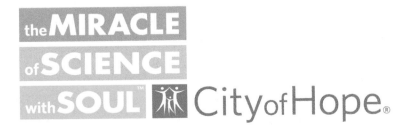

CARDIOLOGY & HEART SURGERY

BRETT ZIEGLER FOR USN&WR

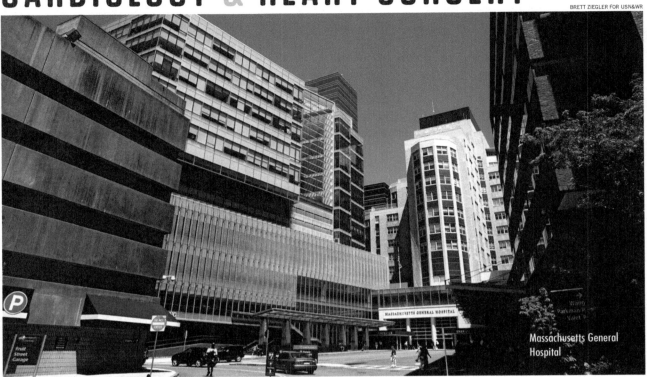

Massachusetts General Hospital

Rank	Hospital	U.S. News score	Survival score (10=best)	Patient safety score (9=best)	Transparency score (3=best)	Number of patients	Nurse staffing score (higher is better)	A Nurse Magnet hospital	Technology score (6=best)	Patient services score (7=best)	Intensivists	% of specialists recommending hospital
1	Cleveland Clinic	100.0	10	6	3	14,254	2.1	Yes	6	7	Yes	47.7%
2	Mayo Clinic, Rochester, Minn.	99.5	10	5	3	11,730	2.7	Yes	6	7	Yes	43.0%
3	New York-Presbyterian Hospital	85.2	10	4	3	17,411	2.8	No	6	7	Yes	15.9%
4	Cedars-Sinai Medical Center, Los Angeles	81.8	10	5	3	11,154	2.6	Yes	6	7	Yes	8.2%
5	Massachusetts General Hospital, Boston	79.0	9	5	3	8,201	2.4	Yes	6	7	Yes	17.6%
6	Johns Hopkins Hospital, Baltimore	77.3	10	5	3	4,270	2.2	Yes	6	7	Yes	15.4%
7	Northwestern Memorial Hospital, Chicago	76.7	10	6	3	4,493	1.6	Yes	6	7	Yes	4.9%
8	Hosps. of the Univ. of Pennsylvania-Penn Presby., Philadelphia	75.4	10	5	2	10,867	2.3	Yes	6	7	Yes	8.4%
9	Mount Sinai Hospital, New York	75.1	10	7	3	8,927	2.0	Yes	6	7	Yes	4.6%
10	Univ. of Michigan Hospitals and Health Centers, Ann Arbor	74.5	10	6	3	5,833	2.8	Yes	6	7	Yes	4.3%
11	Duke University Hospital, Durham, N.C.	74.4	9	5	3	5,865	2.1	Yes	6	7	Yes	13.2%
12	Brigham and Women's Hospital, Boston	73.5	10	5	3	6,247	2.4	No	6	7	Yes	17.9%
13	Barnes-Jewish Hospital, St. Louis, Mo.	72.6	10	5	3	7,865	2.4	Yes	6	7	Yes	3.5%
14	Ronald Reagan UCLA Medical Center, Los Angeles	72.3	10	5	3	5,145	3.0	Yes	6	7	Yes	3.7%
15	Stanford Health Care-Stanford Hospital, Stanford, Calif.	70.0	9	6	3	4,230	2.5	Yes	6	7	Yes	6.3%
16	Houston Methodist Hospital	67.7	10	6	2	7,862	2.0	Yes	6	7	Yes	3.5%
16	The Heart Hospital Baylor Plano, Texas	67.7	10	6	3	4,495	2.4	Yes	5	7	Yes	2.5%
18	Loyola University Medical Center, Maywood, Ill.	67.4	10	6	3	3,263	2.4	Yes	6	7	Yes	1.2%
19	NYU Langone Medical Center, New York	67.3	9	5	3	6,968	2.6	Yes	5	7	Yes	2.7%
20	UPMC Presbyterian Shadyside, Pittsburgh	67.0	10	5	3	10,416	1.9	Yes	6	7	Yes	1.6%
21	Scripps La Jolla Hospitals, La Jolla, Calif.	66.7	9	6	3	4,984	3.1	Yes	5	7	Yes	2.1%
22	Ohio State University Wexner Medical Center, Columbus	66.0	10	5	3	6,910	2.0	Yes	6	7	Yes	1.2%
23	UCSF Medical Center, San Francisco	65.7	10	6	3	2,529	2.4	Yes	5	6	Yes	2.9%
24	Sentara Norfolk Gen. Hosp.-Sentara Heart Hosp., Norfolk, Va.	65.4	10	5	3	5,780	1.6	Yes	6	7	Yes	0.4%

(CONTINUED ON PAGE 112)

Terms are explained on Page 102.

▶ **More @ usnews.com/besthospitals**

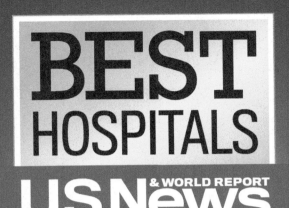
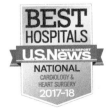
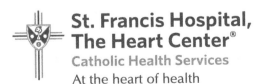
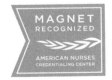

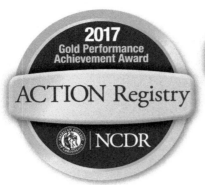
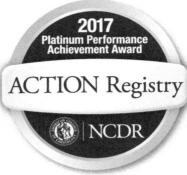
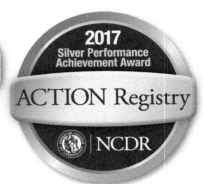

Congratulations
to recipients of the

ACTION Registry®
2017 Performance Achievement Award
Rewarding Excellence. Driving Success. Saving Lives.

The ACTION Registry® Performance Achievement Award recognizes a hospital's success in implementing a higher standard of care for heart attack patients by meeting aggressive performance measures as outlined by the American College of Cardiology (ACC) and the American Heart Association (AHA) clinical guidelines and recommendations.

The ACTION Registry helps hospitals:
- Improve patient outcomes by using clinically and scientifically relevant data to drive decision making
- Apply the ACC/AHA clinical guidelines
- Achieve quality improvement goals through the measurement of care provided
- Advance cardiovascular patient care through clinical peer-reviewed research
- Improve the quality of care for heart attack patients through hospital-wide evaluation of performance standards

The ACTION Registry is the leading source for quality data you can trust, offering clinically and scientifically relevant data driving positive health outcomes for patients.

**To view hospitals participating in the ACTION Registry,
visit ACC's Find Your Heart a Home website at *Cardiosmart.org/ACTION*.**

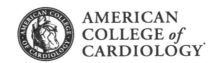

AMERICAN
COLLEGE *of*
CARDIOLOGY®

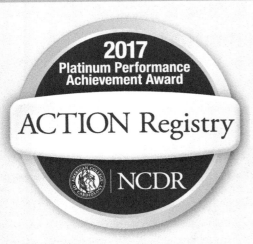

2017
Platinum Performance
Achievement Award

ACTION Registry

NCDR

Flowers Hospital – AL

Providence Alaska
Medical Center – AK

San Joaquin Community
Hospital – CA

John Muir Medical
Center – Concord
Campus – CA

Los Robles Hospital
& Medical Center – CA

Bakersfield
Memorial Hospital – CA

Salinas Valley Memorial
Healthcare System – CA

California Pacific
Medical Center– CA

Doctors Medical Center
of Modesto – CA

Memorial Medical Center
Modesto – CA

Palomar Medical
Center – CA

John Muir Medical
Center – Walnut Creek
Campus – CA

North Colorado
Medical Center – CO

Penrose Hospital – CO

Mercy Regional
Medical Center – CO

Littleton Adventist
Hospital – CO

Memorial Health
System – CO

St. Francis
Medical Center – CO

Medical Center
of the Rockies – CO

St. Anthony Hospital – CO

Porter Adventist
Hospital – CO

Parker Adventist
Hospital – CO

Sky Ridge
Medical Center – CO

St. Vincent's Medical
Center – CT

Saint Francis Hospital
& Medical Center – CT

West Florida Hospital – FL

Emory University Hospital
Midtown – GA

Emory University
Hospital – GA

Gwinnett Hospital
System – GA

West Georgia Health – GA

Emory Johns Creek
Hospital – GA

Redmond Regional
Medical Center – GA

St. Joseph's Hospital – GA

Emory Saint Josephs
Hospital of Atlanta – GA

Piedmont Fayette
Hospital – GA

Saint Alphonsus Regl
Medical Center – ID

Advocate Illinois Masonic
Medical Center – IL

Memorial Hospital
Carbondale – IL

Advocate Sherman
Hospital – IL

Prairie Heart Institute at
St. John's Hospital – IL

OSF Saint Francis
Medical Center – IL

Advocate Good Shepherd
Hospital – IL

Carle Foundation
Hospital – IL

OSF Saint Anthony
Medical Center – IL

Adventist La Grange
Memorial Hospital – IL

Mount Sinai Hospital – IL

Methodist Medical Center
of Illinois – IL

Advocate BroMenn
Medical Center – IL

Presence Resurrection
Medical Center – IL

Advocate Lutheran
General Hospital – IL

Adventist Hinsdale
Hospital – IL

Indiana University Health
Saxony Hospital – IN

Indiana University
Health Ball Memorial
Hospital – IN

Riverview Health – IN

Goshen Hospital – IN

Columbus Regional
Hospital – IN

Community Hospital – IN

Indiana University Health
Methodist Hospital – IN

Mercy Medical Center –
Des Moines – IA

UnityPoint Health, St
Luke's Sioux City – IA

Mercy Iowa City – IA

Saint Lukes Hospital – IA

Olathe
Medical Center – KS

Menorah
Medical Center – KS

St. Francis
Health Center – KS

The University of
Kansas Hospital – KS

Stormont–Vail
HealthCare – KS

Baptist Health
Paducah – KY

St. Francis
Medical Center – LA

University of Maryland
Saint Joseph
Medical Center – MD

Adventist HealthCare
Shady Grove
Medical Center – MD

UM Baltimore Washington
Medical Center – MD

Saint Agnes Hospital – MD

Holy Cross Hospital of
Silver Spring, Inc. – MD

MetroWest
Medical Center – MA

Metro Health Hospital – MI

St. Luke's Hospital – MN

Essentia Health –
Innovis Health – MN

CentraCare Heart &
Vascular Center – MN

Essentia Health – St. Mary's
Medical Center – MN

Mayo Clinic Health System
Mankato – MN

Forrest
General Hospital – MS

Southwest MS Regional
Medical Center – MS

North Mississippi
Medical Center – MS

Ocean Springs Hospital – MS

University of Mississippi
Medical Center – MS

Magnolia Regional Health
Center – MS

St. Dominic – Jackson
Memorial Hospital – MS

Saint Francis Medical
Center – MO

Barnes Jewish
Hospital/Washington
University – MO

Southeast Missouri
Hospital – MO

Truman Medical
Centers – MO

MERCY Hospital
Springfield – MO

SSM Health St. Mary's
Hospital – Madison – MO

Mercy Hospital
Joplin – MO

North Kansas City
Hospital – MO

Research Medical
Center – MO

Centerpoint Medical
Center – MO

Bozeman Health
Deaconess Hospital – MT

Kalispell Regional
Medical Center Inc. – MT

Providence St. Patrick
Hospital – MT

Nebraska Methodist
Hospital – NE

Dignity Health St. Rose
Dominican Siena – NV

Riverview
Medical Center – NJ

Jersey Shore University
Medical Center – NJ

Bayshore
Community Hospital – NJ

Inspira Medical Center –
Woodbury – NJ

Ocean Medical Center – NJ

Presbyterian Healthcare
Services – NM

Mercy Hospital
of Buffalo – NY

The Mount Sinai
Medical Center – NY

Duke University
Hospital – NC

New Hanover Regional
Medical Center – NC

Mission Hospital, Inc. – NC

Frye Regional
Medical Center – NC

Carolinas Medical
Center – Pineville – NC

Novant Health Matthews
Medical Center – NC

Carolinas Medical
Center – NC

CaroMont Regional
Medical Center – NC

Novant Health
Presbyterian Medical
Center – NC

Carolinas HealthCare
System – NorthEast – NC

CarolinaEast
Medical Center – NC

Moses Cone HEALTH – NC

Altru Health System – ND

Aultman Hospital – OH

University Hospitals St.
John Medical Center – OH

Licking Memorial
Hospital – OH

Platinum *continues on next page*

Platinum *continued from previous page*

EMH Regional Medical Center – OH

The Ohio State University Medical Center – OH

The Christ Hospital Health Network – OH

Southwest General Health Center – OH

The MetroHealth System – OH

Akron General Health System – OH

Jane Phillips Memorial Medical Center – OK

Oregon Health & Science University – OR

Jefferson Regional Medical Center – PA

Pinnacle Health System: West Shore Hospital – PA

Doylestown Hospital – PA

Butler Memorial Hospital – PA

Meadville Medical Center – PA

Pinnacle Health System: Harrisburg Hospital – PA

Sharon Regional Health System – PA

Trident Medical Center – SC

AnMed Health – SC

Spartanburg Regional Healthcare System – SC

Rapid City Regional Hospital – SD

Avera Heart Hospital of South Dakota – SD

Sanford USD Medical Center – SD

Holston Valley Medical Center – TN

Bristol Regional Medical Center – TN

Jackson Madison County General Hospital – TN

Baptist Memorial Hospital Memphis – TN

Chattanooga – Hamilton County Hospital Authority – TN

University of Tennessee Medical Center (UHS) – TN

Baptist Memorial Hospital – Golden Triangle – TN

Baptist Memorial Hospital – Desoto – TN

Baylor Jack and Jane Hamilton Heart and Vascular Hospital – TX

Cypress Fairbanks Medical Center – TX

Baylor Scott & White Medical Center – Garland – TX

Houston Northwest Medical Center – TX

Christus Spohn Hospital Corpus Christi – Shoreline – TX

Shannon Medical Center – TX

Methodist Charlton Medical Center – TX

Ben Taub General Hospital – TX

Baylor Scott & White Medical Center – Round Rock – TX

Hendrick Medical Center – TX

Baylor Scott & White Medical Center Irving – TX

Sentara Princess Anne Hospital – VA

Sentara Careplex Hospital – VA

Centra Lynchburg General Hospital – VA

Sentara Martha Jefferson Hospital – VA

Sentara Williamsburg Regional Medical Center – VA

Winchester Medical Center Inc. – VA

Inova Alexandria Hospital – VA

Sentara Leigh Hospital – VA

Inova Fairfax Hospital/ Inova Heart & Vascular Institute – VA

Danville Regional Medical Center – VA

Sentara Norfolk General Hospital – VA

Inova Loudoun Hospital – VA

University of Virginia Medical Center – VA

Sentara Virginia Beach General Hospital – VA

Sentara Northern Virginia Medical Center – VA

Providence Sacred Heart Medical Center – WA

Saint Mary's Medical Center – WV

Wheeling Hospital – WV

University of Wisconsin Hospital & Clinics – WI

Aurora BayCare Medical Center – WI

Aurora Grafton – WI

Holy Family Memorial – WI

Aurora St. Lukes Medical Center – WI

Aspirus Wausau Hospital – WI

Cheyenne Regional Medical Center – WY

Wyoming Medical Center – WY

Hospital totalCor – Brazil

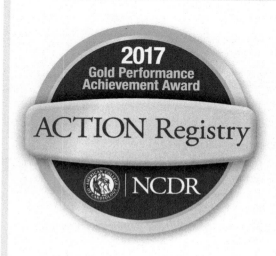

2017 Gold Performance Achievement Award — ACTION Registry — NCDR

NorthBay Medical Center – CA

French Hospital Medical Center – CA

Rose Medical Center – CO

University of CT Health Center/John Dempsey Hospital – CT

Christiana Care Health System – DE

Northside Hospital – Cherokee – GA

Northside Hospital – Forsyth – GA

Northside Hospital – Atlanta – GA

Memorial Medical Center – IL

Rush University Medical Center – IL

Edward Hospital – IL

Elmhurst Memorial Healthcare – IL

Franciscan Health Indianapolis – IN

Terrebonne General Medical Center – LA

Frederick Memorial Hospital – MD

Holland Hospital – MI

Lima Memorial Health System – OH

Fairview Hospital – OH

Mercy Hospital Anderson – OH

Legacy Good Samaritan – OR

The Williamsport Hospital – PA

Mercy Fitzgerald Hospital – PA

Greenville Memorial Hospital – SC

Fort Sanders Regional Medical Center – TN

Methodist Hospital – TX

Seton Medical Center Austin – TX

Seton Medical Center Williamson – TX

CHI St. Joseph Health Regional Hospital – TX

CHRISTUS Hospital – St Elizabeth – TX

Harrison Medical Center – WA

Congratulations to recipients of the *ACTION* Registry°

2017 Performance Achievement Award

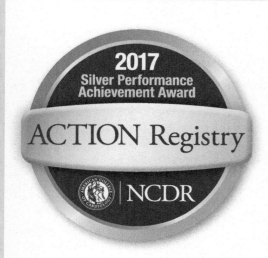

2017 Silver Performance Achievement Award
ACTION Registry
NCDR

Mayo Clinic
Arizona – AZ

St. Bernards
Medical Center – AR

El Camino Hospital – CA

Tri – City
Medical Center – CA

St. Josephs Medical
Center of Stockton – CA

Presbyterian/St.Luke's
Medical Center – CO

University of Colorado
Hospital Authority – CO

Medical Center
of Aurora – CO

Parkview
Medical Center – CO

Stamford Hospital
Health Sciences
Library – CT

Mount Sinai
Medical Center – FL

Florida Hospital – FL

Baptist Hospital,
Inc. – FL

Athens Regional
Medical Center – GA

Dekalb
Medical Center – GA

Northeast Georgia
Medical Center – GA

Riverside
Medical Center – IL

Northwestern
Medicine Central
DuPage Hospital – IL

Loyola University
Medical Center – IL

Trinity Medical Center –
Rock Island – IL

OSF Saint Joseph
Medical Center – IL

Northwestern Medicine
Delnor Hospital – IL

Rush – Copley
Medical Center – IL

The Heart Hospital
at Deaconess
Gateway, LLC – IN

Saint Marys
Health, Inc – IN

Deaconess Hospital – IN

Mercy
Medical Center – IA

Genesis Medical Center,
Davenport – IA

Saint Elizabeth
Healthcare
Edgewood – KY

Washington Adventist
Hospital – MD

Johns Hopkins Bayview
Medical Center – MD

Edward W
Sparrow Hospital
Association – MI

Mayo Clinic
Hospital – Saint
Marys Campus – MN

North Memorial
Medical Center – MN

Saint Luke's East
Hospital – MO

Saint Luke's
North Hospital –
Barry Road – MO

Saint Luke's Hospital
of Kansas City – MO

Capital Region Medical
Center – MO

Community Medical
Center – MT

Billings Clinic (formerly
Deaconess) – MT

Faith Regional Health
Services – NE

Great Plains Health – NE

Kearney Regional
Medical Center – NE

Northern Nevada
Medical Center – NV

Saint Mary's Regional
Medical Center – NV

Newark Beth Israel
Medical Center – NJ

Morristown
Medical Center – NJ

San Juan Regional
Medical Center – NM

Lovelace
Medical Center – NM

Jamaica Hospital
Medical Center – NY

Westchester County
Medical Center – NY

Bronx – Lebanon
Hospital Center – NY

Novant Health Forsyth
Medical Center – NC

Vidant
Medical Center – NC

NC Novant
Health – Rowan
Medical Center – NC

Nash UNC
Healthcare – NC

North Carolina
Baptist Hospital – NC

University of North
Carolina Hospitals – NC

Sanford Fargo
Medical Center – ND

Hillcrest Hospital – OH

Affinity
Medical Center – OH

Adena Regional
Medical Center – OH

Knox Community
Hospital – OH

Mercy
Medical Center – OH

Saint Ritas
Medical Center – OH

St. Anthony
Hospital – OK

Hillcrest
Medical Center – OK

Legacy Emanuel
Medical Center – OR

St. Charles Health
System – OR

Legacy Meridian
Park – OR

Crozer Chester Medical
Center – PA

Aria Health – PA

Lankenau Medical
Center – PA

McLeod Regional
Medical Center – SC

Bon Secours St. Francis
Health System – SC

Beaufort Memorial
Hospital – SC

Blount Memorial
Hospital – TN

CHRISTUS Good
Shepherd Medical
Center – TX

Metroplex Hospital – TX

East Texas Medical
Center – TX

St. David's Medical
Center – TX

Texas Health Huguley
Hospital – TX

Methodist Stone Oak
Hospital – TX

Seton Medical Center
Hays – TX

Memorial Hermann
The Woodlands
Hospital – TX

Metropolitan Methodist
Hospital – TX

Parkland Health &
Hospital System – TX

St. David's South Austin
Medical Center – TX

North Cypress
Medical Center – TX

Medical City
North Hills – TX

University
Medical Center
Brackenridge – TX

Baylor Scott & White
Health (Temple) – TX

Northeast Methodist
Hospital – TX

Heart Hospital
of Austin – TX

University of Texas
Southwestern Medical
Center – TX

Methodist Mansfield
Medical Center – TX

Chesapeake General
Hospital – VA

St. Anthony
Hospital – WA

St. Joseph Medical
Center – WA

Northwest Hospital – WA

Yakima Regional
Medical and Cardiac
Center – WA

HSHS St. Vincent
Hospital – WI

Meriter Hospital – WI

HSHS St. Mary's
Hospital – WI

Campbell County
Memorial – WY

CARDIOLOGY & HEART SURGERY (CONTINUED)

Rank	Hospital	U.S. News score	Survival score (10=best)	Patient safety score (9=best)	Trans-parency score (3=best)	Number of patients	Nurse staffing score (higher is better)	A Nurse Magnet hospital	Technology score (6=best)	Patient services score (7=best)	Intensivists	% of specialists recom-mending hospital
24	Texas Heart Institute at Baylor St. Luke's Medical Cen., Houston	65.4	9	5	3	6,708	1.5	Yes	5	6	Yes	8.9%
26	Beaumont Hospital-Royal Oak, Mich.	65.3	9	6	3	9,692	1.9	Yes	5	7	Yes	1.2%
27	Minneapolis Heart Institute at Abbott Northwestern Hospital	65.1	9	5	3	11,438	2.2	Yes	6	7	Yes	0.8%
28	Vanderbilt University Medical Center, Nashville	64.7	9	5	3	6,243	1.9	Yes	6	7	Yes	3.1%
29	Memorial Hermann-Texas Medical Center, Houston	64.4	10	5	3	3,874	2.1	Yes	6	7	Yes	1.2%
30	University of Alabama at Birmingham Hospital, Birmingham	64.3	10	6	3	5,765	1.8	Yes	6	7	Yes	0.7%
30	University of California, Davis Medical Center, Sacramento	64.3	10	5	3	3,730	2.7	Yes	5	7	Yes	0.2%
32	University of Colorado Hospital, Aurora	64.1	9	5	3	4,201	2.3	Yes	6	7	Yes	1.0%
33	St. Francis Hospital, Roslyn, N.Y.	64.0	9	5	3	9,028	1.7	Yes	5	7	Yes	1.0%
34	St. Luke's Hospital of Kansas City, Mo.	63.9	10	5	3	5,236	1.5	Yes	6	7	Yes	1.7%
35	Morristown Medical Center, Morristown, N.J.	63.8	9	4	3	7,862	2.1	Yes	5	7	Yes	0.5%
36	University of Kansas Hospital, Kansas City	63.2	10	5	3	3,970	2.0	Yes	5	7	Yes	0.4%
37	Aurora St. Luke's Medical Center, Milwaukee	63.1	10	3	3	9,399	2.0	Yes	6	7	Yes	0.9%
38	Advocate Christ Medical Center, Oak Lawn, Ill.	62.4	9	5	3	5,777	2.4	Yes	5	7	Yes	1.2%
39	Mayo Clinic Jacksonville, Fla.	61.9	10	6	2	2,583	2.1	Yes	6	7	Yes	1.2%
40	UC San Diego Health-Sulpizio Cardiovascular Center	61.6	9	5	3	3,236	2.1	Yes	6	7	Yes	0.8%
41	Thomas Jefferson University Hospitals, Philadelphia	61.5	8	6	3	4,697	2.2	Yes	6	7	Yes	0.8%
42	OHSU Hospital, Portland, Ore.	60.9	10	5	3	3,760	2.0	Yes	6	7	Yes	0.5%
43	Rush University Medical Center, Chicago	60.5	9	5	3	2,515	2.3	Yes	5	7	Yes	1.1%
44	Cleveland Clinic Fairview Hospital, Cleveland	60.4	10	6	2	3,606	1.9	Yes	5	7	Yes	0.0%
45	Tampa General Hospital	60.1	9	4	3	5,162	2.2	Yes	6	6	Yes	0.2%
45	University of Washington Medical Center, Seattle	60.1	10	5	2	2,632	2.1	Yes	6	7	Yes	1.4%
47	Mayo Clinic Phoenix	59.7	10	6	2	3,824	2.9	No	6	7	Yes	1.3%
47	MedStar Washington Hospital Center, Washington, D.C.	59.7	9	4	3	8,917	2.3	No	6	7	Yes	1.6%
49	Indiana University Health University Hospital, Indianapolis	59.6	9	5	3	4,600	2.0	Yes	6	7	Yes	0.3%
50	University of Virginia Medical Center, Charlottesville	59.5	9	5	3	3,825	2.0	Yes	6	7	Yes	1.0%

Terms are explained on Page 102.

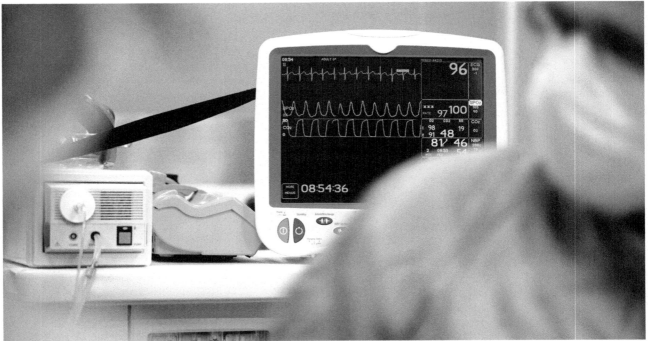

GETTY IMAGES

▶ More @ usnews.com/besthospitals

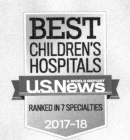

BEST CHILDREN'S HOSPITALS
U.S.News & WORLD REPORT
RANKED IN 7 SPECIALTIES
2017-18

ONE OF THE NATION'S BEST CHILDREN'S HOSPITALS.

One of only a few hospitals in the U.S. performing surgeries on babies before they're born. Our children's hospital is recognized by U.S. News as one of the nation's best To learn how we're doing more for children go to **doingmoremontefiore.org.**

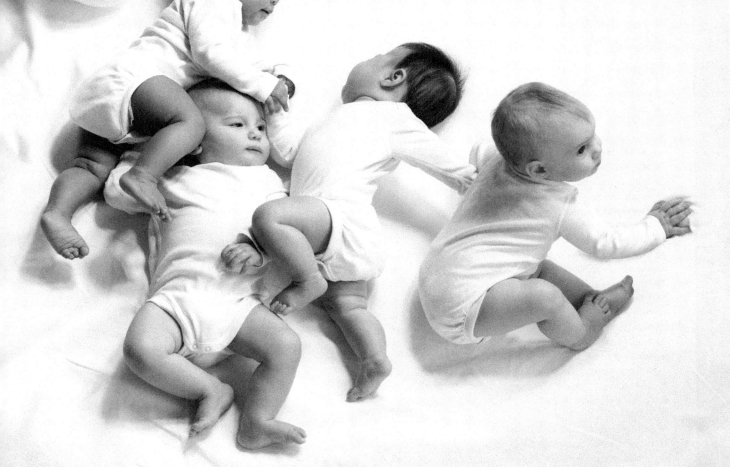

Children's Hospital at Montefiore is ranked nationally by *U.S. News & World Report* in Cancer, Diabetes and Endocrinology, Gastroenterology and Gastrointestinal Surgery, Neonatology, Nephrology, Orthopaedics and Urology.

Montefiore
DOING MORE℠

DIABETES & ENDOCRINOLOGY

Rank	Hospital	U.S. News score	Survival score (10=best)	Patient safety score (9=best)	Number of patients	Nurse staffing score (higher is better)	A Nurse Magnet hospital	Technology score (4=best)	Patient services score (8=best)	Intensivists	% of specialists recom-mending hospital
1	Mayo Clinic, Rochester, Minn.	100.0	8	5	690	2.7	Yes	4	8	Yes	50.5%
2	Massachusetts General Hospital, Boston	84.1	7	5	465	2.4	Yes	4	8	Yes	34.0%
3	Cleveland Clinic	82.2	8	6	702	2.1	Yes	4	8	Yes	16.7%
3	Johns Hopkins Hospital, Baltimore	82.2	8	5	356	2.2	Yes	4	8	Yes	21.7%
5	New York-Presbyterian Hospital	78.6	8	4	1,365	2.8	No	4	8	Yes	10.2%
6	University of Colorado Hospital, Aurora	77.0	9	5	516	2.3	Yes	4	8	Yes	4.4%
7	UCSF Medical Center, San Francisco	74.8	8	6	348	2.4	Yes	4	8	Yes	9.1%
8	Hosps. of the Univ. of Pennsylvania-Penn Presby., Philadelphia	74.4	8	5	578	2.3	Yes	4	8	Yes	8.9%
8	UPMC Presbyterian Shadyside, Pittsburgh	74.4	9	5	736	1.9	Yes	4	8	Yes	3.7%
10	Stanford Health Care-Stanford Hospital, Stanford, Calif.	73.7	9	6	396	2.5	Yes	4	8	Yes	1.5%
11	Abbott Northwestern Hospital, Minneapolis	72.9	10	5	385	2.2	Yes	4	8	Yes	0.0%
12	DMC Harper University Hospital, Detroit	72.8	10	5	224	1.7	Yes	4	8	Yes	0.1%
13	Tampa General Hospital	72.5	10	4	412	2.2	Yes	4	7	Yes	0.0%
14	Beaumont Hospital-Royal Oak, Mich.	72.4	9	6	875	1.9	Yes	4	8	Yes	0.0%
14	Scripps La Jolla Hospitals, La Jolla, Calif.	72.4	9	6	321	3.1	Yes	4	8	Yes	0.3%
16	Ronald Reagan UCLA Medical Center, Los Angeles	71.7	7	5	478	3.0	Yes	4	8	Yes	6.2%
17	Univ. of Michigan Hospitals and Health Centers, Ann Arbor	71.6	7	6	382	2.8	Yes	4	8	Yes	6.0%
18	Cedars-Sinai Medical Center, Los Angeles	71.5	8	5	846	2.6	Yes	4	8	Yes	2.7%
19	Mount Sinai Hospital, New York	70.9	7	7	625	2.0	Yes	4	8	Yes	4.6%
20	OHSU Hospital, Portland, Ore.	70.8	10	5	237	2.0	Yes	4	8	Yes	2.4%
21	University of Alabama at Birmingham Hospital, Birmingham	70.5	9	6	404	1.8	Yes	4	8	Yes	0.7%
22	Brigham and Women's Hospital, Boston	70.3	8	5	389	2.4	No	4	8	Yes	9.5%
23	Houston Methodist Hospital	69.9	8	6	570	2.0	Yes	4	8	Yes	1.2%
24	MedStar Georgetown University Hospital, Washington, D.C.	69.7	10	5	138	1.1	Yes	4	8	Yes	1.1%
25	UT Southwestern Medical Center, Dallas	69.6	8	5	311	2.1	Yes	4	8	Yes	3.3%
26	Ohio State University Wexner Medical Center, Columbus	69.4	8	5	581	2.0	Yes	4	8	Yes	1.8%
26	Thomas Jefferson University Hospitals, Philadelphia	69.4	8	6	616	2.2	Yes	4	8	Yes	1.4%
28	Montefiore Medical Center, Bronx, N.Y.	69.3	9	5	1,042	2.4	No	4	8	Yes	1.8%
29	Yale-New Haven Hospital, New Haven, Conn.	69.0	7	4	799	2.0	Yes	4	8	Yes	6.8%
30	Barnes-Jewish Hospital, St. Louis, Mo.	68.8	7	5	593	2.4	Yes	4	8	Yes	5.6%
31	Northwestern Memorial Hospital, Chicago	67.5	8	6	365	1.6	Yes	4	8	Yes	3.8%
31	UF Health Shands Hospital, Gainesville, Fla.	67.5	9	5	269	1.9	Yes	4	8	Yes	0.4%
33	Providence Portland Medical Center, Portland, Ore.	67.4	10	4	228	1.5	Yes	3	7	Yes	0.0%
34	Christiana Care Hospitals, Newark, Del.	67.3	8	5	811	2.0	Yes	4	8	Yes	0.1%
35	Flagstaff Medical Center, Flagstaff, Ariz.	67.1	10	4	152	1.7	No	4	7	Yes	0.0%
36	NYU Langone Medical Center, New York	66.9	7	5	584	2.6	Yes	4	8	Yes	2.1%
37	University of Kentucky Albert B. Chandler Hospital, Lexington	66.6	9	6	208	1.9	Yes	4	8	Yes	0.1%
38	Duke University Hospital, Durham, N.C.	66.2	8	5	268	2.1	Yes	4	8	Yes	4.2%
39	Queen's Medical Center, Honolulu	65.7	9	5	325	1.8	Yes	4	8	Yes	0.0%
40	St. Cloud Hospital, St. Cloud, Minn.	65.5	9	5	382	1.9	Yes	3	8	Yes	0.0%
40	University of Washington Medical Center, Seattle	65.5	7	5	144	2.1	Yes	4	8	Yes	8.2%
42	Hillcrest Hospital, Cleveland	65.3	9	6	285	1.7	Yes	4	8	Yes	0.0%
43	Sentara Norfolk General Hospital, Norfolk, Va.	65.0	9	5	254	1.6	Yes	4	8	Yes	0.9%
44	University of Virginia Medical Center, Charlottesville	64.9	7	5	239	2.0	Yes	4	8	Yes	4.1%
45	Tufts Medical Center, Boston	64.8	10	5	146	1.6	No	4	8	Yes	0.9%
46	St. Luke's Regional Medical Center, Boise, Idaho	64.3	8	6	345	2.2	Yes	4	6	Yes	0.0%
47	University of Maryland Medical Center, Baltimore	64.2	9	2	150	2.1	Yes	4	7	Yes	0.2%
47	Vanderbilt University Medical Center, Nashville	64.2	7	5	436	1.9	Yes	4	8	Yes	3.2%
49	Advocate Christ Medical Center, Oak Lawn, Ill.	64.1	8	5	331	2.4	Yes	4	8	Yes	0.0%
49	University of California, Davis Medical Center, Sacramento	64.1	8	5	277	2.7	Yes	4	8	Yes	0.5%

Terms are explained on Page 102.

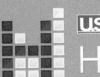
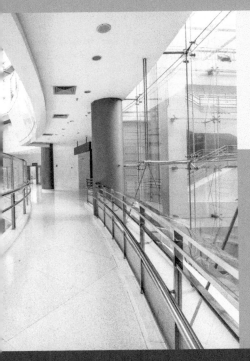
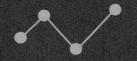

EAR, NOSE & THROAT

Rank	Hospital	U.S. News score	Survival score (10=best)	Patient safety score (9=best)	Number of patients	Nurse staffing score (higher is better)	A Nurse Magnet hospital	Patient services score (8=best)	Trauma center	Intensivists	% of specialists recom-mending hospital
1	Johns Hopkins Hospital, Baltimore	100.0	8	5	183	2.2	Yes	8	Yes	Yes	28.6%
2	Massachusetts Eye and Ear Infirmary, Mass. Gen. Hosp., Boston	98.7	8	5	380	2.4	Yes	8	Yes	Yes	22.6%
2	Ronald Reagan UCLA Medical Center, Los Angeles	98.7	10	5	421	3.0	Yes	8	Yes	Yes	5.9%
4	Mayo Clinic, Rochester, Minn.	96.5	9	5	312	2.7	Yes	8	Yes	Yes	12.7%
5	University of Iowa Hospitals and Clinics, Iowa City	95.9	10	5	170	1.8	Yes	8	Yes	Yes	13.3%
6	Ohio State University Wexner Medical Center, Columbus	93.4	10	5	410	2.0	Yes	8	Yes	Yes	5.9%
6	Univ. of Michigan Hospitals and Health Centers, Ann Arbor	93.4	8	6	310	2.8	Yes	8	Yes	Yes	12.8%
8	Thomas Jefferson University Hospitals, Philadelphia	92.1	10	6	384	2.2	Yes	8	Yes	Yes	2.8%
9	Stanford Health Care-Stanford Hospital, Stanford, Calif.	91.2	9	6	292	2.5	Yes	8	Yes	Yes	9.3%
10	UCSF Medical Center, San Francisco	88.4	9	6	204	2.4	Yes	8	Yes	Yes	7.1%
11	MUSC Health-University Medical Center, Charleston, S.C.	87.6	10	5	196	2.0	Yes	8	Yes	Yes	6.5%
12	University Hospitals Cleveland Medical Center	86.1	10	5	228	2.4	Yes	8	Yes	Yes	2.2%
13	Hosps. of the Univ. of Pennsylvania-Penn Presby., Philadelphia	85.9	8	5	403	2.3	Yes	8	Yes	Yes	9.0%
14	University of North Carolina Hospitals, Chapel Hill	85.3	10	5	203	2.0	Yes	8	Yes	Yes	3.3%
15	University of Texas MD Anderson Cancer Center, Houston	83.1	7	5	602	1.9	Yes	8	No	Yes	9.3%
16	Cleveland Clinic	81.5	8	6	252	2.1	Yes	8	No	Yes	10.6%
17	University of Cincinnati Medical Center	81.1	10	5	235	1.7	No	8	Yes	Yes	5.6%
18	OHSU Hospital, Portland, Ore.	81.0	9	5	235	2.0	Yes	8	Yes	Yes	3.3%
18	University of Utah Health Care-Hosp. and Clinics, Salt Lake City	81.0	10	5	124	2.2	No	8	Yes	Yes	1.6%
20	Memorial Sloan Kettering Cancer Center, New York	80.5	9	6	310	2.1	Yes	8	No	Yes	3.3%
21	Reading Hospital, West Reading, Pa.	80.4	10	4	121	1.2	Yes	7	Yes	Yes	0.0%
22	Yale-New Haven Hospital, New Haven, Conn.	80.0	9	4	358	2.0	Yes	8	Yes	Yes	1.0%
23	Barnes-Jewish Hospital, St. Louis, Mo.	78.4	7	5	314	2.4	Yes	8	Yes	Yes	6.7%
24	Porter Adventist Hospital, Denver	77.7	10	5	194	1.8	Yes	8	No	Yes	0.1%
25	Henry Ford Hospital, Detroit	77.4	10	5	123	1.9	No	8	Yes	Yes	0.9%
26	Cedars-Sinai Medical Center, Los Angeles	76.8	9	5	155	2.6	Yes	8	Yes	Yes	0.9%
27	Ochsner Medical Center, New Orleans	76.7	10	5	155	2.1	Yes	8	Yes	Yes	0.9%
28	Mayo Clinic Phoenix	76.2	10	6	271	2.9	No	8	No	Yes	1.6%
29	UPMC Presbyterian Shadyside, Pittsburgh	76.0	5	5	448	1.9	Yes	8	Yes	Yes	11.9%
30	Queen's Medical Center, Honolulu	75.5	10	5	100	1.8	Yes	8	Yes	Yes	0.0%
31	University of Washington Medical Center, Seattle	75.2	8	5	172	2.1	Yes	8	No	Yes	6.5%
32	University of Virginia Medical Center, Charlottesville	74.8	9	5	107	2.0	Yes	8	Yes	Yes	3.0%
33	Rush University Medical Center, Chicago	74.6	9	5	114	2.3	Yes	8	Yes	Yes	1.1%
34	Wake Forest Baptist Medical Center, Winston-Salem, N.C.	74.1	8	5	367	1.6	Yes	8	Yes	Yes	1.3%
35	University of Miami Hospital	73.4	10	4	522	1.5	No	8	Yes	Yes	0.8%
36	New York-Presbyterian Hospital	73.2	8	4	301	2.8	No	8	Yes	Yes	4.0%
37	Our Lady of the Lake Regional Medical Center, Baton Rouge, La.	72.5	10	4	150	1.3	Yes	7	Yes	Yes	0.6%
37	UF Health Jacksonville, Fla.	72.5	10	5	116	1.3	Yes	8	Yes	Yes	0.0%
39	Carolinas Medical Center, Charlotte, N.C.	71.5	9	6	146	1.9	Yes	8	Yes	Yes	0.0%
40	Fox Chase Cancer Center, Philadelphia	71.3	10	5	106	1.8	Yes	8	No	Yes	0.1%
41	Baylor University Medical Center, Dallas	71.0	9	5	190	1.8	Yes	8	Yes	Yes	0.4%
41	Froedtert Hospital and the Medical College of Wis., Milwaukee	71.0	9	5	116	1.8	Yes	8	Yes	Yes	1.5%
41	University of California, Davis Medical Center, Sacramento	71.0	8	5	153	2.7	Yes	8	Yes	Yes	0.9%
44	Scott and White Memorial Hospital, Temple, Texas	70.5	10	3	87	1.1	No	8	Yes	Yes	0.0%
45	Mayo Clinic Jacksonville, Fla.	70.2	9	6	97	2.1	Yes	8	No	Yes	0.7%
45	Providence Portland Medical Center, Portland, Ore.	70.2	10	4	119	1.5	Yes	7	No	Yes	0.0%
47	Baylor All Saints Medical Center at Fort Worth	67.9	10	5	178	1.6	No	7	No	Yes	0.3%
47	St. Joseph Mercy Ann Arbor Hospital, Ypsilanti, Mich.	67.9	10	5	79	1.8	No	8	Yes	Yes	0.2%
49	Nebraska Medicine-Nebraska Medical Center, Omaha	67.3	8	5	119	2.6	Yes	8	Yes	Yes	0.1%
50	New York Eye and Ear Infirmary of Mount Sinai, N.Y.	66.9	10	5	10	1.2	Yes	8	No	Yes	1.5%
50	UT Southwestern Medical Center, Dallas	66.9	8	5	139	2.1	Yes	8	No	Yes	1.2%
50	University of Alabama at Birmingham Hospital, Birmingham	66.9	6	6	432	1.8	Yes	8	Yes	Yes	1.6%

Terms are explained on Page 102.

More @ usnews.com/besthospitals

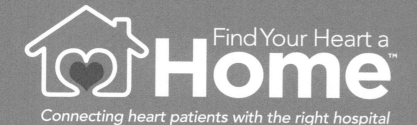

Find Your Heart a Home™

Connecting heart patients with the right hospital

Is **Your Heart** In The **Right Hands?**

Search
local hospitals

Compare
services and
performances

Select
the right
hospital for you

Get Started at *FindYourHeartaHome.org*

Powered by ACC's NCDR®
and CardioSmart®

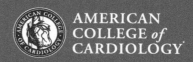

AMERICAN COLLEGE *of* CARDIOLOGY

GASTROENTEROLOGY & GI SURGERY

Rank	Hospital	U.S. News score	Survival score (10=best)	Patient safety score (9=best)	Number of patients	Nurse staffing score (higher is better)	A Nurse Magnet hospital	Technology score (7=best)	Patient services score (8=best)	Trauma center	Intensivists	% of specialists recommending hospital
1	Mayo Clinic, Rochester, Minn.	100.0	10	5	6,881	2.7	Yes	7	8	Yes	Yes	46.5%
2	Cleveland Clinic	88.4	9	6	5,744	2.1	Yes	7	8	No	Yes	30.3%
3	Johns Hopkins Hospital, Baltimore	83.6	8	5	3,097	2.2	Yes	7	8	Yes	Yes	23.3%
4	Cedars-Sinai Medical Center, Los Angeles	78.7	8	5	7,005	2.6	Yes	7	8	Yes	Yes	7.8%
5	Massachusetts General Hospital, Boston	78.5	7	5	4,684	2.4	Yes	7	8	Yes	Yes	17.4%
6	UPMC Presbyterian Shadyside, Pittsburgh	77.2	8	5	7,548	1.9	Yes	7	8	Yes	Yes	8.5%
7	Mayo Clinic Jacksonville, Fla.	76.0	10	6	2,302	2.1	Yes	7	8	No	Yes	5.6%
8	Mount Sinai Hospital, New York	75.3	7	7	4,782	2.0	Yes	7	8	Yes	Yes	11.1%
9	Univ. of Michigan Hospitals and Health Centers, Ann Arbor	74.7	8	6	3,657	2.8	Yes	7	8	Yes	Yes	6.7%
10	Mayo Clinic Phoenix	74.4	10	6	3,372	2.9	No	7	8	No	Yes	4.6%
11	Ronald Reagan UCLA Medical Center, Los Angeles	73.7	7	5	3,839	3.0	Yes	7	8	Yes	Yes	9.3%
12	Hosps. of the Univ. of Pennsylvania-Penn Presby., Philadelphia	73.1	7	5	3,773	2.3	Yes	7	8	Yes	Yes	8.6%
12	Houston Methodist Hospital	73.1	10	6	4,425	2.0	Yes	7	8	No	Yes	1.7%
14	New York-Presbyterian Hospital	71.8	8	4	7,913	2.8	No	7	8	Yes	Yes	6.5%
15	Beaumont Hospital-Royal Oak, Mich.	70.8	8	6	5,663	1.9	Yes	7	8	Yes	Yes	0.7%
16	University of Colorado Hospital, Aurora	70.5	9	5	2,800	2.3	Yes	7	8	Yes	Yes	2.0%
17	Thomas Jefferson University Hospitals, Philadelphia	70.3	7	6	4,559	2.2	Yes	7	8	Yes	Yes	3.4%
17	UCSF Medical Center, San Francisco	70.3	7	6	2,293	2.4	Yes	7	8	Yes	Yes	6.7%
19	NYU Langone Medical Center, New York	70.2	8	5	3,713	2.6	Yes	7	8	Yes	Yes	3.0%
20	Barnes-Jewish Hospital, St. Louis, Mo.	70.0	7	5	5,137	2.4	Yes	7	8	Yes	Yes	5.0%
21	Stanford Health Care-Stanford Hospital, Stanford, Calif.	69.9	7	6	3,263	2.5	Yes	7	8	Yes	Yes	3.9%
22	Indiana University Health University Hospital, Indianapolis	69.7	8	5	4,085	2.0	Yes	7	8	Yes	Yes	2.5%
22	Northwestern Memorial Hospital, Chicago	69.7	8	6	2,707	1.6	Yes	7	8	Trauma	Yes	3.8%
22	Ochsner Medical Center, New Orleans	69.7	9	5	3,810	2.1	Yes	7	8	Yes	Yes	1.4%
25	Scripps La Jolla Hospitals, La Jolla, Calif.	69.2	8	6	2,588	3.1	Yes	7	8	Yes	Yes	0.6%
26	University Hospitals Cleveland Medical Center	68.8	8	5	2,436	2.4	Yes	7	8	Yes	Yes	2.1%
27	Hoag Memorial Hospital Presbyterian, Newport Beach, Calif.	68.7	9	7	4,284	2.3	Yes	6	8	No	Yes	0.0%
27	Tampa General Hospital	68.7	9	4	2,919	2.2	Yes	7	7	Yes	Yes	0.7%
29	Baylor University Medical Center, Dallas	67.7	7	5	4,007	1.8	Yes	7	8	Yes	Yes	2.9%
30	University of North Carolina Hospitals, Chapel Hill	67.6	7	5	2,011	2.0	Yes	7	8	Yes	Yes	5.2%
31	Cleveland Clinic Fairview Hospital, Cleveland	67.0	9	6	1,871	1.9	Yes	6	8	Yes	Yes	0.1%
32	Sanford USD Medical Center, Sioux Falls, S.D.	66.9	9	5	2,219	2.5	Yes	6	8	Yes	Yes	0.0%
33	Yale-New Haven Hospital, New Haven, Conn.	66.7	6	4	5,495	2.0	Yes	7	8	Yes	Yes	3.3%
34	University of Kansas Hospital, Kansas City	66.2	8	5	2,370	2.0	Yes	7	8	Yes	Yes	0.2%
35	Penn State Milton S. Hershey Medical Center, Hershey	66.1	8	5	2,398	2.1	Yes	7	8	Yes	Yes	0.7%
36	Loyola University Medical Center, Maywood, Ill.	66.0	8	6	1,918	2.4	Yes	7	8	Yes	Yes	0.1%
37	Christiana Care Hospitals, Newark, Del.	65.5	7	5	5,104	2.0	Yes	6	8	Yes	Yes	0.3%
37	University of Wisconsin Hospitals, Madison	65.5	8	5	2,439	2.5	Yes	7	8	Trauma	Yes	0.5%
39	Lehigh Valley Hospital, Allentown, Pa.	65.4	8	5	3,872	1.7	Yes	6	8	Yes	Yes	0.1%
40	Duke University Hospital, Durham, N.C.	65.3	6	5	2,729	2.1	Yes	7	8	Yes	Yes	6.3%
41	DMC Harper University Hospital, Detroit	65.1	10	5	1,149	1.7	Yes	7	8	No	Yes	0.0%
42	Advocate Lutheran General Hospital, Park Ridge, Ill.	65.0	8	6	2,451	1.7	Yes	6	8	Yes	Yes	0.0%
42	Cleveland Clinic Florida, Weston	65.0	9	5	2,060	2.2	No	6	8	No	Yes	4.0%
42	University of Chicago Medical Center	65.0	6	6	1,998	2.4	No	7	8	Yes	Yes	9.1%
45	University of Washington Medical Center, Seattle	64.9	8	5	1,487	2.1	Yes	7	8	No	Yes	1.6%
46	Aurora St. Luke's Medical Center, Milwaukee	64.8	9	3	3,970	2.0	Yes	7	8	No	Yes	0.3%
46	St. Francis Hospital, Roslyn, N.Y.	64.8	8	5	2,381	1.7	Yes	6	8	Yes	Yes	0.1%
46	UC San Diego Medical Center	64.8	7	5	2,067	2.1	Yes	7	8	Yes	Yes	1.5%
49	Brigham and Women's Hospital, Boston	64.7	7	5	3,634	2.4	No	6	8	Yes	Yes	5.9%
50	Emory University Hospital, Atlanta	64.5	8	5	2,374	1.9	Yes	7	8	No	Yes	2.5%

Terms are explained on Page 102.

GERIATRICS

Rank	Hospital	U.S. News score	Survival score (10=best)	Patient safety score (9=best)	Number of patients	Nurse staffing score (higher is better)	A Nurse Magnet hospital	NIA Alzheimer's center	Patient services score (9=best)	Intensivists	% of specialists recommending hospital
1	Mayo Clinic, Rochester, Minn.	100.0	10	5	28,071	2.7	Yes	Yes	9	Yes	15.6%
2	Johns Hopkins Hospital, Baltimore	96.1	10	5	8,461	2.2	Yes	Yes	9	Yes	23.0%
3	Mount Sinai Hospital, New York	94.3	8	7	21,517	2.0	Yes	Yes	9	Yes	23.4%
4	Ronald Reagan UCLA Medical Center, Los Angeles	89.0	9	5	18,572	3.0	Yes	No	9	Yes	26.3%
5	Cleveland Clinic	87.1	10	6	20,515	2.1	Yes	No	9	Yes	11.4%
6	New York-Presbyterian Hospital	85.4	9	4	43,729	2.8	No	Yes	9	Yes	6.8%
7	Univ. of Michigan Hospitals and Health Centers, Ann Arbor	85.3	9	6	11,562	2.8	Yes	Yes	9	Yes	5.4%
8	Massachusetts General Hospital, Boston	85.1	9	5	21,378	2.4	Yes	Yes	9	Yes	7.4%
9	Northwestern Memorial Hospital, Chicago	84.0	10	6	11,395	1.6	Yes	Yes	9	Yes	2.2%
10	UCSF Medical Center, San Francisco	83.8	8	6	9,184	2.4	Yes	Yes	9	Yes	8.7%
11	UPMC Presbyterian Shadyside, Pittsburgh	82.4	8	5	28,907	1.9	Yes	Yes	9	Yes	7.9%
12	NYU Langone Medical Center, New York	81.9	8	5	22,965	2.6	Yes	Yes	9	Yes	2.8%
13	Hosps. of the Univ. of Pennsylvania-Penn Presby., Philadelphia	80.5	9	5	15,849	2.3	Yes	Yes	9	Yes	3.1%
14	Rush University Medical Center, Chicago	79.5	9	5	7,724	2.3	Yes	Yes	9	Yes	2.2%
15	Mayo Clinic Phoenix	79.3	10	6	13,354	2.9	No	Yes	9	Yes	1.0%
15	Yale-New Haven Hospital, New Haven, Conn.	79.3	7	4	30,787	2.0	Yes	Yes	9	Yes	6.2%
17	Barnes-Jewish Hospital, St. Louis, Mo.	78.7	9	5	17,654	2.4	Yes	Yes	9	Yes	1.6%
18	University of Kansas Hospital, Kansas City	78.1	9	5	9,031	2.0	Yes	Yes	9	Yes	0.9%
19	University of California, Davis Medical Center, Sacramento	77.8	9	5	9,938	2.7	Yes	Yes	9	Yes	0.6%
20	University of Washington Medical Center, Seattle	77.5	9	5	4,419	2.1	Yes	Yes	9	Yes	1.6%
21	Cedars-Sinai Medical Center, Los Angeles	77.1	9	5	34,389	2.6	Yes	No	8	Yes	2.4%
22	Stanford Health Care-Stanford Hospital, Stanford, Calif.	76.4	8	6	13,481	2.5	Yes	Yes	9	Yes	1.1%
23	Houston Methodist Hospital	76.3	10	6	20,619	2.0	Yes	No	9	Yes	2.2%
24	UT Southwestern Medical Center, Dallas	75.7	9	5	6,206	2.1	Yes	Yes	9	Yes	0.8%
25	Indiana University Health University Hospital, Indianapolis	74.9	8	5	12,676	2.0	Yes	Yes	9	Yes	2.4%
26	Mayo Clinic Jacksonville, Fla.	74.8	8	6	8,774	2.1	Yes	Yes	9	Yes	1.8%
27	Keck Hospital of USC, Los Angeles	74.7	10	6	5,116	3.0	No	Yes	9	Yes	0.9%
28	Beaumont Hospital-Royal Oak, Mich.	74.3	9	6	32,637	1.9	Yes	No	9	Yes	1.4%
29	Banner University Medical Center Phoenix	74.0	9	5	7,750	1.9	Yes	Yes	9	Yes	0.2%
30	OHSU Hospital, Portland, Ore.	72.6	9	5	7,848	2.0	Yes	Yes	9	Yes	0.2%
31	University of Wisconsin Hospitals, Madison	72.4	7	5	8,856	2.5	Yes	Yes	9	Yes	1.9%
32	University of Colorado Hospital, Aurora	72.2	10	5	10,255	2.3	Yes	No	9	Yes	1.7%
33	Wake Forest Baptist Medical Center, Winston-Salem, N.C.	72.0	7	5	15,773	1.6	Yes	Yes	9	Yes	3.2%
34	UC San Diego Medical Center	71.7	7	5	8,503	2.1	Yes	Yes	9	Yes	1.5%
35	Emory Wesley Woods Geriatric Hospital, Atlanta	70.5	7	5	9,270	1.9	Yes	Yes	8	Yes	2.4%
36	Scripps La Jolla Hospitals, La Jolla, Calif.	69.5	9	6	15,123	3.1	Yes	No	7	Yes	0.8%
37	Abbott Northwestern Hospital, Minneapolis	69.2	9	5	23,544	2.2	Yes	No	9	Yes	0.0%
38	Brigham and Women's Hospital, Boston	68.9	8	5	13,948	2.4	No	Yes	9	Yes	1.2%
38	Thomas Jefferson University Hospitals, Philadelphia	68.9	8	6	16,997	2.2	Yes	No	9	Yes	2.7%
40	Duke University Hospital, Durham, N.C.	68.2	7	5	10,584	2.1	Yes	No	9	Yes	9.2%
41	Aurora St. Luke's Medical Center, Milwaukee	67.8	9	3	23,393	2.0	Yes	No	9	Yes	0.6%
42	UF Health Shands Hospital, Gainesville, Fla.	67.7	7	5	9,875	1.9	Yes	Yes	9	Yes	0.2%
43	University of Kentucky Albert B. Chandler Hospital, Lexington	67.4	7	6	7,521	1.9	Yes	Yes	9	Yes	0.0%
44	University Hospitals Cleveland Medical Center	67.2	9	5	10,755	2.4	Yes	No	9	Yes	1.6%
45	St. Cloud Hospital, St. Cloud, Minn.	67.1	9	5	21,526	1.9	Yes	No	8	Yes	0.0%
46	Banner University Medical Center Tucson, Ariz.	67.0	7	4	7,143	1.8	Yes	Yes	7	Yes	0.5%
47	Hoag Memorial Hospital Presbyterian, Newport Beach, Calif.	66.6	8	7	22,196	2.3	Yes	No	9	Yes	0.0%
47	University of Alabama at Birmingham Hospital, Birmingham	66.6	8	6	13,067	1.8	Yes	No	8	Yes	3.4%
49	UC Irvine Medical Center, Orange, Calif.	66.4	7	5	7,059	2.1	Yes	Yes	7	Yes	0.3%
50	Boston Medical Center	66.2	9	5	4,547	1.3	No	Yes	7	Yes	1.9%

Terms are explained on Page 102.

GYNECOLOGY

Rank	Hospital	U.S. News score	Survival score (10=best)	Patient safety score (9=best)	Number of patients	Nurse staffing score (higher is better)	A Nurse Magnet hospital	Technology score (5=best)	Patient services score (9=best)	Intensivists	% of specialists recommending hospital
1	Mayo Clinic, Rochester, Minn.	100.0	10	5	444	2.7	Yes	5	9	Yes	13.4%
2	Memorial Sloan Kettering Cancer Center, New York	91.6	10	6	586	2.1	Yes	5	8	Yes	6.8%
3	Univ. of Michigan Hospitals and Health Centers, Ann Arbor	90.3	10	6	188	2.8	Yes	5	9	Yes	2.5%
4	Brigham and Women's Hospital, Boston	90.2	10	5	302	2.4	No	5	9	Yes	12.2%
5	Cleveland Clinic	89.4	10	6	257	2.1	Yes	5	9	Yes	11.2%
6	Johns Hopkins Hospital, Baltimore	88.7	10	5	145	2.2	Yes	5	9	Yes	12.7%
7	Stanford Health Care-Stanford Hospital, Stanford, Calif.	86.8	10	6	178	2.5	Yes	5	9	Yes	4.0%
8	UCSF Medical Center, San Francisco	86.6	10	6	171	2.4	Yes	5	9	Yes	9.9%
9	Huntington Memorial Hospital, Pasadena, Calif.	84.9	10	6	135	2.5	Yes	4	9	Yes	0.7%
10	Scripps La Jolla Hospitals, La Jolla, Calif.	83.1	10	6	153	3.1	Yes	5	8	Yes	1.2%
11	Massachusetts General Hospital, Boston	82.5	9	5	310	2.4	Yes	5	9	Yes	6.0%
12	University of California, Davis Medical Center, Sacramento	82.4	10	5	263	2.7	Yes	5	9	Yes	1.4%
13	University of Wisconsin Hospitals, Madison	81.4	10	5	352	2.5	Yes	5	9	Yes	0.4%
14	Ronald Reagan UCLA Medical Center, Los Angeles	80.3	9	5	135	3.0	Yes	5	9	Yes	4.7%
14	Vanderbilt University Medical Center, Nashville	80.3	10	5	138	1.9	Yes	5	9	Yes	2.1%
16	New York-Presbyterian Hospital	79.6	9	4	286	2.8	No	5	9	Yes	7.8%
17	University of Texas MD Anderson Cancer Center, Houston	78.6	8	5	465	1.9	Yes	5	9	Yes	10.4%
18	Barnes-Jewish Hospital, St. Louis, Mo.	78.5	8	5	484	2.4	Yes	5	9	Yes	4.1%
19	Medical City Dallas Hospital	78.2	10	5	154	2.0	Yes	4	8	Yes	0.4%
19	University Hospitals Cleveland Medical Center	78.2	10	5	245	2.4	Yes	5	9	Yes	0.9%
21	Duke University Hospital, Durham, N.C.	78.0	9	5	144	2.1	Yes	5	9	Yes	7.2%
22	City of Hope, Duarte, Calif.	77.8	10	5	174	2.2	No	5	8	Yes	0.1%
23	Mount Sinai Hospital, New York	77.1	9	7	288	2.0	Yes	5	9	Yes	2.5%
23	Queen's Medical Center, Honolulu	77.1	10	5	123	1.8	Yes	5	8	Yes	0.0%
25	Abbott Northwestern Hospital, Minneapolis	76.7	9	5	358	2.2	Yes	5	9	Yes	0.1%
26	University of Alabama at Birmingham Hospital, Birmingham	76.4	9	6	471	1.8	Yes	5	9	Yes	2.9%
27	Sharp Memorial Hospital, San Diego	76.3	10	5	132	2.3	Yes	5	7	Yes	0.5%
28	Cedars-Sinai Medical Center, Los Angeles	76.0	8	5	313	2.6	Yes	5	9	Yes	3.4%
28	University of North Carolina Hospitals, Chapel Hill	76.0	9	5	216	2.0	Yes	5	9	Yes	4.4%
30	Aurora St. Luke's Medical Center, Milwaukee	75.9	10	3	198	2.0	Yes	5	9	Yes	0.3%
30	MUSC Health-University Medical Center, Charleston, S.C.	75.9	10	5	200	2.0	Yes	5	9	Yes	0.8%
32	St. Joseph's Hospital and Medical Center, Phoenix	75.5	10	6	127	1.8	No	5	8	Yes	0.1%
33	Wake Forest Baptist Medical Center, Winston-Salem, N.C.	75.4	10	5	276	1.6	Yes	5	9	Yes	1.4%
34	Rush University Medical Center, Chicago	75.3	9	5	272	2.3	Yes	5	9	Yes	0.4%
35	UF Health Shands Hospital, Gainesville, Fla.	75.1	10	5	147	1.9	Yes	5	9	Yes	1.0%
36	Northwestern Memorial Hospital, Chicago	74.4	9	6	102	1.6	Yes	5	9	Yes	5.1%
37	Memorial Medical Center, Modesto, Calif.	74.3	10	5	100	2.0	No	5	9	Yes	0.0%
38	Banner University Medical Center Tucson, Ariz.	74.2	10	4	170	1.8	Yes	5	9	Yes	0.0%
39	University Hospital, San Antonio	74.0	10	5	89	1.7	Yes	5	9	Yes	0.2%
40	Rose Medical Center, Denver	73.8	10	5	117	1.9	Yes	5	8	Yes	0.0%
41	Nebraska Medicine-Nebraska Medical Center, Omaha	73.6	10	5	76	2.6	Yes	5	9	Yes	1.1%
42	UC San Diego Medical Center	73.5	10	5	79	2.1	Yes	5	9	Yes	1.2%
43	Northwestern Medicine Central DuPage Hospital, Winfield, Ill.	73.3	10	5	91	1.8	Yes	5	9	Yes	0.1%
43	University of Colorado Hospital, Aurora	73.3	9	5	280	2.3	Yes	5	9	Yes	0.7%
45	Christ Hospital, Cincinnati	73.2	10	5	85	1.9	Yes	5	8	Yes	0.9%
46	University of Chicago Medical Center	73.1	10	6	124	2.4	No	5	9	Yes	1.4%
47	OSF St. Francis Medical Center, Peoria, Ill.	73.0	9	5	196	2.1	Yes	5	9	Yes	0.0%
48	St. Luke's Hospital of Kansas City, Mo.	72.7	10	5	207	1.5	Yes	5	8	Yes	0.1%
49	Froedtert Hospital and the Medical College of Wis., Milwaukee	72.6	10	5	98	1.8	Yes	5	9	Yes	0.2%
50	John Muir Medical Center, Walnut Creek, Calif.	71.9	9	4	228	2.3	Yes	5	8	Yes	0.9%

Terms are explained on Page 102.

More @ usnews.com/besthospitals

NEPHROLOGY

Rank	Hospital	U.S. News score	Survival score (10=best)	Patient safety score (9=best)	Number of patients	Nurse staffing score (higher is better)	A Nurse Magnet hospital	Technology score (7=best)	Patient services score (8=best)	Intensivists	% of specialists recommending hospital
1	Mayo Clinic, Rochester, Minn.	100.0	10	5	1,930	2.7	Yes	7	8	Yes	23.7%
2	Cleveland Clinic	94.7	10	6	2,019	2.1	Yes	7	8	Yes	21.2%
3	Johns Hopkins Hospital, Baltimore	89.3	9	5	1,087	2.2	Yes	7	8	Yes	14.8%
4	New York-Presbyterian Hospital	88.7	8	4	3,298	2.8	No	7	8	Yes	19.5%
5	UCSF Medical Center, San Francisco	87.3	10	6	1,033	2.4	Yes	7	8	Yes	8.2%
6	Ronald Reagan UCLA Medical Center, Los Angeles	86.2	9	5	1,392	3.0	Yes	7	8	Yes	7.2%
7	Hosps. of the Univ. of Pennsylvania-Penn Presby., Philadelphia	83.5	9	5	1,180	2.3	Yes	7	8	Yes	8.7%
8	Massachusetts General Hospital, Boston	82.8	7	5	1,453	2.4	Yes	7	8	Yes	12.5%
9	Barnes-Jewish Hospital, St. Louis, Mo.	82.2	8	5	1,882	2.4	Yes	7	8	Yes	6.2%
10	Mount Sinai Hospital, New York	82.0	8	7	1,394	2.0	Yes	7	8	Yes	7.8%
11	University of Colorado Hospital, Aurora	81.7	10	5	1,035	2.3	Yes	7	8	Yes	3.0%
12	Vanderbilt University Medical Center, Nashville	81.3	8	5	1,502	1.9	Yes	7	8	Yes	9.1%
13	Univ. of Michigan Hospitals and Health Centers, Ann Arbor	80.7	9	6	1,312	2.8	Yes	7	8	Yes	3.2%
14	University of Alabama at Birmingham Hospital, Birmingham	80.4	9	6	1,183	1.8	Yes	7	8	Yes	6.1%
15	Cedars-Sinai Medical Center, Los Angeles	79.8	9	5	2,233	2.6	Yes	7	8	Yes	2.5%
16	Stanford Health Care-Stanford Hospital, Stanford, Calif.	79.4	8	6	1,004	2.5	Yes	7	8	Yes	5.5%
17	Ohio State University Wexner Medical Center, Columbus	79.1	9	5	1,628	2.0	Yes	7	8	Yes	3.6%
18	Tampa General Hospital	79.0	10	4	1,493	2.2	Yes	7	7	Yes	1.3%
19	Indiana University Health University Hospital, Indianapolis	78.9	9	5	1,670	2.0	Yes	7	8	Yes	2.4%
20	University of North Carolina Hospitals, Chapel Hill	78.2	9	5	785	2.0	Yes	7	8	Yes	5.6%
21	Duke University Hospital, Durham, N.C.	77.9	8	5	935	2.1	Yes	7	8	Yes	7.1%
22	OHSU Hospital, Portland, Ore.	76.8	10	5	647	2.0	Yes	7	8	Yes	0.4%
23	Northwestern Memorial Hospital, Chicago	76.4	9	6	1,235	1.6	Yes	7	8	Yes	2.7%
24	Brigham and Women's Hospital, Boston	76.2	7	5	1,021	2.4	No	7	8	Yes	15.5%
25	UF Health Shands Hospital, Gainesville, Fla.	75.2	9	5	1,132	1.9	Yes	7	8	Yes	2.0%
26	University of California, Davis Medical Center, Sacramento	75.0	9	5	1,069	2.7	Yes	7	8	Yes	1.1%
27	Wake Forest Baptist Medical Center, Winston-Salem, N.C.	74.9	8	5	1,860	1.6	Yes	7	8	Yes	3.3%
28	Beaumont Hospital-Royal Oak, Mich.	74.5	8	6	2,172	1.9	Yes	7	8	Yes	0.4%
28	Ochsner Medical Center, New Orleans	74.5	9	5	1,584	2.1	Yes	7	8	Yes	0.7%
28	University of Wisconsin Hospitals, Madison	74.5	9	5	815	2.5	Yes	7	8	Yes	0.5%
31	Yale-New Haven Hospital, New Haven, Conn.	74.1	7	4	2,387	2.0	Yes	7	8	Yes	3.3%
32	Mayo Clinic Phoenix	74.0	10	6	1,293	2.9	No	7	8	Yes	2.6%
32	University Hospitals Cleveland Medical Center	74.0	9	5	914	2.4	Yes	7	8	Yes	0.9%
34	Miami Valley Hospital, Dayton, Ohio	73.7	9	5	1,429	2.6	Yes	6	8	Yes	0.0%
35	UPMC Presbyterian Shadyside, Pittsburgh	73.5	6	5	2,481	1.9	Yes	7	8	Yes	4.3%
36	Banner University Medical Center Phoenix	72.5	9	5	599	1.9	Yes	7	8	Yes	0.8%
36	Christiana Care Hospitals, Newark, Del.	72.5	8	5	1,990	2.0	Yes	7	8	Yes	0.2%
36	Loyola University Medical Center, Maywood, Ill.	72.5	8	6	881	2.4	Yes	7	8	Yes	0.4%
39	Houston Methodist Hospital	72.3	9	6	1,607	2.0	Yes	7	8	Intensivists	1.0%
39	Scripps La Jolla Hospitals, La Jolla, Calif.	72.3	8	6	534	3.1	Yes	7	8	Yes	0.3%
39	UT Southwestern Medical Center, Dallas	72.3	9	5	1,036	2.1	Yes	7	8	Yes	1.1%
42	Froedtert Hospital and the Medical College of Wis., Milwaukee	72.1	9	5	790	1.8	Yes	7	8	Yes	1.4%
43	Queen's Medical Center, Honolulu	71.7	9	5	868	1.8	Yes	7	8	Yes	0.0%
44	Rush University Medical Center, Chicago	71.5	8	5	733	2.3	Yes	7	8	Yes	2.1%
44	University of Washington Medical Center, Seattle	71.5	8	5	579	2.1	Yes	7	8	Yes	4.2%
46	University of Kansas Hospital, Kansas City	71.4	8	5	1,172	2.0	Yes	7	8	Yes	0.4%
47	NYU Langone Medical Center, New York	71.3	7	5	1,582	2.6	Yes	7	8	Yes	0.9%
48	Thomas Jefferson University Hospitals, Philadelphia	71.1	8	6	1,296	2.2	Yes	7	8	Yes	0.8%
49	DMC Harper University Hospital, Detroit	70.8	10	5	799	1.7	Yes	7	8	Yes	0.1%
49	VCU Medical Center, Richmond, Va.	70.8	9	5	555	2.1	Yes	7	8	Yes	0.3%

Terms are explained on Page 102.

NEUROLOGY & NEUROSURGERY

Rank	Hospital	U.S. News score	Survival score (10=best)	Patient safety score (9=best)	Number of patients	Nurse staffing score (higher is better)	A Nurse Magnet hospital	NAEC epilepsy center	Technology score (5=best)	Patient services score (9=best)	Intensivists	% of specialists recommending hospital
1	Mayo Clinic, Rochester, Minn.	100.0	8	5	4,598	2.7	Yes	Yes	5	9	Yes	37.8%
2	Johns Hopkins Hospital, Baltimore	92.0	8	5	2,307	2.2	Yes	Yes	5	9	Yes	28.6%
3	Massachusetts General Hospital, Boston	85.8	6	5	4,529	2.4	Yes	Yes	5	9	Yes	27.5%
4	New York-Presbyterian Hospital	85.3	8	4	6,627	2.8	No	Yes	5	9	Yes	17.4%
5	UCSF Medical Center, San Francisco	84.7	7	6	2,618	2.4	Yes	Yes	4	9	Yes	21.1%
6	Cleveland Clinic	83.7	9	6	3,879	2.1	Yes	Yes	5	9	Yes	21.0%
7	Barnes-Jewish Hospital, St. Louis, Mo.	77.6	7	5	4,534	2.4	Yes	Yes	5	9	Yes	8.1%
8	Univ. of Michigan Hospitals and Health Centers, Ann Arbor	76.7	8	6	2,118	2.8	Yes	Yes	5	9	Yes	5.5%
9	Northwestern Memorial Hospital, Chicago	76.6	9	6	2,117	1.6	Yes	Yes	5	9	Yes	2.7%
10	NYU Langone Medical Center, New York	75.8	8	5	3,277	2.6	Yes	Yes	5	9	Yes	4.2%
11	Ronald Reagan UCLA Medical Center, Los Angeles	75.7	7	5	3,145	3.0	Yes	Yes	5	9	Yes	9.5%
12	Hosps. of the Univ. of Pennsylvania-Penn Presby., Philadelphia	73.4	6	5	2,808	2.3	Yes	Yes	5	9	Yes	8.4%
13	Stanford Health Care-Stanford Hospital, Stanford, Calif.	72.3	7	6	2,458	2.5	Yes	Yes	5	9	Yes	5.8%
14	Cedars-Sinai Medical Center, Los Angeles	72.0	9	5	4,485	2.6	Yes	Yes	5	9	Yes	2.1%
15	St. Joseph's Hospital and Medical Center, Phoenix	71.4	8	6	4,449	1.8	No	Yes	5	9	Yes	6.7%
16	Mount Sinai Hospital, New York	71.3	8	7	2,554	2.0	Yes	Yes	5	9	Yes	2.4%
17	Rush University Medical Center, Chicago	70.6	9	5	2,086	2.3	Yes	Yes	5	9	Yes	2.9%
18	Houston Methodist Hospital	70.1	9	6	3,959	2.0	Yes	Yes	5	9	Yes	2.6%
19	Brigham and Women's Hospital, Boston	69.4	7	5	3,101	2.4	No	Yes	5	9	Yes	8.2%
20	UPMC Presbyterian Shadyside, Pittsburgh	67.5	6	5	7,454	1.9	Yes	Yes	5	9	Yes	3.1%
21	Thomas Jefferson University Hospitals, Philadelphia	66.9	7	6	5,097	2.2	Yes	Yes	5	9	Yes	2.8%
22	Ohio State University Wexner Medical Center, Columbus	66.7	8	5	3,490	2.0	Yes	Yes	5	9	Yes	1.7%
23	DMC Harper University Hospital, Detroit	66.0	10	5	676	1.7	Yes	Yes	5	8	Yes	0.1%
24	Ochsner Medical Center, New Orleans	65.2	8	5	2,899	2.1	Yes	Yes	5	9	Yes	0.4%
25	Beaumont Hospital-Royal Oak, Mich.	65.1	8	6	4,473	1.9	Yes	Yes	5	9	Yes	0.1%
26	University of California, Davis Medical Center, Sacramento	64.0	7	5	1,911	2.7	Yes	Yes	5	9	Yes	0.3%
26	University of Kansas Hospital, Kansas City	64.0	7	5	2,136	2.0	Yes	Yes	5	9	Yes	1.3%
28	University of Colorado Hospital, Aurora	63.6	8	5	2,055	2.3	Yes	Yes	5	9	Yes	1.6%
28	Yale-New Haven Hospital, New Haven, Conn.	63.6	6	4	4,162	2.0	Yes	Yes	5	9	Yes	2.5%
30	Indiana University Health University Hospital, Indianapolis	63.5	7	5	3,133	2.0	Yes	Yes	5	9	Yes	1.1%
31	Mayo Clinic Jacksonville, Fla.	63.4	6	6	1,707	2.1	Yes	Yes	5	9	Yes	3.7%
32	University Hospitals Cleveland Medical Center	63.0	8	5	2,861	2.4	Yes	Yes	5	9	Yes	1.1%
33	Mayo Clinic Phoenix	62.9	7	6	2,070	2.9	No	Yes	5	9	Yes	3.6%
34	Emory University Hospital, Atlanta	62.8	6	5	2,209	1.9	Yes	Yes	5	9	Yes	3.6%
34	University of Alabama at Birmingham Hospital, Birmingham	62.8	7	6	3,966	1.8	Yes	Yes	5	8	Yes	1.6%
36	UF Health Shands Hospital, Gainesville, Fla.	62.7	6	5	2,847	1.9	Yes	Yes	5	9	Yes	3.1%
37	Wake Forest Baptist Medical Center, Winston-Salem, N.C.	62.0	6	5	3,703	1.6	Yes	Yes	5	9	Yes	1.5%
38	UT Southwestern Medical Center, Dallas	61.4	8	5	1,636	2.1	Yes	No	5	9	Yes	2.4%
39	UR Medicine Strong Memorial Hospital, Rochester, N.Y.	60.7	6	5	3,299	1.8	Yes	Yes	5	9	Yes	2.5%
40	Baylor St. Luke's Medical Center, Houston	60.6	8	5	2,126	1.5	Yes	Yes	5	8	Yes	2.2%
40	UC San Diego Medical Center	60.6	6	5	1,617	2.1	Yes	Yes	5	9	Yes	1.1%
42	Abbott Northwestern Hospital, Minneapolis	60.0	8	5	3,928	2.2	Yes	Yes	5	9	Yes	0.1%
43	University of Wisconsin Hospitals, Madison	59.7	6	5	2,215	2.5	Yes	Yes	5	9	Yes	1.3%
44	University of Kentucky Albert B. Chandler Hospital, Lexington	59.6	6	6	2,716	1.9	Yes	Yes	5	9	Yes	0.4%
45	OHSU Hospital, Portland, Ore.	59.4	5	5	2,483	2.0	Yes	Yes	5	9	Yes	1.8%
46	Duke University Hospital, Durham, N.C.	59.0	5	5	2,236	2.1	Yes	Yes	5	9	Yes	5.2%
46	St. Luke's Hospital of Kansas City, Mo.	59.0	7	5	3,256	1.5	Yes	Yes	5	9	Yes	0.1%
48	Memorial Hermann-Texas Medical Center, Houston	58.9	6	5	4,148	2.1	Yes	Yes	5	9	Yes	2.0%
49	OhioHealth Riverside Methodist Hospital, Columbus	58.8	6	5	6,159	2.0	Yes	Yes	5	9	Yes	0.2%
50	Hackensack University Medical Center, Hackensack, N.J.	58.7	7	5	2,462	2.4	Yes	Yes	5	9	Yes	0.4%

Terms are explained on Page 102.

More @ usnews.com/besthospitals

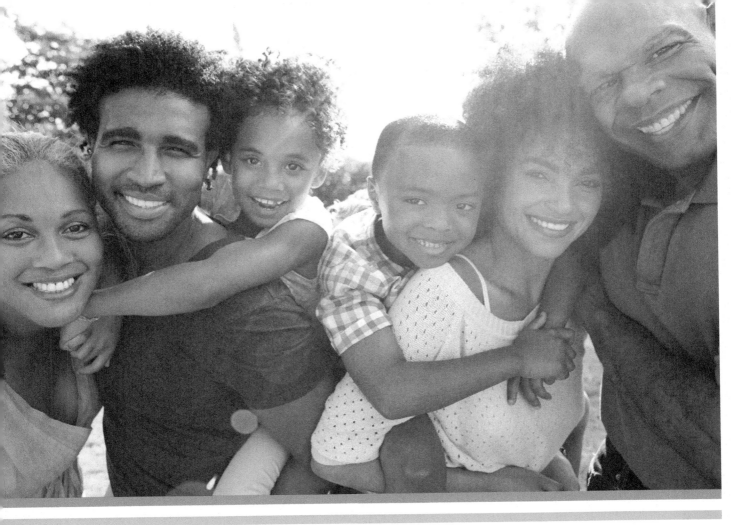

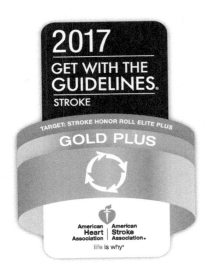

2017
GET WITH THE GUIDELINES.
STROKE

TARGET: STROKE HONOR ROLL ELITE PLUS
GOLD PLUS

American **Heart** Association | American **Stroke** Association.

life is why*

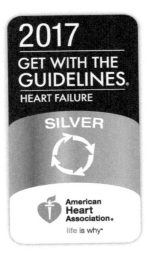

2017
GET WITH THE GUIDELINES.
HEART FAILURE

SILVER

American **Heart** Association.

life is why*

UI Health's Neurology and Cardiology programs are recognized by the American Heart Association/American Stroke Association, so our patients know they will receive the best care.

We are proud to have received Get With The Guidelines™ recognitions for both Stroke and Heart Failure care.

Visit us at UIHealth.Care

✚ UI Health | UIC

ORTHOPEDICS

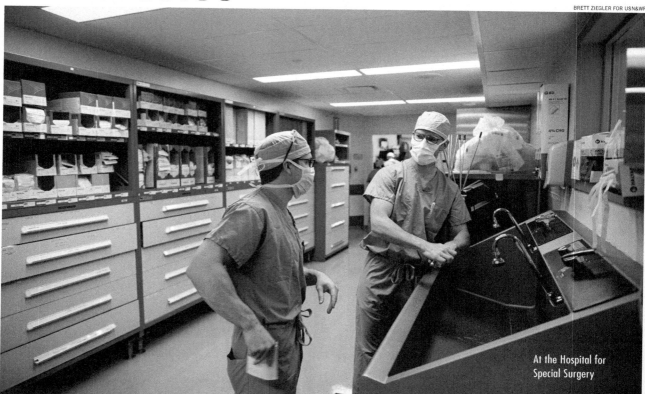

BRETT ZIEGLER FOR USN&WR

At the Hospital for
Special Surgery

Rank	Hospital	U.S. News score	Survival score (10=best)	Patient safety score (9=best)	Number of patients	Nurse staffing score (higher is better)	A Nurse Magnet hospital	Technology score (2=best)	Patient services score (7=best)	Intensivists	% of specialists recommending hospital
1	Hospital for Special Surgery, New York	100.0	10	9	14,152	3.3	Yes	2	7	Yes	36.0%
2	Mayo Clinic, Rochester, Minn.	82.4	9	5	7,791	2.7	Yes	2	7	Yes	30.7%
3	Cleveland Clinic	73.6	10	6	3,230	2.1	Yes	2	7	Yes	18.7%
4	Rothman Institute at Thomas Jefferson Univ. Hosps., Philadelphia	72.2	10	6	5,438	2.2	Yes	2	7	Yes	8.6%
5	Rush University Medical Center, Chicago	71.0	10	5	2,623	2.3	Yes	2	7	Yes	9.6%
6	UCSF Medical Center, San Francisco	69.5	10	6	2,798	2.4	Yes	2	7	Yes	4.0%
7	Massachusetts General Hospital, Boston	68.6	9	5	3,318	2.4	Yes	2	7	Yes	11.7%
8	Hosp. for Joint Diseases, NYU Langone Med. Center, New York	66.8	9	5	5,435	2.6	Yes	2	7	Yes	6.6%
9	Northwestern Memorial Hospital, Chicago	66.7	10	6	2,917	1.6	Yes	2	7	Yes	2.7%
10	Cedars-Sinai Medical Center, Los Angeles	66.5	10	5	5,948	2.6	Yes	2	7	Yes	2.3%
11	Johns Hopkins Hospital, Baltimore	65.8	10	5	1,128	2.2	Yes	2	7	Yes	6.5%
12	Stanford Health Care-Stanford Hospital, Stanford, Calif.	64.8	9	6	4,194	2.5	Yes	2	7	Yes	2.1%
13	Barnes-Jewish Hospital, St. Louis, Mo.	64.1	9	5	4,114	2.4	Yes	2	7	Yes	6.0%
14	Santa Monica-UCLA Medical Center and Orthopedic Hospital	62.8	9	5	2,344	3.0	Yes	2	7	Yes	2.2%
15	New England Baptist Hospital, Boston	62.4	10	6	4,494	2.3	No	2	7	Yes	1.2%
16	Hosps. of the Univ. of Pennsylvania-Penn Presby., Philadelphia	62.1	9	5	2,242	2.3	Yes	2	7	Yes	2.9%
17	University of Iowa Hospitals and Clinics, Iowa City	62.0	10	5	1,899	1.8	Yes	2	7	Yes	5.6%
18	University of Colorado Hospital, Aurora	61.9	10	5	2,236	2.3	Yes	2	7	Yes	1.1%
19	Abbott Northwestern Hospital, Minneapolis	61.8	10	5	6,545	2.2	Yes	2	7	Yes	0.5%
20	UC San Diego Medical Center	61.7	10	5	1,791	2.1	Yes	2	7	Yes	0.9%
21	Houston Methodist Hospital	61.2	9	6	4,549	2.0	Yes	2	7	Yes	2.6%
22	Duke University Hospital, Durham, N.C.	60.7	8	5	2,360	2.1	Yes	2	7	Yes	6.1%

(CONTINUED ON PAGE 126)

Terms are explained on Page 102.

More @ usnews.com/besthospitals

Thank you to everyone who helped us earn our **eighth consecutive #1 ranking.**

Sustained success is not something we take for granted. HSS has been among the top-rated institutions for orthopedics and rheumatology in the U.S. for 26 consecutive years. Whether we're conducting industry-leading research or delivering new levels of highly personalized musculoskeletal care, we remain steadfast in our commitment to always leading the way.

ORTHOPEDICS (CONTINUED)

Rank	Hospital	U.S. News score	Survival score (10=best)	Patient safety score (9=best)	Number of patients	Nurse staffing score (higher is better)	A Nurse Magnet hospital	Technology score (2=best)	Patient services score (7=best)	Intensivists	% of specialists recommending hospital
22	UPMC Presbyterian Shadyside, Pittsburgh	60.7	7	5	5,124	1.9	Yes	2	7	Yes	6.9%
24	Keck Hospital of USC, Los Angeles	60.3	10	6	2,116	3.0	No	2	7	Yes	2.5%
25	Hoag Memorial Hospital Presbyterian, Newport Beach, Calif.	59.8	9	7	6,768	2.3	Yes	2	7	Yes	0.0%
26	Magee-Womens Hospital of UPMC, Pittsburgh	59.7	10	5	1,090	0.8	No	2	7	Yes	0.0%
27	Pennsylvania Hospital, Philadelphia	59.3	10	5	1,578	1.6	Yes	2	7	Yes	0.6%
28	Beaumont Hospital-Royal Oak, Mich.	59.2	8	6	5,754	1.9	Yes	2	7	Yes	1.1%
28	Univ. of Michigan Hospitals and Health Centers, Ann Arbor	59.2	8	6	1,619	2.8	Yes	2	7	Yes	2.1%
30	Northwestern Medicine Central DuPage Hospital, Winfield, Ill.	59.1	9	5	2,503	1.8	Yes	2	7	Yes	0.1%
31	Cleveland Clinic Florida, Weston	59.0	10	5	1,183	2.2	No	2	7	Yes	0.4%
31	University of California, Davis Medical Center, Sacramento	59.0	9	5	2,037	2.7	Yes	2	7	Yes	0.9%
33	University of Virginia Medical Center, Charlottesville	58.5	9	5	1,862	2.0	Yes	2	7	Yes	1.6%
34	Carolinas Medical Center, Charlotte, N.C.	58.1	8	6	3,718	1.9	Yes	2	7	Yes	2.8%
34	Emory University Hospital, Atlanta	58.1	9	5	2,225	1.9	Yes	2	6	Yes	1.1%
34	Scripps La Jolla Hospitals, La Jolla, Calif.	58.1	8	6	3,824	3.1	Yes	2	6	Yes	1.2%
37	Porter Adventist Hospital, Denver	57.9	10	5	3,560	1.8	Yes	2	6	Yes	0.3%
38	Mercy Medical Center, Baltimore	57.8	10	5	2,429	1.3	Yes	2	6	Yes	0.0%
39	Loyola University Medical Center, Maywood, Ill.	57.7	9	6	1,147	2.4	Yes	2	7	Yes	0.6%
39	Mayo Clinic Phoenix	57.7	10	6	3,487	2.9	No	2	7	Yes	1.2%
41	UW Medicine/Harborview Medical Center, Seattle	57.4	10	6	1,565	1.9	No	2	6	Yes	3.3%
42	VCU Medical Center, Richmond, Va.	57.2	9	5	1,414	2.1	Yes	2	7	Yes	0.8%
43	University Hospitals Cleveland Medical Center	57.1	8	5	1,480	2.4	Yes	2	7	Yes	2.5%
44	Mount Sinai Hospital, New York	57.0	8	7	2,493	2.0	Yes	2	7	Yes	0.5%
45	University of Washington Medical Center, Seattle	56.9	10	5	793	2.1	Yes	1	7	Yes	2.3%
45	University of Wisconsin Hospitals, Madison	56.9	8	5	1,691	2.5	Yes	2	7	Yes	0.9%
47	Hackensack University Medical Center, Hackensack, N.J.	56.8	8	5	2,296	2.4	Yes	2	7	Yes	0.4%
48	Penn State Milton S. Hershey Medical Center, Hershey	56.5	8	5	1,870	2.1	Yes	2	7	Yes	0.3%
49	Morristown Medical Center, Morristown, N.J.	56.4	8	4	3,936	2.1	Yes	2	7	Yes	0.3%
50	Brigham and Women's Hospital, Boston	56.3	8	5	2,380	2.4	No	2	7	Yes	5.8%

Terms are explained on Page 102.

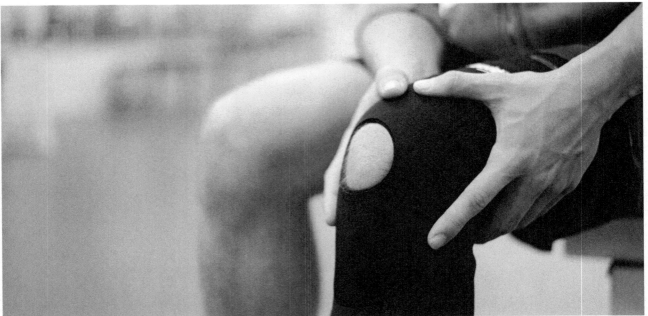

GETTY IMAGES

▶ **More** @ usnews.com/besthospitals

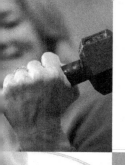

OUTSTANDING HOSPITALS DON'T SIMPLY TREAT FRAGILITY FRACTURES—
THEY PREVENT FRACTURES FROM RECURRING

THE BEST HOSPITALS AND PRACTICES OWN THE BONE.

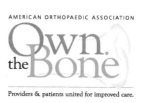

AMERICAN ORTHOPAEDIC ASSOCIATION

Own.
the Bone

Providers & patients united for improved care.

The American Orthopaedic Association applauds the following institutions for their achievements and participation in the Own the Bone® quality improvement program:

STAR PERFORMERS

Institutions are recognized for at least 75% compliance on 5 of the 10 recommended measures over the last year.

Akron General Medical Center - Akron, OH

Allina Health-Buffalo Hospital - Buffalo, MN

Anne Arundel Medical Group Orthopedics and Sports Medicine Specialists - Annapolis, MD

Berkshire Medical Center - Pittsfield, MA

Chippenham & Johnston Willis Hospitals/CJW Medical Center - Richmond, VA

^**Christiana Hospital** - Greenville, DE

Coastal Fracture Prevention Center - Sebastian, FL

Colorado Spine Institute PLLC - Loveland, CO

Concord Hospital - Concord, NH

Cooper Health System - Camden, NJ

Cox Medical Center Branson - Branson, MO

Crystal Clinic Orthopaedic Center - Akron, OH

Doylestown Health - Doylestown, PA

ETMC First Physicians Orthopedic Institute - Tyler, TX

Forsyth Medical Center - Winston Salem, NC

Good Samaritan Hospital - San Jose - San Jose, CA

^**Greenville Hospital System University Medical Center** - Greenville, SC

Herrin Hospital - Herrin, IL

Hoag Orthopedic Institute - Irvine, CA

Huntington Hospital - Northwell Health - Huntington, NY

^**Huntsville Hospital** - Huntsville, AL

Illinois Bone & Joint Institute, LLC - Morton Grove, IL

Jefferson Hospital - Pittsburgh, PA

JPS Health Network - Fort Worth, TX

Lakeshore Bone and Joint Institute - Chesterton, IN

LewisGale Medical Center - Salem, VA

MaineGeneral Medical Center - Augusta, ME

Marshfield Clinic - Marshfield, WI

Medical Center Arlington - Arlington, TX

Medical University of South Carolina - Charleston, SC

Memorial Regional Hospital - Hollywood, FL

Mercy Regional Medical Center - Durango, CO

Michigan Neurosurgical Institute - Grand Blanc, MI

Mission Hospital - Asheville, NC

NewYork-Presbyterian/Queens - Flushing, NY

Northwestern Medicine Central DuPage Hospital - Winfield, IL

Northwestern Medicine Delnor Hospital - Geneva, IL

Norton Women's and Children's Hospital - Louisville, KY

Norwalk Hospital - Norwalk, CT

NWIA Bone, Joint & Sports Surgeons - Spencer, IA

OhioHealth Grant Medical Center - Columbus, OH

^**Oklahoma Sports and Orthopedics Institute - Bone Health Clinic** - Norman, OK

Orthopaedic Associates of Michigan - Grand Rapids, MI

Palmetto Health - Columbia, SC

Paramount Care, Inc. - Maumee, OH

^**Park Nicollet Methodist Hospital** - Minneapolis, MN

Parkview Regional Medical Center - Fort Wayne, IN

Peninsula Regional Medical Center - Salisbury, MD

ProMedica Toledo Hospital - Toledo, OH

Regions Hospital/HealthPartners Orthopaedic and Sports Medicine - Minneapolis, MN

Sacred Heart Hospital - Pensacola - Pensacola, FL

^**Sanford Medical Center Fargo** - Fargo, ND

Southeast Georgia Health System - Brunswick, GA

St. Luke's Boise Medical Center - Boise, ID

St. Luke's University Hospital and Health Network - Bethlehem, PA

St. Vincent's Medical Center - Bridgeport, CT

Tahoe Forest Health System - Truckee, CA

Tallahassee Memorial HealthCare - Tallahassee, FL

The CORE Institute - Arizona - Phoenix, AZ

The Medical Center of Aurora - Aurora, CO

The Methodist Hospitals Spine Care Center - Merrillville, IN

The Ohio State University Medical Center - Columbus, OH

^**The Queen's Medical Center** - Honolulu, HI

University Hospital - San Antonio, TX

University of Michigan Hospitals & Health Centers - Ann Arbor, MI

University of Wisconsin Hospitals and Clinics - Madison, WI

UW Medicine Northwest Hospital and Medical Center - Seattle, WA

VCU HealthSystem - Richmond, VA

Western Reserve Hospital - Cuyahoga Falls, OH

^**Wilmington Hospital** - Wilmington, DE

Winthrop-University Hospital - Mineola, NY

^**WVU Hospitals, Department of Orthopaedics** - Morgantown, WV

NEWLY ENROLLED INSTITUTIONS

Eastern Maine Medical Center - Bangor, ME

Florida Hospital Flagler Orthopedics & Sports Medicine - Palm Coast, FL

Heiden Orthopedics - Cottonwood Heights, UT

Hilo Medical Center - Hilo, HI

Mendelson Kornblum Orthopedic & Spine Specialists - Livonia, MI

^**Mountain View Regional Hospital & Clinic** - Casper, WY

***Newton Medical Center** - Newton, KS

Northwest Orthopaedic Specialists - Spokane, WA

***NYU Langone Health** - New York City, NY

Providence St. Vincent Medical Center - Portland, OR

Sturgis Orthopedics - Sturgis, MI

^***The University of Vermont Health Network - Central Vermont Medical Center** - Berlin, VT

^First in State to enroll in Own the Bone®
*Also a Star Performer

Own the Bone is a national quality improvement initiative that provides institutions tools to ensure fragility fracture patients receive the heath care to prevent future fractures.

Visit us: www.ownthebone.org

The AOA recognizes **Radius Health** for its 2017 Own the Bone Educational Alliance support

PULMONOLOGY

Rank	Hospital	U.S. News score	Survival score (10=best)	Patient safety score (9=best)	Number of patients	Nurse staffing score (higher is better)	A Nurse Magnet hospital	Technology score (6=best)	Patient services score (8=best)	Intensivists	% of specialists recommending hospital
1	National Jewish Health, Denver-Univ. of Colorado Hosp., Aurora	100.0	9	5	4,102	2.3	Yes	6	8	Yes	46.7%
2	Mayo Clinic, Rochester, Minn.	97.6	9	5	7,609	2.7	Yes	6	8	Yes	31.6%
3	Cleveland Clinic	87.2	8	6	5,313	2.1	Yes	6	8	Yes	26.1%
4	Massachusetts General Hospital, Boston	82.9	8	5	6,099	2.4	Yes	6	8	Yes	12.6%
5	UPMC Presbyterian Shadyside, Pittsburgh	79.5	7	5	8,373	1.9	Yes	6	8	Yes	11.3%
6	UCSF Medical Center, San Francisco	78.8	7	6	3,389	2.4	Yes	6	8	Yes	12.7%
6	Univ. of Michigan Hospitals and Health Centers, Ann Arbor	78.8	8	6	3,930	2.8	Yes	6	8	Yes	6.3%
8	Barnes-Jewish Hospital, St. Louis, Mo.	77.9	7	5	5,471	2.4	Yes	6	8	Yes	9.7%
9	Hosps. of the Univ. of Pennsylvania-Penn Presby., Philadelphia	77.3	7	5	5,612	2.3	Yes	6	8	Yes	10.4%
10	Ronald Reagan UCLA Medical Center, Los Angeles	77.1	7	5	6,755	3.0	Yes	6	8	Yes	4.7%
11	Johns Hopkins Hospital, Baltimore	76.6	6	5	2,501	2.2	Yes	6	8	Yes	17.2%
12	Duke University Hospital, Durham, N.C.	75.9	6	5	4,173	2.1	Yes	6	8	Yes	12.4%
13	UC San Diego Medical Center	74.9	7	5	3,332	2.1	Yes	6	8	Yes	7.3%
14	Mayo Clinic Phoenix	74.7	10	6	5,105	2.9	No	5	8	Yes	2.6%
15	Houston Methodist Hospital	74.6	9	6	6,195	2.0	Yes	6	8	Yes	1.5%
15	Scripps La Jolla Hospitals, La Jolla, Calif.	74.6	9	6	4,439	3.1	Yes	5	8	Yes	0.1%
17	New York-Presbyterian Hospital	74.2	7	4	11,686	2.8	No	6	8	Yes	7.6%
17	University of Alabama at Birmingham Hospital, Birmingham	74.2	8	6	5,531	1.8	Yes	6	8	Yes	2.3%
19	Yale-New Haven Hospital, New Haven, Conn.	74.0	7	4	10,812	2.0	Yes	5	8	Yes	3.8%
20	Cedars-Sinai Medical Center, Los Angeles	73.4	7	5	10,294	2.6	Yes	6	8	Yes	1.5%
21	Northwestern Memorial Hospital, Chicago	73.3	8	6	3,552	1.6	Yes	6	8	Yes	2.8%
22	Beaumont Hospital-Royal Oak, Mich.	73.2	8	6	9,278	1.9	Yes	5	8	Yes	0.1%
23	St. Luke's Regional Medical Center, Boise, Idaho	72.8	10	6	5,028	2.2	Yes	5	6	Yes	0.0%
24	University of California, Davis Medical Center, Sacramento	72.1	9	5	4,348	2.7	Yes	5	8	Yes	0.5%
25	Ohio State University Wexner Medical Center, Columbus	71.9	8	5	5,943	2.0	Yes	6	8	Yes	1.0%
26	Cleveland Clinic Fairview Hospital, Cleveland	71.7	9	6	3,307	1.9	Yes	5	8	Yes	0.1%
26	NYU Langone Medical Center, New York	71.7	7	5	6,950	2.6	Yes	5	8	Yes	2.2%
28	Miami Valley Hospital, Dayton, Ohio	71.1	8	5	6,233	2.6	Yes	5	8	Yes	0.5%
28	Tampa General Hospital	71.1	8	4	3,853	2.2	Yes	6	7	Yes	1.1%
28	University of Wisconsin Hospitals, Madison	71.1	8	5	2,957	2.5	Yes	6	8	Yes	1.2%
31	Cleveland Clinic Akron General Medical Center, Ohio	71.0	9	4	5,218	1.3	Yes	5	8	Yes	0.1%
32	Loyola University Medical Center, Maywood, Ill.	70.9	8	6	2,346	2.4	Yes	6	8	Yes	1.5%
32	University of Kansas Hospital, Kansas City	70.9	9	5	3,452	2.0	Yes	5	8	Yes	1.3%
34	Mayo Clinic Jacksonville, Fla.	70.6	8	6	3,174	2.1	Yes	6	8	Yes	2.4%
34	UF Health Shands Hospital, Gainesville, Fla.	70.6	8	5	3,627	1.9	Yes	6	8	Yes	2.0%
34	Vanderbilt University Medical Center, Nashville	70.6	7	5	4,426	1.9	Yes	6	8	Yes	5.6%
37	Stanford Health Care-Stanford Hospital, Stanford, Calif.	70.5	7	6	4,414	2.5	Yes	6	8	Yes	2.8%
38	Froedtert Hospital and the Medical College of Wis., Milwaukee	70.2	8	5	3,622	1.8	Yes	6	8	Yes	0.9%
39	Brigham and Women's Hospital, Boston	69.8	7	5	4,842	2.4	No	6	8	Yes	8.4%
39	Indiana University Health University Hospital, Indianapolis	69.8	8	5	5,183	2.0	Yes	6	8	Yes	0.5%
39	St. Cloud Hospital, St. Cloud, Minn.	69.8	9	5	6,514	1.9	Yes	4	8	Yes	0.0%
42	Banner University Medical Center Tucson, Ariz.	69.3	9	4	2,809	1.8	Yes	6	7	Yes	0.2%
43	Spectrum Hlth Hosps. Butterworth-Blodgett, Grand Rapids, Mich.	69.1	7	4	9,044	1.6	Yes	6	8	Yes	0.2%
44	Banner Estrella Medical Center, Phoenix	69.0	10	5	2,141	1.8	Yes	5	8	Yes	0.0%
44	Rochester General Hospital, Rochester, N.Y.	69.0	9	4	5,186	1.9	Yes	5	8	Yes	0.0%
46	Hoag Memorial Hospital Presbyterian, Newport Beach, Calif.	68.9	7	7	8,681	2.3	Yes	5	8	Yes	0.0%
47	St. Luke's Hospital of Kansas City, Mo.	68.7	9	5	3,043	1.5	Yes	5	8	Yes	0.1%
48	Intermountain Medical Center, Murray, Utah	68.6	9	5	4,387	2.4	No	5	8	Yes	0.6%
48	University of Washington Medical Center, Seattle	68.6	7	5	1,751	2.1	Yes	6	8	Yes	6.5%
50	Aurora St. Luke's Medical Center, Milwaukee	68.5	9	3	7,122	2.0	Yes	5	8	Yes	0.1%

Terms are explained on Page 102.

▶ **More @ usnews.com/besthospitals**

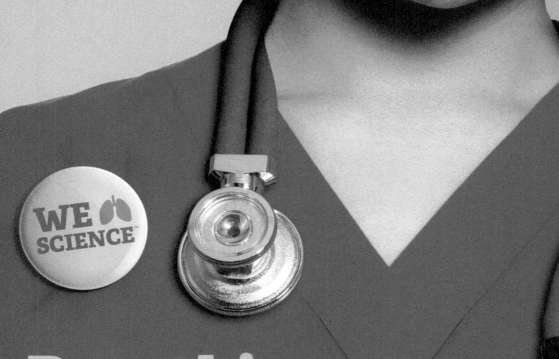

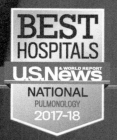

Breathing Science is Life.™

It's easy to take breathing for granted — until you can't.
At National Jewish Health, the nation's leading respiratory hospital, we help people who struggle to breathe get back to living the life they enjoy. For 118 years, our groundbreaking research and personalized care have transformed millions of lives. We breathe science, so you can breathe life. **To make an appointment, call 800.621.0505 or visit njhealth.org.**

National Jewish Health®

UROLOGY

Rank	Hospital	U.S. News score	Survival score (10=best)	Patient safety score (9=best)	Number of patients	Nurse staffing score (higher is better)	A Nurse Magnet hospital	Technology score (6=best)	Patient services score (9=best)	Intensivists	% of specialists recommending hospital
1	Cleveland Clinic	100.0	9	6	888	2.1	Yes	6	9	Yes	45.1%
2	Mayo Clinic, Rochester, Minn.	99.5	10	5	1,094	2.7	Yes	6	9	Yes	25.4%
3	Johns Hopkins Hospital, Baltimore	95.9	9	5	569	2.2	Yes	6	9	Yes	35.4%
4	Ronald Reagan UCLA Medical Center, Los Angeles	86.6	8	5	580	3.0	Yes	6	9	Yes	17.5%
5	Memorial Sloan Kettering Cancer Center, New York	86.3	9	6	999	2.1	Yes	6	8	Yes	12.7%
6	UCSF Medical Center, San Francisco	85.1	8	6	671	2.4	Yes	6	9	Yes	12.2%
7	Univ. of Michigan Hospitals and Health Centers, Ann Arbor	83.7	9	6	743	2.8	Yes	6	9	Yes	6.3%
8	New York-Presbyterian Hospital	80.4	8	4	1,348	2.8	No	6	9	Yes	8.6%
9	Vanderbilt University Medical Center, Nashville	80.2	7	5	828	1.9	Yes	6	9	Yes	12.3%
10	Duke University Hospital, Durham, N.C.	80.1	8	5	448	2.1	Yes	6	9	Yes	10.5%
11	Northwestern Memorial Hospital, Chicago	79.0	10	6	381	1.6	Yes	6	9	Yes	4.7%
12	Cedars-Sinai Medical Center, Los Angeles	78.0	9	5	1,016	2.6	Yes	6	9	Yes	1.4%
13	UPMC Presbyterian Shadyside, Pittsburgh	77.7	8	5	838	1.9	Yes	6	9	Yes	3.6%
14	Stanford Health Care-Stanford Hospital, Stanford, Calif.	77.3	8	6	537	2.5	Yes	6	9	Yes	4.5%
15	NYU Langone Medical Center, New York	76.5	8	5	511	2.6	Yes	6	9	Yes	5.9%
16	University of Wisconsin Hospitals, Madison	76.0	9	5	390	2.5	Yes	6	9	Yes	1.8%
17	University of Kansas Hospital, Kansas City	75.6	9	5	472	2.0	Yes	6	9	Yes	2.0%
18	Barnes-Jewish Hospital, St. Louis, Mo.	74.4	8	5	745	2.4	Yes	6	9	Yes	3.6%
19	UT Southwestern Medical Center, Dallas	74.2	9	5	566	2.1	Yes	6	9	Yes	4.2%
20	University of Alabama at Birmingham Hospital, Birmingham	73.8	9	6	411	1.8	Yes	6	9	Yes	1.2%
21	Beaumont Hospital-Royal Oak, Mich.	73.7	8	6	749	1.9	Yes	6	9	Yes	1.1%
22	Massachusetts General Hospital, Boston	73.4	7	5	583	2.4	Yes	6	9	Yes	5.9%
22	University of California, Davis Medical Center, Sacramento	73.4	9	5	488	2.7	Yes	6	9	Yes	0.8%
24	Tampa General Hospital	73.1	9	4	617	2.2	Yes	6	8	Yes	0.8%
25	Queen's Medical Center, Honolulu	72.7	10	5	393	1.8	Yes	6	8	Yes	0.0%
26	West Virginia University Hospitals, Morgantown	72.6	10	4	139	2.0	Yes	6	9	Yes	0.2%
27	Thomas Jefferson University Hospitals, Philadelphia	72.5	7	6	640	2.2	Yes	6	9	Yes	2.1%
28	University of Maryland Medical Center, Baltimore	72.4	10	2	307	2.1	Yes	6	8	Yes	0.2%
29	Keck Hospital of USC, Los Angeles	72.0	7	6	924	3.0	No	6	9	Yes	8.1%
29	Yale-New Haven Hospital, New Haven, Conn.	72.0	8	4	887	2.0	Yes	6	9	Yes	0.9%
31	University of Iowa Hospitals and Clinics, Iowa City	71.6	9	5	318	1.8	Yes	6	9	Yes	1.3%
32	University of North Carolina Hospitals, Chapel Hill	71.5	8	5	461	2.0	Yes	6	9	Yes	2.8%
33	Christ Hospital, Cincinnati	71.2	10	5	252	1.9	Yes	6	8	Yes	0.8%
33	University of Cincinnati Medical Center	71.2	10	5	127	1.7	No	6	9	Yes	1.5%
35	University of Virginia Medical Center, Charlottesville	70.9	8	5	250	2.0	Yes	6	9	Yes	2.2%
36	Hosps. of the Univ. of Pennsylvania-Penn Presby., Philadelphia	70.7	7	5	635	2.3	Yes	6	9	Yes	3.1%
36	Indiana University Health University Hospital, Indianapolis	70.7	6	5	699	2.0	Yes	6	9	Yes	4.1%
38	University of Colorado Hospital, Aurora	70.6	8	5	529	2.3	Yes	6	9	Yes	0.6%
39	Loyola University Medical Center, Maywood, Ill.	70.5	8	6	402	2.4	Yes	6	8	Yes	2.1%
39	Nebraska Medicine-Nebraska Medical Center, Omaha	70.5	9	5	276	2.6	Yes	6	9	Yes	0.1%
41	Huntington Memorial Hospital, Pasadena, Calif.	70.3	8	6	264	2.5	Yes	6	9	Yes	0.2%
42	Hahnemann University Hospital, Philadelphia	69.8	10	5	114	1.7	Yes	6	9	No	0.0%
42	Moffitt Cancer Center and Research Institute, Tampa	69.8	10	4	578	1.2	Yes	6	9	Yes	1.7%
44	Banner University Medical Center Phoenix	69.7	9	5	232	1.9	Yes	6	9	Yes	0.1%
44	St. Patrick Hospital, Missoula, Mont.	69.7	10	5	108	1.6	Yes	6	8	Yes	0.0%
46	MUSC Health-University Medical Center, Charleston, S.C.	69.6	9	5	264	2.0	Yes	6	9	Yes	0.6%
47	Mayo Clinic Phoenix	69.5	9	6	827	2.9	No	6	8	Yes	2.7%
48	Mount Sinai Hospital, New York	69.4	6	7	620	2.0	Yes	6	9	Yes	2.3%
49	Hackensack University Medical Center, Hackensack, N.J.	69.3	8	5	433	2.4	Yes	6	9	Yes	0.7%
50	Advocate Illinois Masonic Medical Center, Chicago	69.0	10	4	81	1.8	Yes	5	8	Yes	0.1%
50	St. Cloud Hospital, St. Cloud, Minn.	69.0	9	5	513	1.9	Yes	5	9	Yes	0.0%

Terms are explained on Page 102.

● More @ usnews.com/besthospitals

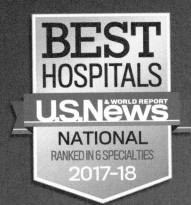
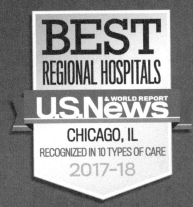
  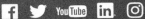
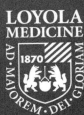

THESE HOSPITALS ARE AMONG THE BEST in their specialty for particularly challenging patients, in the view of at least 5 percent of specialists who responded to the latest three years of U.S. News physician surveys.

Ophthalmology

Rank	Hospital	% of specialists recommending hospital
1	Bascom Palmer Eye Institute-Anne Bates Leach Eye Hosp., Miami	59.6%
2	Wills Eye Hospital, Thomas Jefferson U. Hospitals, Philadelphia	53.0%
3	Wilmer Eye Institute, Johns Hopkins Hospital, Baltimore	43.1%
4	Massachusetts Eye and Ear Infirmary, Mass. General Hosp., Boston	29.1%
5	Stein and Doheny Eye Institutes, UCLA Medical Cen., Los Angeles	23.7%
6	Duke University Hospital, Durham, N.C.	12.6%
6	University of Iowa Hospitals and Clinics, Iowa City	12.6%
8	W.K. Kellogg Eye Center, University of Michigan, Ann Arbor	9.4%
9	Cole Eye Institute, Cleveland Clinic	9.0%
10	UCSF Medical Center, San Francisco	7.0%
11	USC Roski Eye Institute, Los Angeles	5.7%
12	New York Eye and Ear Infirmary of Mount Sinai, N.Y.	5.6%
13	Emory University Hospital, Atlanta	5.1%

Psychiatry

Rank	Hospital	% of specialists recommending hospital
1	McLean Hospital, Belmont, Mass.	23.0%
2	Massachusetts General Hospital, Boston	20.0%
3	Menninger Clinic, Houston	17.7%
4	New York-Presbyterian Hospital	16.8%
5	Johns Hopkins Hospital, Baltimore	16.4%
6	Sheppard and Enoch Pratt Hospital, Baltimore	15.2%
7	Mayo Clinic, Rochester, Minn.	12.0%
8	Resnick Neuropsychiatric Hospital at UCLA, Los Angeles	11.7%
9	Austen Riggs Center, Stockbridge, Mass.	6.9%
10	UCSF Medical Center, San Francisco	6.4%
11	Yale-New Haven Hospital, New Haven, Conn.	5.7%
12	UPMC Presbyterian Shadyside, Pittsburgh	5.2%

Rehabilitation

Rank	Hospital	% of specialists recommending hospital
1	Shirley Ryan AbilityLab, Chicago	39.4%
2	TIRR Memorial Hermann, Houston	22.2%
3	Kessler Institute for Rehabilitation, West Orange, N.J.	20.4%
4	Spaulding Rehabilitation Hospital, Mass. General Hosp., Boston	18.9%
5	University of Washington Medical Center, Seattle	17.9%
6	Mayo Clinic, Rochester, Minn.	15.7%
7	Craig Hospital, Englewood, Colo.	12.6%
8	Rusk Rehabilitation at NYU Langone Medical Center, New York	10.4%
9	Shepherd Center, Atlanta	9.6%
10	MossRehab, Elkins Park, Pa.	7.9%
11	UPMC Presbyterian Shadyside, Pittsburgh	6.0%
12	New York-Presbyterian Hospital	5.6%
13	Magee Rehabilitation Hospital, Philadelphia	5.2%
14	University of Michigan Hospitals and Health Centers, Ann Arbor	5.0%

Rheumatology

Rank	Hospital	% of specialists recommending hospital
1	Johns Hopkins Hospital, Baltimore	43.8%
2	Cleveland Clinic	39.3%
3	Hospital for Special Surgery, New York-Presbyterian Hosp., N.Y.	39.1%
4	Mayo Clinic, Rochester, Minn.	35.8%
5	Brigham and Women's Hospital, Boston	23.1%
6	Ronald Reagan UCLA Medical Center, Los Angeles	18.8%
7	UCSF Medical Center, San Francisco	14.7%
8	Massachusetts General Hospital, Boston	14.1%
9	Hospital for Joint Diseases, NYU Langone Medical Cen., New York	12.6%
10	University of Alabama at Birmingham Hospital, Birmingham	9.7%
11	UPMC Presbyterian Shadyside, Pittsburgh	7.6%
12	University of Michigan Hospitals and Health Centers, Ann Arbor	7.4%
13	Duke University Hospital, Durham, N.C.	6.9%
14	Stanford Health Care-Stanford Hospital, Stanford, Calif.	5.9%

▶ **More** @ usnews.com/besthospitals

Carol Shields, MD,
Chief, Ocular Oncology
and Carter.

We have a way at Wills.

We believe that it is the bond between you
and your doctor that helps turn treatments
into cures. Skill with Compassion –
what our doctors provide every day.

WillsEye Hospital

840 Walnut Street Philadelphia, PA 19107 www.willseye.org 1-877-AT-WILLS

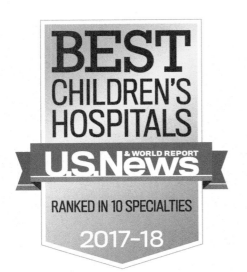

Proudly ranked in all 10 specialties.

We're honored to be the only children's hospital in Northern California to be ranked in all ten pediatric specialties by U.S. News & World Report.

Lucile Packard Children's Hospital Stanford, the centerpiece of Stanford Children's Health, has been **recognized for 13 consecutive years**, affirming the exceptional quality of care our faculty, physicians and staff provide to patients.

Stanford Children's Health

Lucile Packard Children's Hospital Stanford

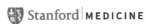

Learn more at stanfordchildrens.org

CHILDREN'S HEALTH

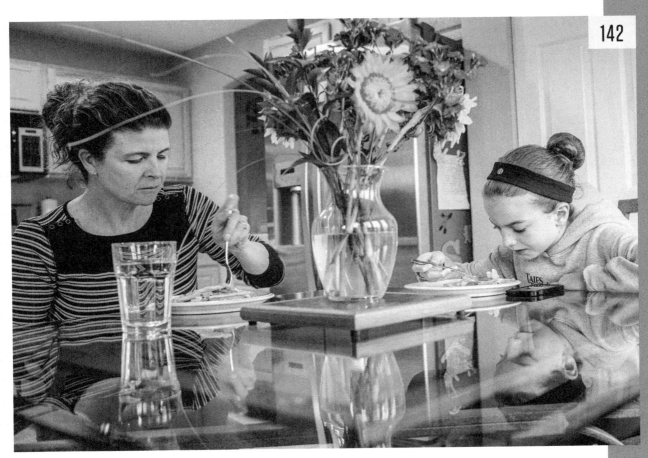

142

IMPROVING CARE OF THE MEDICALLY FRAGILE CHILD

Hospitals are finding better ways to manage and support kids with serious, complex conditions

By Linda Marsa

Victor Zapata seemed like a normal, healthy baby until suddenly, at just under 6 months old, he was gripped by intractable seizures. His condition steadily worsened; he suffered such a severe seizure on his first birthday that he was placed in an induced coma and was not expected to live. Miraculously, he did – although he was blind and partially deaf, and doctors much later diagnosed a rare genetic mutation that causes serious neurological damage, developmental deficits, and digestive issues as well as seizures. Now 16, Victor needs round-the-clock care, including bathing assistance, getting nutrition intravenously, suctioning of his airways, and the aid of a ventilator to help him breathe when he has seizures.

Still, with a lot of support from Nemours/Alfred I. duPont Hospital for Children in Wilmington, Delaware, Victor has always been able to live at home. "I had a child who was almost in a vegetative state," says Olga Zapata, who gave up a career as a chemist to become his full-time caregiver. "There was no way one person could do this." Hospital staffers helped the Zapatas – husband Luis pilots corporate jets – set up a fully equipped room for Victor, fight for insurance coverage, apply for Medicaid to supplement the coverage, and contact local nursing agencies to procure some relief. Now Victor has nursing care 16 hours a day. Teachers and therapists come to the house in the

mornings, and doctors at the hospital are on call in case of a crisis that lands the teen in the emergency room. "We spend a lot of time in the intensive care unit," says Zapata, who lives in nearby Newark. "But the hospital team makes sure he can recover at home. To save a child – that's where their priorities are, and there is never a moment of hesitation."

Victor Zapata is one of about 3 million kids in the United States who are considered medically fragile or medically complex. These youngsters have daunting health needs that may have been caused by a congenital, genetic or developmental disorder; an accident or traumatic brain injury that left them disabled or paralyzed and wheelchair bound; or a debilitating or chronic illness like cancer. What they share is a dependency on life-sustaining medications, treatments and equipment that assist with the activities of daily living, such as tube feedings, oxygen therapy, suctioning, tracheostomy care, and breathing with the aid of a ventilator.

The intense care – and care coordination – these children need are a growing focus of children's hospitals across the country. For one thing, such care is hugely expensive. Medicaid supports the needs of severely disabled children through waivers that disregard family income, and statistics reveal that the 6 percent of youngsters who are medically complex consume about 40 percent of Medicaid

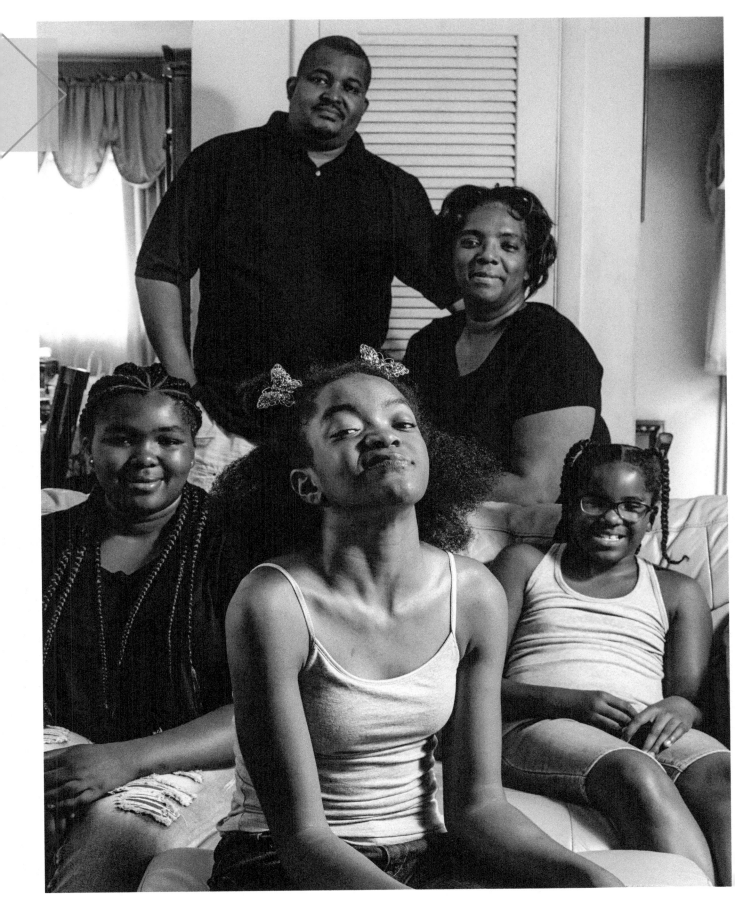

"Ten children's hospitals are testing new care models for 9,000 kids.

funding spent on kids. Programs like the one at Nemours/Alfred I. duPont that help families keep their children at home and cut down on hospital visits can rein in costs considerably.

They also can greatly improve the quality of care – and of families' lives. "These programs can help parents get the maximum benefits for their children and to realize their potential," says Kurt Newman, president and CEO of Children's National Health System in Washington, D.C. "We don't want to lose sight of that potential."

In addition to putting together its own comprehensive medical management program, Children's National developed a robust parent navigator initiative a decade ago. It has grown from a handful of parent volunteers with medically fragile kids to seven full-time staffers who connect families with such community resources as physical therapy, special education programs and summer camps and help them negotiate the maze of regulations involved in applying for assistance. They also provide a sympathetic sounding board. "Who better to assist families than someone who has been through it?" says Newman.

He and other experts worry that changes to Medicaid envisioned by Congress and the new administration would undermine these fledgling initiatives, leaving families in dire straits and hospitals drowning in red ink. In 2016 the Nemours Foundation, which operates a children's hospital in Orlando as well as the one in Delaware, experienced a $73 million gap between reimbursement by Medicaid and other public health programs and what it spent on care for eligible kids; it made up the shortfall via donations and support from the Alfred I. duPont Testamentary Trust. "We are stretched and pushed each year to make ends meet," says David J. Bailey, president and CEO of the Nemours Foundation.

Without aid, a child who has a complex disease or condition "will bankrupt a family in record time even when both parents are working," says Meri Armour, president and CEO of Le Bonheur Children's Hospital in Memphis, Tennessee, where 68 percent of kids are on Medicaid. "These kids count on our hospital as a resource."

Many such initiatives were launched as part of a three-year federally funded demonstration project. In partnership with the Children's Hospital Association, 10 of the nation's children's hospitals and their primary care physician partners are testing new care models for about 9,000 children. (Participants are Children's Hospital Colorado, Children's Mercy Kansas City, Children's National Health System, Cincinnati Children's Hospital Medical Center, Cook Children's Medical Center, Lucile Packard Children's Hospital Stanford, Mattel Children's Hospital UCLA, St. Joseph's Children's Hospital of Tampa, The Children's Hospital of Philadelphia and Wolfson Children's Hospital in Jacksonville, Florida.)

"What we've seen early on is very encouraging," says Mark Wietecha, president and CEO of the Children's Hospital Association. Given that even a minor cold or other manageable conditions can escalate into a full-blown crisis in these patients, for example, hotlines that operate around the clock, providing families with steps they can take at home, can often stave off panicked trips to the ER in the middle of the night. "Keeping parents connected to a network of caregivers [who] can answer their questions can provide reassurance about what to do," says Wietecha. The expectation is that reduced emergency department visits and hospitalizations will trim overall costs while easing stresses on families.

Other innovations include centralized scheduling for each child's doctors. At Children's Hospital Colorado,

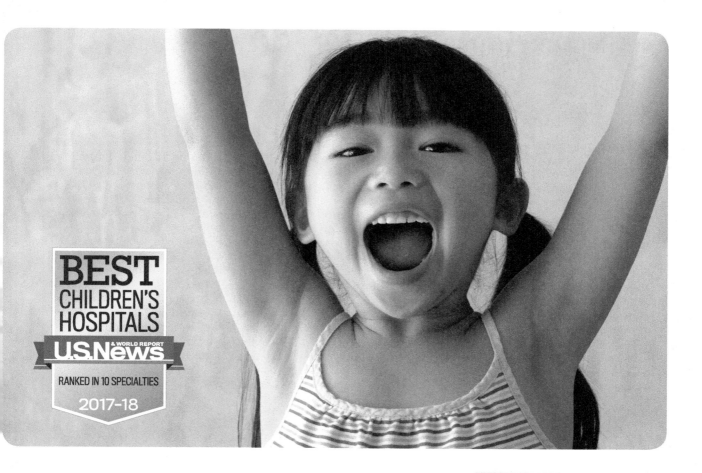

One of the best children's hospitals in the nation. 25 years and counting.

For the first time ever, Seattle Children's received national rankings for all 10 specialty areas, with every one of our programs ranked in the top 20 by *U.S. News & World Report*. We're extremely proud of this honor, and of the additional recognition we've received this year alone. To learn more, visit **seattlechildrens.org/usnews**

Our Research Institute is one of the nation's top five pediatric research centers in National Institutes of Health funding.

Our Hospital and Research Foundation was ranked as a top performing healthcare nonprofit for fundraising, with over $126 million raised for uncompensated care to help families pay for critical services.

Our medical school department of pediatrics was ranked #5 by *U.S. News & World Report*.

Named one of Becker's "100 Great Hospitals in America."

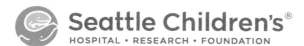

Seattle Children's®
HOSPITAL · RESEARCH · FOUNDATION

Hope. Care. Cure.™

for instance, parents can make multiple appointments at once and take an often difficult-to-transport child to see several specialists in one day. "We coordinate all of the things that need to be done within that visit cycle, from diagnostic testing to receiving lab results and seeing a team of specialists, so they don't have to come in on different days of the week," says Jena Hausmann, the hospital's president and CEO. Families also can call for a same-day appointment in the event of an urgent need.

This program has been a boon for the Fischer family of Denver, whose lives changed dramatically when Cecilia, then 11 months old, choked on a

doctors in Denver to consult 24/7 with local physicians and with families by video; the technology even allows a provider in Denver to listen through a special stethoscope to the distant patient's heartbeat. The hospital also offers clinics in rural areas across a broad swath of the Rocky Mountain region. Families who do have to travel to Denver for extended periods can take advantage of on-site schooling and tutoring to make sure patient and siblings can keep up with their studies.

Helping families put all the pieces in place is the mission of TjaMeika Davenport, a former music teacher in Maryland parochial schools who now is a parent navigator on the staff of

family has private health insurance and a middle-class income, but assistance through Maryland's autism waiver program – which the Davenports qualified for after nine years on the waiting list – has been a huge help since this past January, when they were finally able to gain the help of an autism technician who provides intensive in-home therapy.

Doctors and families alike say that a combination of cuts to Medicaid and a return to the days when patients with pre-existing conditions could be penalized and insurers could cap life-

Without aid, a child who has a complex disease or condition will bankrupt a family in record time.

piece of fruit and suffered severe brain damage that left her a quadriplegic and coping with epilepsy. Now 9, Cecelia is unable to speak or move and requires a gastronomy tube to eat and a tracheostomy to breathe. But the assistance hospital staffers have given to the family, which includes three other children ages 11, 9 and 5, enables them to live a somewhat normal life. "It took a really long time to get her stabilized, but now we don't have to be fighting fires all the time," says Jenny Fischer, who works from home for a management consulting firm while her husband teaches Spanish in junior and senior high school. "Now we're at the hospital maybe four or five times a year, tops."

Because Children's Hospital Colorado mainly serves a wide seven-state region, and patients in those states may travel 800 or 1,000 miles to be seen, a telemedicine option allows

Children's National Medical Center. "I tell them 'it's a new life, but this is doable,'" says Davenport, who speaks from experience. Her 12-year-old daughter, Kennedy, was born with three chromosomal abnormalities and has been a patient at the hospital since she was 3 months old. She suffers from intellectual impairments, gait problems that make it difficult to walk long distances, autism, ADHD and epilepsy. Even though she takes several medications to control what otherwise could be a hundred seizures a day, she wears a helmet because she still often experiences dozens.

Over the years, Kennedy's condition has stabilized, thanks to more than two dozen specialists and intensive physical, occupational and speech therapy, plus an arsenal of medications. Once she started school, her mother was able to return to work part time. The

time payouts would be devastating financially and leave many children without good care. Since qualifying for Medicaid, says Jenny Fischer, "all of a sudden, we can now breathe." The Fischers need home health care as well as a private nurse to suction Cecelia's lungs while she's in school, for example, and they have to replace her $25,000 wheelchair every few years as she grows. Private insurance pays just $2,000. Medicaid also provides an array of services that keep Cecelia healthy and out of the ER, including appointments with nutritionists, orthopedic and rehabilitation doctors, and weekly physical and occupational therapy. If they were to lose the assistance, she says, accessing the best care for Cecelia would become far, far more difficult. ●

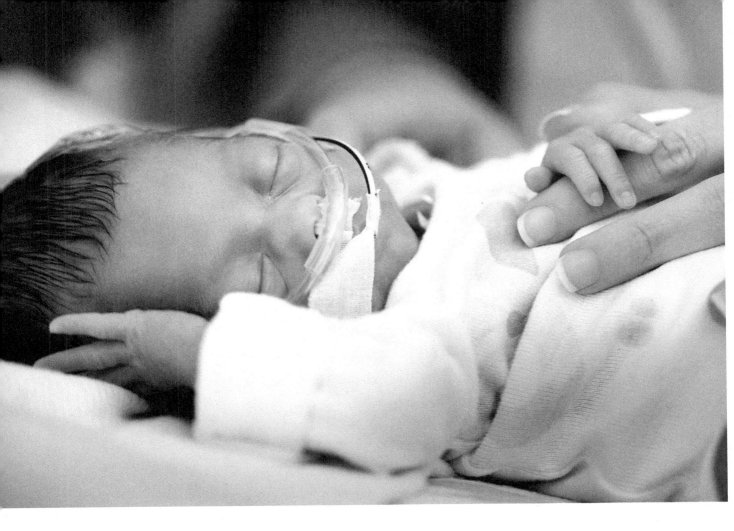

Accelerating the Future of Child Health

A national leader in pediatric medicine.
A global advocate for best outcomes in child health.

Discover more at **NationwideChildrens.org/future-health**

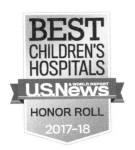

The Honor Roll recognizes
America's Top 10 Children's
Hospitals across all specialties

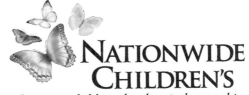

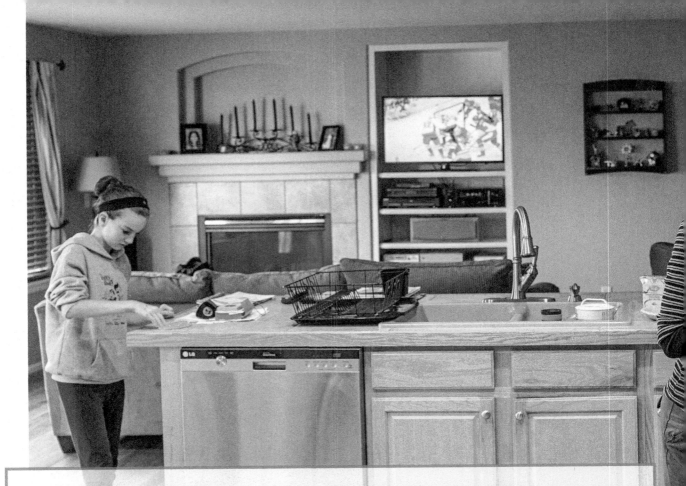

GOING GLUTEN-FREE?
A FEW CAVEATS FOR KIDS

Absent celiac disease, there are good reasons to eat wheat

By Katherine Hobson

Samara Schoch's 5-year-old checkup revealed the worrisome fact that the Centennial, Colorado, youngster wasn't growing as expected. When Samara's mom, Lana, mentioned that the little girl also consistently had stomachaches after eating, the pediatrician immediately prescribed a test for celiac disease. "I thought that was silly, but I was wrong," says Lana. Samara's blood tests for the condition, which causes inflammation of the small intestine when gluten found in wheat, barley and rye is eaten, were "off the charts." The only treatment: a gluten-free diet. "I would go to the grocery store and sit in the parking lot,

almost in tears," says Lana, recalling how overwhelmed she felt realizing that gluten is found in everything from bread to broth to salad dressing.

Samara, now 12, is shunning gluten because it keeps her disease in check. Consultations with a registered dietitian and classes at Children's Hospital Colorado have helped the family learn how to steer clear of problematic ingredients while still planning varied meals. There are separate toasters for Samara and her parents, and when the family eats out, they ask that gluten-free pasta be cooked in fresh water. But about 2.7 million Americans without celiac choose to follow a gluten-free diet, too, according to an analysis published last year. Market research firm NPD Group finds that 28 percent of adults are eliminating the protein or cutting back. And more than a few of them, it seems, are doing the

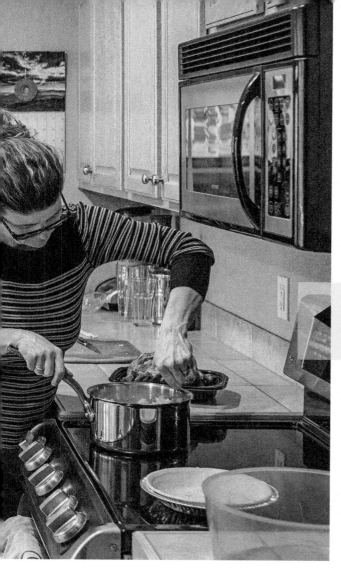

> ## The diet can be low in key nutrients – the B vitamins, vitamin D, iron, zinc, calcium.

Lana Schoch, right, has mastered the art of gluten-free meal prep for Samara, who has celiac disease.

same for the whole family. While there are no hard statistics on how many kids are eating gluten-free for reasons other than celiac disease, pediatricians say they've noticed an uptick in parents putting their kids on the diet.

Most "have heard bad things about gluten and think that going gluten-free is simply healthier," says Claire McCarthy, a pediatrician at Boston Children's Hospital. Some are responding to symptoms like constipation or stomachaches, or have heard it might help their child with autism, she says. Edwin Liu, director of the Colorado Center for Celiac Disease Children's Hospital Colorado, says he sees parents turn to a gluten-free diet for a wide range of symptoms, including belly pain, fatigue and behavioral issues.

But both point out that a gluten-free diet for children isn't a move to be made lightly, before consulting a healthcare provider. Importantly, a child who has symptoms that might indicate celiac disease, such as failure to gain weight, GI upset or chronic diarrhea, can have difficulty being properly diagnosed once gluten has been eliminated. Current methods of testing – blood work and an intestinal biopsy – will produce normal readings if gluten hasn't been eaten in a while. That can lead to medical limbo, says Norelle Reilly, a pediatric gastroenterologist in the department of pediatrics and the Celiac Disease Center at

Columbia University Medical Center. To get a diagnosis, the child might have to go back to eating gluten for a few months – a so-called "gluten challenge."

If your child doesn't have celiac disease or an allergy to wheat, or a different condition known as non-celiac gluten sensitivity that causes discomfort when gluten is eaten, there are no data to support any health benefits of a gluten-free diet, wrote Reilly in a commentary published last year in the Journal of Pediatrics. The U.S. Preventive Services Task Force earlier this year said there's not enough evidence to recommend for or against screening people who don't have symptoms.

"People think a gluten-free diet is inherently healthy. But it's only healthy if you make it healthy," says Liu. All depends on what's replacing those gluten-containing foods. A Canadian study published in 2014 found that many gluten-free packaged foods were similar in calorie count to regular foods but higher in fat and carbohydrates, lower in protein, and lower in some nutrients.

And gluten-free diets can be low in important nutrients, notably most of the B vitamins, vitamin D, iron, zinc and calcium. "Whole wheat has a really nice profile of nutrients," says Melinda Dennis, a registered dietitian and nutrition coordinator at the Celiac Center at Beth Israel Deaconess Medical Center in Boston. And the replacements for wheat, which are often more refined starches from rice, corn and potato, aren't as naturally nutritious, nor are they often enriched and fortified. Much better substitutes are a variety of whole pseudo-grains like quinoa, millet and amaranth, she says.

There is particular concern about rice, which can contain naturally occurring inorganic arsenic. Exposure in utero or in early life can raise the risk of cancer and affect neurological development, among other negative effects. The Food and Drug Administration last year proposed limiting the amount of inorganic arsenic in infant rice cereal.

A study published in February found that Americans

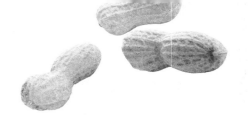

on gluten-free diets had higher concentrations of arsenic and mercury in their urine and blood than people on a regular diet, perhaps from rice consumption. It's unclear whether that is translating to health problems for adults or for children, who are more vulnerable to contaminants because of their developing brains, says Tracy Punshon, a research assistant professor in the department of biological sciences at Dartmouth College. She and her colleagues are trying to find funding to study arsenic exposure in people with celiac disease who are on a gluten-free diet.

If your main goal is to get your kids to eat more healthfully, that can be accomplished (and more easily) without going gluten-free. More cheaply, too: "One grocery bag of gluten-free products costs $80 to $100," says Lana Schoch. The best diet is one that avoids refined carbs, is low in added sugar and is full of fruits, vegetables, a variety of whole grains, nuts, fish and other lean protein, says McCarthy. And yes, that diet would probably be a bit lower in gluten. But that's not what would make it more healthful, she says.

In restaurants, servers often ask Lana if her daughter is gluten-free by choice or because she's ill. She can't quite believe the question. "What kid," she wonders, "would choose to go gluten-free?" ●

AVOIDING A PEANUT ALLERGY

For years, parents worried about the risk of peanut allergies were told to delay introducing their kids to foods containing the nut until age 3. No longer. In the wake of research showing that the opposite approach is called for, the National Institute of Allergy and Infectious Diseases earlier this year came out with new guidance. "The short version is: Eat it before you become allergic to it," says Scott Sicherer, an author of the new guidelines and a professor of pediatrics, allergy and immunology at the Icahn School of Medicine at Mount Sinai.

According to the latest advice, kids are best protected from developing a peanut allergy by exposure in infancy. Kids at highest risk of an allergy – those with severe eczema or an existing egg allergy – should be exposed as early as at 4 or 6 months after consultation with a physician, who may recommend allergy tests and possibly an in-office introduction of the food. Kids with only mild to moderate eczema should try peanut-containing foods at around 6 months. Everyone else can introduce the foods at around the same age.

"There's a significant opportunity that we all have in our hands to potentially decrease the rate of peanut allergies," says Matthew Greenhawt, co-director of the food allergy research and challenge unit at Children's Hospital Colorado and an author of the new guidelines. A survey in 2009 and 2010 found that, based on parents' reports, about 2 percent of U.S. kids younger than 18 were allergic to peanuts, more than reported allergies to milk and shellfish

The guidance on peanuts has been evolving for a while. In 2008, in response to rising rates of peanut allergies, the American Academy of Pediatrics modified its stance recommending delay for high-risk kids until age 3, saying there was no benefit to waiting past the age of 4 to 6 months to introduce any solid foods. Many parents didn't get that message, though, or continued to delay out of an abundance of caution.

Then, in 2015, researchers presented the results of a clinical trial that showed a big benefit from early exposure. Among participants who didn't show any sensitivity to peanuts during a skin test, just 1.9 percent of those who got an early introduction later developed allergies, compared to 13.7 percent of those who avoided peanuts. And among the children who initially showed sensitivity, 10.6 percent of the early group became allergic, compared to 35.3 percent of the avoiders.

Of course, there are some common-sense constraints – namely, don't feed infants or small children whole or partial pieces of peanuts, because of the choking hazard. (One option: smooth peanut butter thinned with water.) And don't make peanuts the first food to be introduced, since the normal coughing and gagging that can happen with first solids might be mistaken as an allergic reaction. It's also important to note that the guidance isn't going to prevent every peanut allergy. "It's not foolproof," says Sicherer. And it doesn't apply to children already diagnosed with a peanut allergy. Once diagnosed as allergic, they'll avoid the food.

For now, the new prevention advice is limited to peanuts. Research is ongoing to see if the same principle would work for eggs, too; a review of five trials published last year in JAMA found "moderate-certainty evidence" that introducing eggs at 4 to 6 months was associated with a lower risk of egg allergy. –K.H.

I choose Orlando's only "Best Children's Hospital" ranked by *U.S. News & World Report.*

I choose Orlando Health Arnold Palmer Hospital for Children.

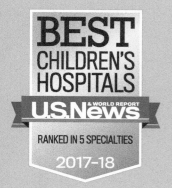

For the eighth year in a row, **Arnold Palmer Hospital** is Orlando's only nationally ranked "Best Children's Hospital" by *U.S. News & World Report.* When it comes to the best care for my kids, **I choose a national leader.**

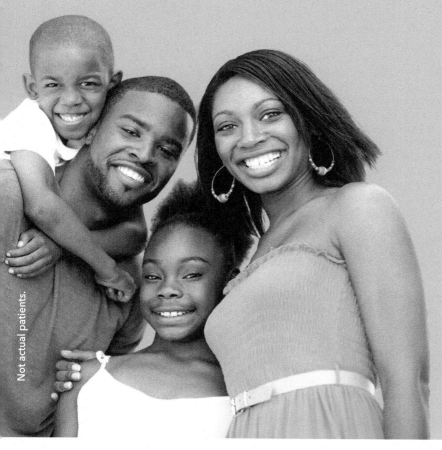

Not actual patients.

ORLANDO HEALTH®

ARNOLD PALMER
HOSPITAL
For Children

Healthier *Kids,*
Stronger *Families.*

ArnoldPalmerHospital.com

A PARENT'S GUIDE TO SOCIAL MEDIA

Expert Devorah Heitner offers tips on helping kids navigate their digital world

A CONVERSATION WITH **Katherine Hobson**

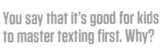

Not so long ago, "screen time" referred to the hours kids spent parked in front of the tube or playing video games. Today, they're also using their tablets and smartphones to swap messages with friends, share music videos, and rack up "likes" by posting photos. These forms of social media, which allow people to broadcast information publicly and make connections far beyond the people they actually know, can be confusing for parents to get a handle on. But you might want to, because according to a 2015 survey by Common Sense Media, 45 percent of teens use social media every day, spending an average of an hour and 11 minutes interacting on their devices.

How can parents make sure kids are using social media safely and appropriately? When the American Academy of Pediatrics issued its latest recommendations on media use by school-aged kids and adolescents last October, it didn't endorse any specific screen time limit. Instead, it said getting enough

sleep and physical activity should take priority, and that family rules should take into account the media being used and the individual child. The pediatricians noted that research has identified both positive and negative effects of social media on physical and mental health. For advice on how you can help keep your own kids' experience positive, U.S. News & World Report consulted **Devorah Heitner**, founder of Raising Digital Natives and author of "Screenwise: Helping Kids Thrive (and Survive) in Their Digital World." This interview was condensed and edited for clarity.

How should parents think about the role of social media in their child's life?

You can argue that social media isn't needed. But it's pretty important. Friends are a huge part of defining one's social identity. And social media is a portal to friends. The same urge that kept you and me up late at night talk-

ing on the phone is now pushing kids to connect on Snapchat or Musical.ly, a platform for creating and sharing short music videos. And social media can support your child's interests. It's a way to hang out without needing adults to drive somewhere or give permission.

You say that it's good for kids to master texting first. Why?

Texting is a crucial skill. If you're going to send your kids to eighth grade or high school without the ability to text, how will they make plans? It would be the modern-day equivalent of the

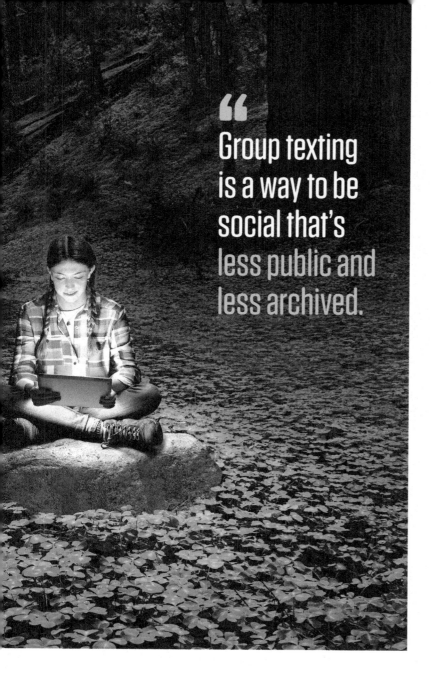

> ## " Group texting is a way to be social that's less public and less archived.

you know all the people they're connected to. At age 12, you could require that the child personally know all of his or her connections. And at an older age, say 16, maybe it's OK to connect online with other people who have shared interests.

What's your thinking about reputation?

We tell kids to be careful about their behavior on social media with warnings like "You won't get into college." That won't work at age 11. What you can say is, "Your friends' parents may check. Will they want you to come to their home for dinner if you've posted a gross joke?" At age 16, it's realistic to say there are implications for colleges and career. And you can say "Yes, you can get kicked off the team for a photo of you appearing to be drinking."

What about time management?

Kids probably need hands-on help with this. You can say no access overnight, no access until homework is done. And think about your own actions. If you're texting your kid during the day, you're undermining the notion that school is a place for school activities.

Should parents monitor their kids' accounts?

There is no advantage to covertly monitoring accounts. What do you do if you see something bad? Say nothing? How bad does it have to get? But you can overtly monitor new users. You can say, "I'm going to spot check your texts for the first year, and here's what I'm looking for." Be clear that you want to make sure she's not using a potty mouth online or passing around inappropriate pictures. You can also control their passwords so you have access to their accounts.

It's better to mentor than to monitor. For example, you can talk about when to share news. Do you share news that's not yours? You can talk about what's public and what's private in general,

family that didn't have a telephone. Also, group texting allows kids to be social online, but in a way that's less public and less archived than social media. There are fewer opportunities to damage your reputation, and it's less consuming than social media, which is more of a rabbit hole of possible distractions.

How old should kids be when they venture into social media?

The minimum age for many apps is 13, although many kids are using them at 10, 11 and 12. The rule is broken in a widespread way. At younger ages, it's more important that parents mentor and supervise.

You want your children to be mature enough to understand the concepts of relationships, reputation and time management. With relationships, kids need to understand the difference between a friend and someone who follows them on social media. You can talk to them about people in your life who were there when a sibling was born, or who traveled with you. Those are real friends. If your child is 8 years old and going on Musical.ly, you could require that what doesn't go outside the family. You can set an example by letting your kids share their own college acceptances and not doing it yourself.

And we can say that it isn't rude to choose not to connect with someone. You don't have to say yes. We can also talk about time boundaries. Help them tell their friends that they can't text after 9 p.m. Otherwise they might feel anxiety if friends text at 10 p.m., and they don't text back. And ask them to find out what their friends' boundaries are too, so they can be respectful.

We also want to teach kids when it's time to go speak with someone in person. If there's a conflict with a friend, it's best to go see that friend; the more important the relationship, the more important it is to have face-to-face contact. Kids can find that awkward. But they need to learn that anything really important can be awkward, and that firing back on the keyboard can have negative consequences.

How can parents stay current on what their kids are doing online?

It's good to understand what apps they're on, so you'll know what they're talking about when they say they are staying up late to maintain their Snapstreak on Snapchat. But some adults are full abstainers. At that point, you might see if you have a niece or a nephew willing to get in the sandbox with them. That can be a good reminder for kids that someone trusted is watching and may talk to their parents. It's also someone they can go to for advice or help. I don't think we want them to be out there without guidance as new users.

Parents may want to let their kids know that they can always use them as an excuse. That's not going to work past a certain age. But for younger kids, it can be very helpful to say, "My dad looks at my phone, and I don't want to get grounded." It's a positive way for kids to not get in over their heads.

If a child is being harassed, or someone is asking him or her to cheat, those are situations we want kids to come to us to get help with. And we need to be

> ## "
> # It isn't rude to choose not to connect with someone. You don't have to say yes.

clear that anytime someone is telling them not to tell their parents something, that's a huge red flag.

Some research has connected social media use by tweens and teens with reduced life satisfaction and depression. What do you make of this?

We know some of the ways that social media can affect kids – and all of us. Norms can make us feel bad. If the norm seems to be that everyone in our community goes on spring break because the five people we see the most on social media are going, we might feel deprived. There's also exclusion, seeing things we are left out of. We need to help kids get perspective. They need to learn how to unfollow someone. We can support and mentor kids in reflecting on, "Is this making me feel good to spend hours looking at parties I wasn't invited to?"

If kids are anxious and social media seems to increase their anxiety, I would address that with them directly and try to help them find a balance. If your child is especially impulsive or struggles to manage aggression, I'd see how long you can hold off on social media and then start with baby steps, like texting from a shared device. The challenge

with mental health issues like self-harm or eating disorders is that in a worst-case scenario, kids can find "how-to" information on social media or websites.

Kids who are socially on the outs won't necessarily have their lives improved by being on social media. So don't force a child who is struggling to get on social media in the hopes it will improve his or her popularity. It's important for all of us to remember that social media is a performance. Other people are sharing a tiny slice of experience – the slice they think will generate the most approval.

Kids need to understand they might unintentionally make people feel excluded, too.

As much as possible, try to help kids get there themselves. Ask them what a good rule for birthday parties might be. I wouldn't ground them for posting a birthday photo on Instagram, but talk about your own experiences: "I loved seeing Aunt Lucy's destination wedding on social media, but it was a little hard because we weren't invited." Ask them to share with you what kind of photos might be best not to post to avoid making others feel excluded.

What about the implications of being constantly engaged with a device in general?

Research shows that having a phone out makes the conversational quality decline. Anecdotally, a lot of us have experienced this. My own research is qualitative, and when I ask kids to design apps to solve problems, many say they want an app to keep their parents off the phone!

When I'm home working on my laptop, I close it to talk, or I make it clear I'm working and can talk later. In my family, we call it "turning into a screen monster" when someone isn't really listening. But you can also have fun on the screen – by reading together on a Kindle or an iPad, say, or by playing games together. Screen time can be positive family time. ●

BLOCKING CANCER WITH A SHOT

The HPV vaccine has proven to be effective. But it's underused

By Mariya Greeley

Jason Terk, a pediatrician at Cook Children's Health Care System in Keller, Texas, was pleased when the U.S. Food and Drug Administration approved the use of a new vaccine series in 2006 for children to protect them from the potentially dangerous consequences of the human papillomavirus. HPV is extremely common. About 1 in 4 people in the United States are infected with the sexually transmitted virus currently. Most infections go away naturally, but in more than 30,000 cases every year, HPV causes various forms of cancer. "We're talking about cancers that can be very difficult to treat," notes Terk. Cervical cancer is the most common HPV-associated disease for women, while cancers of the throat, tongue and tonsils most commonly afflict men.

Despite its potential benefits, public suspicion toward the HPV vaccine mounted quickly, based on alarming stories alleging serious side effects and parental fears of encouraging early sexual activity. Even today, after 10 years of experience have shown the vaccine to be safe and effective against the strains of HPV it targets, fewer than half of youngsters are fully protected – and instances of HPV-associated cancers are on the rise. As a result, cancer centers across the country have issued a plea for parents to get their children vaccinated, which should be a bit easier than in the past thanks to a revised recommendation that the Centers for Disease Control and Prevention put out late last year. The new guidance calls for two shots of the vaccine for 11- and 12-year-olds (the second dose coming six to 12 months after the first) instead of three shots in six months.

Fears about side effects, and the belief that tweens who are not sexually active don't need the vaccine, are misguided, experts say. The millions of doses given show that the most serious side effect is fainting, according to the CDC – a concern for any vaccine or medical procedure. Jessica Cataldi, a pediatrician at Children's Hospital Colorado, frames the vaccine to parents as a way to prevent cancer rather than sexually transmitted infection, and explains that "this earlier age is actually when you have the strongest and most lasting immune response." Plus, patients need to be armed against HPV long before they are exposed to risk. "If [parents] try to wait until they think it's a relevant issue then most of the time it's too late," Terk says.

Surprisingly, it may be doctors rather than parents who present the biggest obstacle to wider use. Studies show that a lackluster provider recommendation is often to blame for HPV vaccine refusal: Physicians tend to overestimate how resistant parents will be to the HPV vaccine and either overexplain the details or recommend it less forcefully than the other common tween vaccines – Tdap, which protects against tetanus, diphtheria and pertussis, and one that protects against meningococcal disease, including meningitis. "[Parents] pick up that it's being talked about differently and sort of pull back," says Melinda Wharton, director of the Immunization Services Division in CDC's National Center of Immunization and Respiratory Diseases. "There's sort of a feedback loop that's not very good between providers and families." When doctors recommend the three vaccines as a bundle, parents are much more likely to vaccinate against HPV.

Recently, health professionals have seen reason for optimism. HPV vaccination rates are inching upwards as health care organizations put more resources into advocating for the vaccine and providers make more effective recommendations. The new, easier vaccination schedule may help, too. Females who miss the 11- to 12-year-old window can still benefit by getting vaccinated up until age 26; young men, up to age 21. Gay, bisexual and transgender males can benefit up till age 26.

The medical community has no illusions about the potential cost of slow progress. "My worst nightmare is that one of my former patients will end up with one of these cancers that I could have prevented," Terk says. ●

> ## Fears about side effects are
> ## misguided, experts say.

Together

we're raising the bar.

Let's continue to make a better future for every child and every family.

To learn more, visit cincinnatichildrens.org/usnews

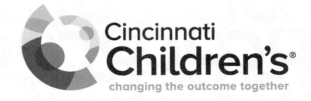

BEST CHILDREN'S HOSPITALS

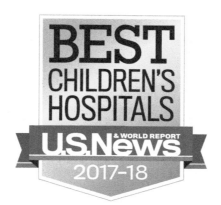

THE HONOR ROLL

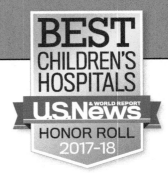

Hospitals on this year's elite list excelled in every pediatric specialty. All hospitals received Honor Roll points for a specialty ranking – 25 points for No. 1, 24 for No. 2 and so on; hospitals ranked 21-50 received 5 points. The 10 hospitals with the most points defined the Honor Roll.

1 Boston Children's Hospital
244 points

2 Children's Hospital of Philadelphia
234 points

3 Cincinnati Children's Hospital Medical Center
209 points

4 Texas Children's Hospital
Houston, 202 points

5 Johns Hopkins Children's Center
Baltimore
165 points

6 Children's Hospital Los Angeles
157 points

7* Ann and Robert H. Lurie Children's Hospital of Chicago
144 points

7* Nationwide Children's Hospital
Columbus, Ohio
144 points

9 Children's Hospital of Pittsburgh of UPMC
141 points

10 Children's National Medical Center
Washington, D.C.
138 points

*Denotes a tie

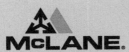

CLOCKWISE FROM LEFT: KATHERINE C. COHEN — BOSTON
CHILDREN'S HOSPITAL; BRETT ZIEGLER FOR USN&WR;
RYAN KURTZ — CINCINATTI CHILDREN'S HOSPITAL

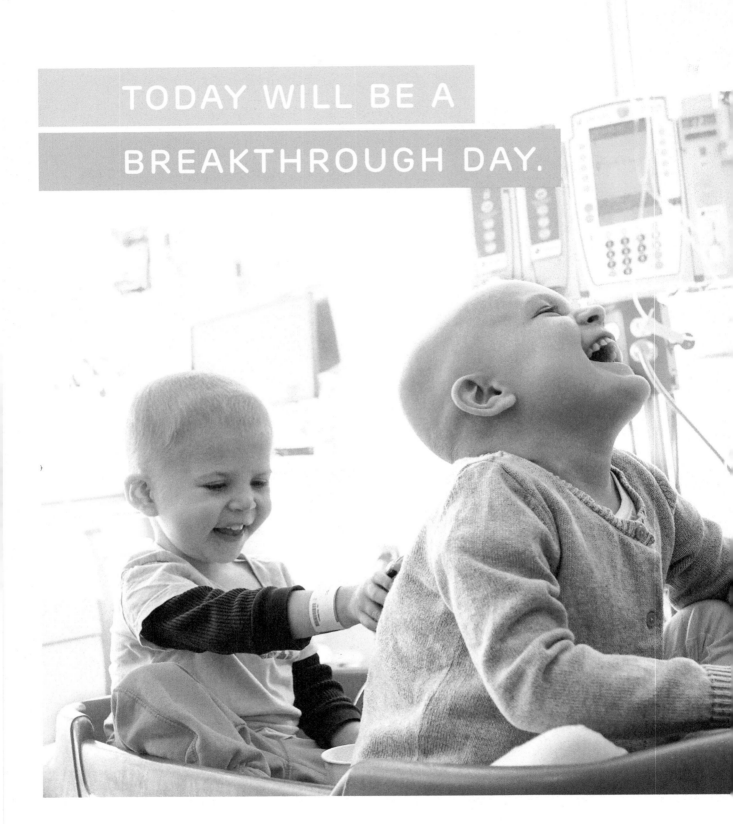

TODAY WILL BE A
BREAKTHROUGH DAY.

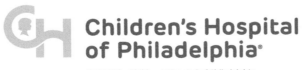

Children's Hospital
of Philadelphia®

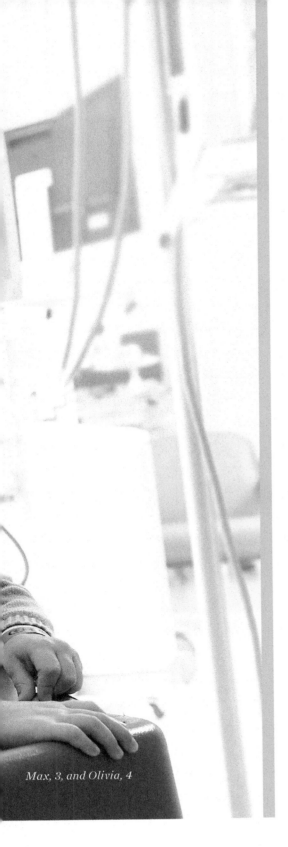

Max, 3, and Olivia, 4

TODAY AT CHILDREN'S HOSPITAL OF PHILADELPHIA:

We will battle the diseases that rob children of childhood — armed with therapies unheard of just a few years ago.

We will relentlessly pursue the next breakthrough in the lab, at the bedside and in the OR.

We will touch the lives of families in our community and around the world.

We will train future leaders to re-imagine what is possible.

We will serve as a voice for the most vulnerable in our society.

We will transform lives — and lifetimes.

At Children's Hospital of Philadelphia, more than 14,000 of us will come to work with one purpose: improving the health of children. It's going to be quite a day.

Breakthroughs. Every day.

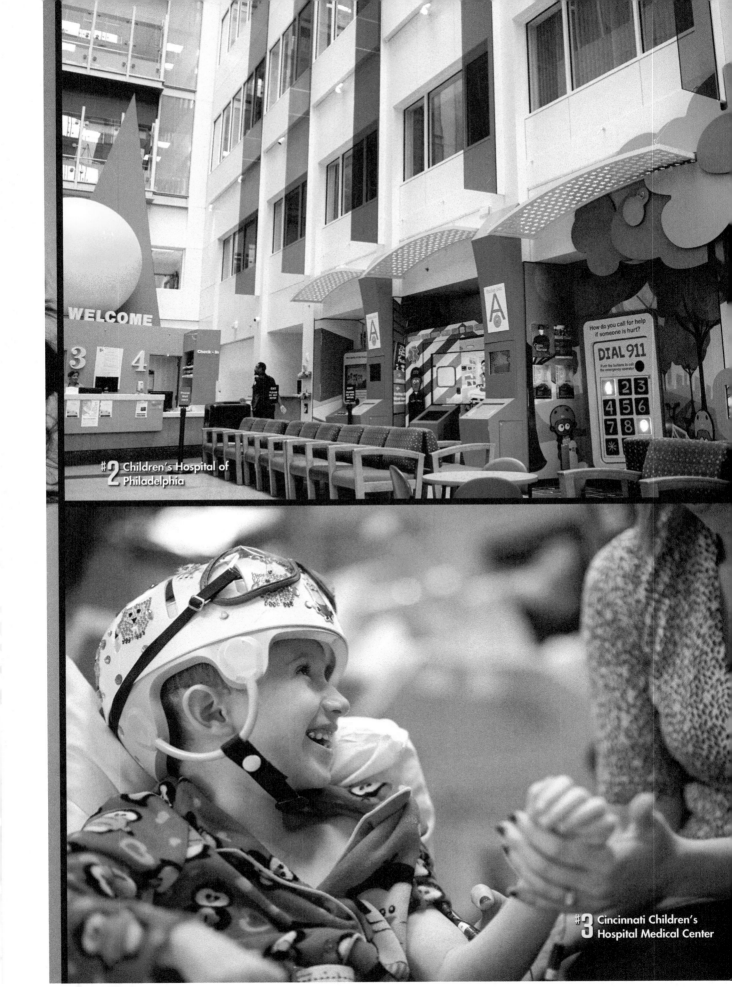

WELCOME

3 4

Check - In

How do you call for help
if someone is hurt?

DIAL 911
Push the buttons to call
the emergency operator

1 2 3
4 5 6
7 8 0

#2 Children's Hospital of
Philadelphia

#3 Cincinnati Children's
Hospital Medical Center

A KEY TO THE RANKINGS

How we identified 82 outstanding hospitals in 10 specialties

By Avery Comarow

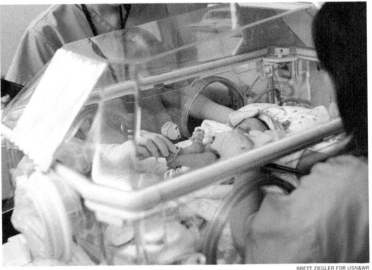

BRETT ZIEGLER FOR USN&WR

Where should desperate parents take a newborn with a life-threatening heart defect, or find ongoing care for a child with failing kidneys or lung-clogging cystic fibrosis? The local hospital's pediatric department might see plenty of kids, but won't likely have the expertise to treat the sickest children. Even within the compact universe of fewer than 200 children's hospitals, some are better than others. U.S. News created the Best Children's Hospitals rankings to help parents find the ones best suited to help their child.

The 2017-18 rankings highlight top children's centers in 10 specialties: cancer, cardiology and heart surgery, diabetes and endocrinology, gastroenterology and GI surgery, neonatology, nephrology, neurology and neurosurgery, orthopedics, pulmonology and urology. This year, 82 hospitals ranked in at least one specialty. The 2017-18 Honor Roll recognizes 10 standouts that scored at or near the top in all or most specialties. Many ranked hospitals are independent centers. Most of the rest are pediatric departments so big they are very much like their stand-alone brethren.

Judging children's hospitals is far more challenging than evaluating hospitals in adult care (as U.S. News has done since 1990 in Best Hospitals for high-risk patients in 16 specialties, page 96). Which information to collect, and even agreement on standards for interpreting it, are a constant source of debate. Nor is there a pediatric version of the federal Medicare database that U.S. News draws on for the adult rankings.

Almost all of the medical data used in these rankings are therefore obtained by asking hospitals to complete a lengthy online survey. This year, 113 of the 187 hospitals surveyed by U.S. News provided enough data to be evaluated in at least one specialty. Most surveyed hospitals are members of the Children's Hospital Association; a few are specialty centers or non-CHA hospitals that were previously ranked or were recommended by trusted sources.

This year's survey was updated with the help of 126 medical directors, clinical specialists and other pediatric experts who served as advisers on 12 U.S. News specialty task forces. RTI International, a North Carolina-based research and consulting firm, ran the survey and analyzed the findings.

Whether and how high an institution was ranked depended on three elements: its clinical outcomes (such as survival and surgical complications), its delivery of care (how well a hospital synchronizes all that must be done to treat patients effectively and keep them safe), and its resources (such as staffing and technology). A detailed rankings FAQ is available at usnews.com/aboutchildrens.

Each element contributed one-third of a hospital's overall score. Here are the basics:

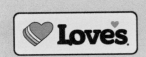

Clinical outcomes. These reveal a hospital's success at keeping kids alive after their treatment or surgery, protecting them from infections and complications, and improving their quality of life.

Delivery of care. How well a hospital handles day-to-day care was determined in part by compliance with accepted "best practices," such as having a full-time infection preventionist and holding regular conferences to discuss unexpected deaths and complications. U.S. News also surveys pediatric specialists annually, asking them to identify up to 10 hospitals they consider best in their area of expertise for children with serious or difficult medical problems, ignoring distance and cost. Results from surveys in 2015, 2016 and 2017 were factored into a hospital's score. More than 3,000 physicians responded to the 2017 survey.

Resources. Surgical volume, nurse-patient ratio, and clinics and programs for conditions such as asthma were among the 37 measures and hundreds of submeasures involved in the rankings. ●

A WORD ON THE TERMS

USED IN MORE THAN ONE SPECIALTY

A Nurse Magnet hospital: hospital recognized by American Nurses Credentialing Center as meeting standards for nursing excellence.
Infection prevention score, ICU: ability to prevent central-line bloodstream infections and urinary tract infections in intensive care units.
Infection prevention score, overall: ability to prevent infections through measures such as hand hygiene and vaccination.
No. of best practices: how well hospital adheres to recommended ways of diagnosing and treating patients, such as documenting blood sugar levels for a high percentage of outpatients (diabetes & endocrinology) and conducting hip exams with ultrasound specialists (orthopedics).
Nurse-patient ratio: balance of full-time registered nurses to inpatients.
Patient volume score: relative number of patients in past year with specified disorders.
% of specialists recommending hospital: percentage of physician specialists responding to surveys in 2015, 2016 and 2017 who named hospital among best for very challenging patients.
Procedure volume score: relative number of tests and nonsurgical procedures in past one, two or three years, such as implanting radioactive seeds in a cancerous thyroid (diabetes & endocrinology) and using an endoscope for diagnosis (gastroenterology). Surgical procedures are included in orthopedics.
Surgery volume score: relative number of patients who had specified surgical procedures in past year.
Surgical complications prevention score: ability to prevent surgery-related complications and readmissions within 30 days (neurology & neurosurgery, orthopedics, urology).
U.S. News score: 0 to 100 summary of overall performance in specialty.
NA: not applicable; service not provided by hospital.
NR: data not reported or unavailable.

USED IN ONE SPECIALTY

CANCER
Bone marrow transplant survival score: survival of stem cell recipients at 100 days.
Five-year survival score: survival five years after treatment for acute lymphoblastic leukemia, acute myeloid leukemia, and neuroblastoma.
Palliative care score: how well program meets specified training and staffing standards for children with terminal or life-limiting conditions, and number of cancer patients referred to program.

CARDIOLOGY & HEART SURGERY
Catheter procedure volume score: relative number of specified catheter-based procedures in past year, such as inserting stents and treating heart rhythm problems.
Norwood/hybrid surgery survival score: survival at one year after the first in a series of reconstructive surgeries, evaluated over past four years.
Risk-adjusted surgical survival

score: survival in the hospital and 30 days from discharge after congenital heart surgery, adjusted for operative and patient risk, evaluated over past four years.

DIABETES & ENDOCRINOLOGY
Diabetes management score: ability to prevent serious problems in children with Type 1 diabetes and to keep blood sugar levels in check.
Hypothyroid management score: relative proportions of children treated for underactive thyroid who test normal and of infants who begin treatment by three weeks of age.

GASTROENTEROLOGY & GI SURGERY
Liver transplant survival score: relative survival one year after liver transplant.
Nonsurgical procedure volume score: relative number of tests and noninvasive procedures.
Selected treatments success score: shown, for example, by high remission rates for inflammatory bowel disease and few complications from endoscopic procedures.

NEONATOLOGY
Infection prevention score, NICU: ability to prevent central-line bloodstream infections in neonatal ICU.
Leaves NICU on breast milk score: relative percentage of infants discharged from NICU receiving some nutrition from breast milk.
Readmissions prevention score: ability to minimize unplanned readmissions to NICU within seven days after discharge.

NEPHROLOGY
Biopsy complications prevention score: ability to minimize complications after kidney biopsy.
Dialysis management score: relative proportion of dialysis patients in

past two years who tested normal.
Infection prevention score, dialysis: ability to minimize dialysis-related infection.
Kidney transplant survival score: based on patient survival and functioning kidney at one and three years.

NEUROLOGY & NEUROSURGERY
Clinic patient volume score: relative number of clinic patients in past year with specified disorders or procedures.
Epilepsy management score: ability to treat children with epilepsy.
Surgical survival score: survival at 30 days after complex surgery and procedures, such as those involving brain tumors, epilepsy and head trauma.

ORTHOPEDICS
Fracture repair score: ability to treat complex leg and forearm fractures efficiently.

PULMONOLOGY
Asthma inpatient care score: ability to minimize asthmatic children's asthma-related deaths, length of stay, and readmissions.
Cystic fibrosis management score: ability to improve lung function and nutritional status.
Lung transplant survival score: reflects number of transplants in past two years, one-year survival, and recognition by United Network for Organ Sharing.

UROLOGY
Minimally invasive volume score: relative number of patients in past year who had specified nonsurgical procedures.
Testicular torsion care score: promptness of emergency surgery to correct twisted spermatic cord.

WHERE THE MIRACLES ARE.

Because you give, our member hospitals are the best of the best.

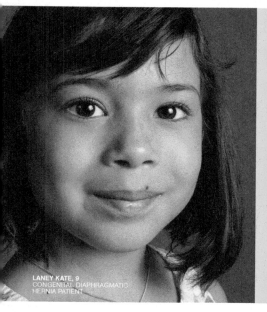

LANEY KATE, 9
CONGENITAL DIAPHRAGMATIC
HERNIA PATIENT

TOP 10

The top 10 *U.S. News* children's hospitals are all Children's Miracle Network Hospitals

1. Boston Children's Hospital, Boston, MA
2. Children's Hospital of Philadelphia, Philadelphia, PA
3. Cincinnati Children's Hospital Medical Center, Cincinnati, OH
4. Texas Children's Hospital, Houston, TX
5. Johns Hopkins Children's Center, Baltimore, MD
6. Children's Hospital Los Angeles, Los Angeles, CA
7. Ann and Robert H. Lurie Children's Hospital of Chicago, Chicago, IL*
7. Nationwide Children's Hospital, Columbus, Ohio*
9. Children's Hospital of Pittsburgh of UPMC, Pittsburgh, PA
10. Children's National Health System, Washington, DC

*Tied for 7th place

Coincidence? We think not.

Thanks to local donations, Children's Miracle Network Hospitals® are able to provide the best care for kids. Congratulations to the following member hospitals on being recognized among the best children's hospitals in the country.

Akron Children's Hospital, Akron, OH

Ann and Robert H. Lurie Children's Hospital of Chicago, Chicago, IL

Arkansas Children's Hospital, Little Rock, AR

Arnold Palmer Children's Hospital, Orlando, FL

Boston Children's Hospital, Boston, MA

Children's Healthcare of Atlanta, Atlanta, GA

Children's Hospital and Medical Center, Omaha, NE

Children's Hospital Colorado, Aurora, CO

Children's Hospital Los Angeles, Los Angeles, CA

Children's Hospital of Alabama, Birmingham, AL

Children's Hospital of Illinois, Peoria, IL

Children's Hospital of Philadelphia, Philadelphia, PA

Children's Hospital of Pittsburgh of UPMC, Pittsburgh, PA

Children's Hospital of Richmond at VCU, Richmond, VA

Children's Hospital of Wisconsin, Milwaukee, WI

Children's Health Children's Medical Center, Dallas, TX

Children's Mercy Kansas City, Kansas City, MO

Children's National Health System, Washington, DC

CHOC Children's, Orange, CA

Cincinnati Children's, Cincinnati, OH

Cohen Children's Medical Center of New York, New Hyde Park, NY

Connecticut Children's Medical Center, Hartford, CT

Cook Children's Medical Center, Fort Worth, TX

Dell Children's Medical Center of Central Texas, Austin, TX

OHSU Doernbecher Children's Hospital, Portland, OR

Duke Children's, Durham, NC

Johns Hopkins All Children's Hospital, Tampa-St. Petersburg, FL

Johns Hopkins Children's Center, Baltimore, MD

Le Bonheur Children's Hospital, Memphis, TN

Levine Children's Hospital, Charlotte, NC

Medical University of South Carolina Shawn Jenkins Children's Hospital, Charleston, SC

Monroe Carell Jr. Children's Hospital at Vanderbilt, Nashville, TN

Nationwide Children's Hospital, Columbus, OH

Nicklaus Children's Hospital, Miami, FL

Penn State Children's Hospital, Hershey, PA

Phoenix Children's Hospital, Phoenix, AZ

Primary Children's Hospital, Salt Lake City, UT

Rady Children's Hospital-San Diego, San Diego, CA

University Hospitals Rainbow Babies & Children's Hospital, Cleveland, OH

Riley Hospital for Children, Indianapolis, IN

Seattle Children's Hospital, Seattle, WA

Helen DeVos Children's Hospital, Grand Rapids, MI

SSM Health Cardinal Glennon Children's Hospital, St. Louis, MO

St. Louis Children's Hospital, St. Louis, MO

Texas Children's Hospital, Houston, TX

UCSF Benioff Children's Hospitals, San Francisco, CA

UF Health Shands Children's Hospital, Gainesville, FL

UC Davis Children's Hospital, Sacramento, CA

University of Iowa Stead Family Children's Hospital, Iowa City, IA

Golisano Children's Hospital at the University of Rochester Medical Center, Rochester, NY

University of Virginia Children's Hospital, Charlottesville, VA

Valley Children's Hospital, Madera, CA

Give Today

to your children's hospital

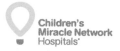

Children's
Miracle Network
Hospitals®

CMNHospitals.org

A NEW VOICE FOR CHILDREN'S HOSPITALS

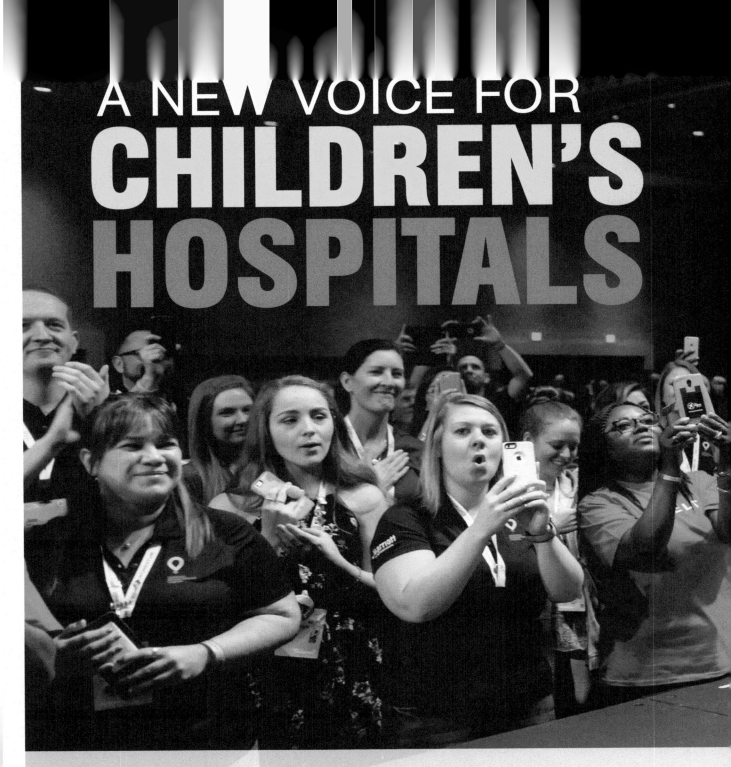

Born without a jaw, 17-year-old Isaiah Acosta has never spoken a word. Yet, he just released his first rap song, "Oxygen to Fly." The song speaks to his struggles being born without the pathways needed for oxygen to enter his body and his survival despite huge doubts.

Isaiah has found his voice and is using it to advocate for children's hospitals.

This year, Isaiah is sharing his story across the United States as a Champion for Children's Miracle Network Hospitals. He is one of 52 kids — representing each state, Washington, D.C. and Puerto Rico — advocating for local donations to children's hospitals. Medicaid and insurance programs do not cover the full cost of caring for kids. Children's hospitals rely on donations to provide critical care for more than 10 million kids each year.

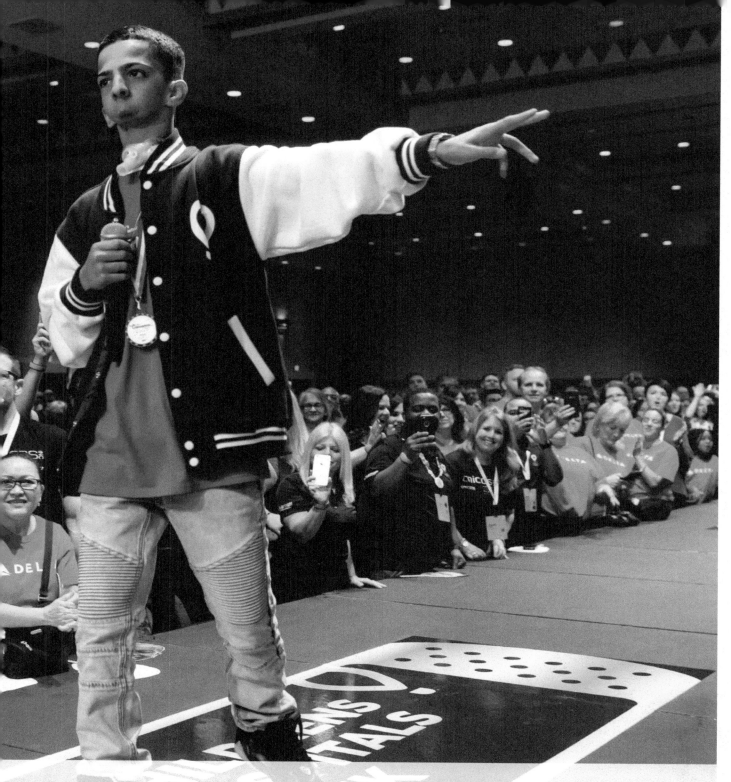

At Isaiah's hospital, donations support the Hope Fund, which helps launch new programs, purchase essential equipment, conduct cutting-edge research, provide charitable care and more.

To help children's hospitals across the country, Isaiah is donating the proceeds of his first song to Children's Miracle Network Hospitals. Download the song and learn more at **oxygentofly.org**.

Children's Miracle Network Hospitals®

Champions

The Children's Miracle Network Hospitals Champions program is possible thanks to these generous partners:

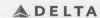

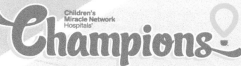

CANCER

Rank	Hospital	U.S. News score	Five-year survival score (15=best)	Bone marrow transplant survival score (6=best)	Infection prevention score, overall (32=best)	Infection prevention score, ICU (15=best)	Patient volume score (21=best)	Nurse-patient ratio (higher is better)	A Nurse Magnet hospital	Palliative care score (8=best)	% of specialists recommending hospital
1	St. Jude Children's Research Hospital, Memphis, Tenn.	100.0	14	4	31	15	21	4.7	Yes	8	48.7%
2	Dana-Farber/Boston Children's Cancer and Blood Disorders Center	99.9	14	5	31	7	21	4.5	Yes	8	65.4%
3	Children's Hospital of Philadelphia	98.4	13	5	30	7	18	3.5	Yes	8	69.6%
4	Texas Children's Hospital, Houston	95.6	11	5	32	9	21	3.7	Yes	8	43.5%
5	Cincinnati Children's Hospital Medical Center	95.3	15	3	30	9	21	4.4	Yes	8	54.2%
6	Johns Hopkins Children's Center, Baltimore	92.5	14	6	32	9	17	3.4	Yes	8	17.3%
7	Children's National Medical Center, Washington, D.C.	92.4	13	4	32	14	21	3.2	Yes	8	15.0%
8	Children's Hospital Colorado, Aurora	91.8	13	5	30	12	21	3.3	Yes	8	23.3%
9	Children's Hospital Los Angeles	91.7	12	6	29	9	19	3.3	Yes	8	30.3%
10	Nationwide Children's Hospital, Columbus, Ohio	91.1	14	6	31	9	21	3.2	Yes	8	15.4%
11	Seattle Children's Hospital	87.5	10	6	28	7	20	2.8	Yes	8	38.9%
12	Ann and Robert H. Lurie Children's Hospital of Chicago	86.9	11	4	32	10	21	3.2	Yes	8	19.2%
13	Children's Healthcare of Atlanta	86.2	13	5	31	9	21	4.1	No	8	18.4%
14	UCSF Benioff Children's Hospitals, San Francisco and Oakland	84.4	12	5	29	9	20	3.6	Yes	8	13.7%
15	Memorial Sloan Kettering Cancer Center, New York	83.1	12	4	29	8	14	4.6	Yes	8	17.7%
16	Monroe Carell Jr. Children's Hospital at Vanderbilt, Nashville, Tenn.	80.8	14	5	29	9	20	3.1	Yes	8	1.9%
17	Lucile Packard Children's Hospital Stanford, Palo Alto, Calif.	79.7	14	6	30	7	21	3.9	No	8	9.1%
18	Children's Medical Center Dallas	78.4	9	5	25	10	21	3.0	Yes	7	8.0%
19	Mayo Clinic Children's Center, Rochester, Minn.	77.8	10	6	32	7	18	3.8	Yes	8	2.1%
20	Cohen Children's Center, New Hyde Park, N.Y.	76.8	10	5	32	14	11	3.3	Yes	8	1.4%
21	Children's Hospital of Pittsburgh of UPMC	76.3	12	4	30	7	21	3.4	Yes	8	5.5%
21	Rainbow Babies and Children's Hospital, Cleveland	76.3	9	5	30	10	12	3.0	Yes	8	3.8%
23	Rady Children's Hospital, San Diego	76.2	11	6	31	8	15	3.1	Yes	8	2.2%
24	North Carolina Children's Hospital at UNC, Chapel Hill	75.6	10	5	30	11	18	3.9	Yes	7	0.7%
25	Nemours Alfred I. duPont Hosp. for Children, Wilmington, Del.	75.2	10	5	31	11	7	4.3	Yes	8	1.0%
25	Primary Children's Hospital, Salt Lake City	75.2	14	5	30	9	18	3.9	No	8	1.7%
27	NY-Presby. Morgan Stanley-Komansky Children's Hospital, N.Y.	75.0	11	4	32	12	18	2.8	No	6	5.1%
28	Yale-New Haven Children's Hospital, New Haven, Conn.	74.9	8	6	30	11	17	2.5	Yes	7	0.9%
29	Phoenix Children's Hospital	74.6	14	4	30	11	21	2.8	No	8	2.7%
30	University of Michigan C.S. Mott Children's Hospital, Ann Arbor	74.1	12	4	27	10	16	3.7	Yes	8	4.1%
31	Duke Children's Hospital and Health Center, Durham, N.C.	73.9	11	5	28	9	18	3.2	Yes	7	7.6%
32	St. Louis Children's Hospital-Washington University	73.6	9	5	32	9	17	3.4	Yes	8	5.1%
33	Spectrum Hlth. Helen DeVos Children's Hosp., Grand Rapids, Mich.	73.1	13	5	27	13	8	2.8	Yes	7	1.0%
34	University of Iowa Children's Hospital, Iowa City	72.9	12	6	30	11	15	3.0	Yes	8	0.7%
35	American Family Children's Hospital, Madison, Wis.	72.5	14	6	22	9	7	4.7	Yes	5	0.7%
36	MUSC Health-Children's Hospital, Charleston, S.C.	71.8	14	5	29	10	7	2.8	Yes	8	0.3%
37	Children's Hospital at Montefiore, New York	71.6	10	4	32	13	8	3.5	No	8	1.8%
37	Levine Children's Hospital, Charlotte, N.C.	71.6	9	6	25	12	7	3.1	Yes	8	0.2%
39	Children's Hospital of Wisconsin, Milwaukee	71.3	8	2	25	13	19	4.5	Yes	8	3.6%
40	Children's Hospital of Alabama at UAB, Birmingham	70.2	13	3	24	13	21	3.0	No	8	2.6%
40	Riley Hospital for Children at IU Health, Indianapolis	70.2	11	5	24	6	10	4.1	Yes	8	2.5%
42	Children's Mercy Kansas City, Mo.	69.7	11	5	30	7	19	4.3	Yes	6	2.9%
43	CHOC Children's Hospital, Orange, Calif.	68.3	12	4	29	8	9	2.9	Yes	8	1.6%
44	Cleveland Clinic Children's Hospital	67.6	7	5	31	6	17	3.5	Yes	8	0.6%
45	UCLA Mattel Children's Hospital, Los Angeles	67.3	7	5	27	7	15	3.7	Yes	8	3.4%
46	UF Health Shands Children's Hospital, Gainesville, Fla.	66.8	11	5	25	8	13	2.6	Yes	8	0.7%
47	Doernbecher Children's Hospital, Portland, Ore.	66.7	11	4	27	7	11	3.7	Yes	6	2.7%
48	Cook Children's Medical Center, Fort Worth	66.6	14	3	24	9	21	2.6	Yes	8	1.5%
49	Children's Hospital of Michigan, Detroit	66.4	9	6	29	9	19	2.9	No	8	0.7%
50	MD Anderson Children's Cancer Hospital, Houston	66.2	4	5	18	15	17	2.8	Yes	6	6.0%
50	Penn State Children's Hospital, Hershey, Pa.	66.2	6	5	28	8	14	3.1	Yes	8	1.6%

Terms are explained on Page 158.

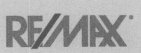

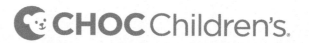
CHOC Children's.

350 CLINICAL TRIALS
1 GOAL

Research can save lives. Charlotte's rare disease went undiagnosed until she was 3½ years old when CHOC metabolic specialists discovered she had glycogen storage disease 1a. That's why the Research Institute at CHOC Children's has over 350 research studies, including Phase 1 research, in more than 30 specialties to provide patients, like Charlotte, with access to new treatment options. Our scientists work to translate the latest advances in molecular profiling — including whole genome sequencing — to meet the individual needs of their patients at every stage of their young lives. At CHOC, every study, every specialist, every person works toward a common goal.

Learn more at choc.org/research

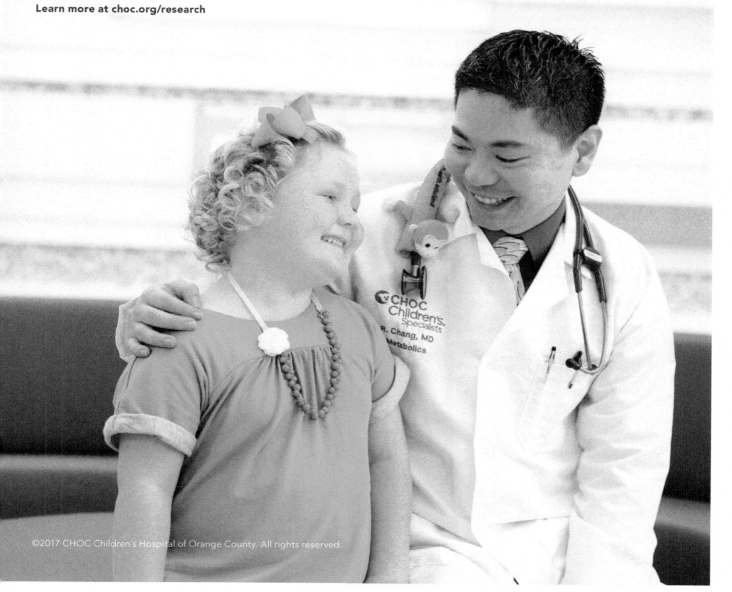

CARDIOLOGY & HEART SURGERY

Rank	Hospital	U.S. News score	Risk-adjusted surgical survival score (21=best)	Norwood/hybrid surgery survival score (12=best)	Infection prevention score, overall (38=best)	Infection prevention score, ICU (5=best)	Surgery volume score (12=best)	Catheter procedure volume score (33=best)	Nurse-patient ratio (higher is better)	A Nurse Magnet hospital	% of specialists recommending hospital
1	Texas Children's Hospital, Houston	100.0	17	9	37	3	10	33	3.7	Yes	55.6%
2	Boston Children's Hospital	97.3	14	9	37	1	12	33	4.5	Yes	80.2%
3	Ann and Robert H. Lurie Children's Hospital of Chicago	92.6	18	11	38	2	6	18	3.2	Yes	14.9%
3	University of Michigan C.S. Mott Children's Hospital, Ann Arbor	92.6	15	10	32	4	11	28	3.7	Yes	46.1%
5	Children's Hospital of Wisconsin, Milwaukee	91.2	18	12	30	5	9	19	4.5	Yes	16.5%
6	Cincinnati Children's Hospital Medical Center	90.7	15	10	36	1	8	28	4.4	Yes	31.4%
7	Children's Hospital Colorado, Aurora	88.4	15	9	36	4	9	32	3.3	Yes	11.4%
8	Children's Hospital Los Angeles	88.1	14	12	36	3	10	29	3.3	Yes	18.9%
9	Children's Hospital of Philadelphia	86.5	11	9	36	1	11	33	3.5	Yes	73.5%
10	NY-Presby. Morgan Stanley-Komansky Children's Hospital, N.Y.	86.4	13	11	38	4	10	32	2.8	No	19.9%
11	MUSC Children's Heart Network of South Carolina, Charleston	85.7	17	10	35	4	7	26	2.8	Yes	7.7%
12	Children's Hospital of Pittsburgh of UPMC	85.4	17	12	36	1	6	19	3.4	Yes	9.4%
13	Children's Medical Center Dallas	83.3	15	12	31	2	8	27	3.0	Yes	3.5%
14	Primary Children's Hospital, Salt Lake City	83.2	15	10	37	3	9	31	3.9	No	6.9%
15	Lucile Packard Children's Hospital Stanford, Palo Alto, Calif.	82.7	12	9	36	1	11	32	3.9	No	47.3%
16	Seattle Children's Hospital	81.6	15	8	35	1	9	25	2.8	Yes	12.9%
17	Rady Children's Hospital, San Diego	79.6	16	11	37	2	6	30	3.1	Yes	4.7%
18	Phoenix Children's Hospital	79.1	18	9	35	3	7	27	2.8	No	2.2%
19	Children's Healthcare of Atlanta	79.0	10	8	37	3	11	33	4.1	No	31.2%
19	Children's Mercy Kansas City, Mo.	79.0	17	10	36	1	8	25	4.3	Yes	3.1%
21	UF Health Shands Children's Hospital, Gainesville, Fla.	78.2	17	12	31	2	5	11	2.6	Yes	1.0%
22	Mayo Clinic Children's Center, Rochester, Minn.	77.7	13	11	38	1	7	21	3.8	Yes	8.0%
23	Monroe Carell Jr. Children's Hospital at Vanderbilt, Nashville, Tenn.	77.6	12	9	34	3	9	32	3.1	Yes	5.5%
24	Levine Children's Hospital, Charlotte, N.C.	77.5	15	10	31	4	6	19	3.1	Yes	2.2%
25	Riley Hospital for Children at IU Health, Indianapolis	76.8	14	10	31	2	7	26	4.1	Yes	3.3%
26	Nationwide Children's Hospital, Columbus, Ohio	76.3	9	9	37	3	8	27	3.2	Yes	19.4%
27	Cleveland Clinic Children's Hospital	76.0	15	12	38	0	4	21	3.5	Yes	2.6%
28	Advocate Children's Heart Institute, Oak Lawn and Park Ridge, Ill.	75.7	18	9	32	3	7	24	3.7	Yes	1.2%
29	Le Bonheur Children's Hospital, Memphis, Tenn.	75.3	17	9	34	3	6	18	3.2	Yes	2.2%
30	Johns Hopkins All Children's Hospital, St. Petersburg, Fla.	74.9	16	11	35	1	7	18	3.2	No	2.1%
31	St. Louis Children's Hospital-Washington University	74.8	11	9	37	3	6	31	3.4	Yes	5.4%
32	Children's National Medical Center, Washington, D.C.	74.4	10	10	37	4	6	29	3.2	Yes	10.8%
33	Nemours Alfred I. duPont Hosp. for Children, Wilmington, Del.	73.5	14	11	37	3	5	15	4.3	Yes	0.3%
34	Johns Hopkins Children's Center, Baltimore	72.6	12	9	38	3	6	20	3.4	Yes	2.8%
35	UCLA Mattel Children's Hospital, Los Angeles	72.5	12	9	33	3	5	30	3.7	Yes	6.5%
36	UCSF Benioff Children's Hospitals, San Francisco and Oakland	70.2	13	9	37	3	6	27	3.6	Yes	7.8%
37	Arkansas Children's Hospital, Little Rock	70.1	14	10	33	4	6	18	3.2	Yes	1.7%
38	Duke Children's Hospital and Health Center, Durham, N.C.	69.6	10	10	35	3	6	20	3.2	Yes	3.9%
39	Penn State Children's Hospital, Hershey, Pa.	69.5	18	11	33	2	4	15	3.1	Yes	0.8%
40	Children's Hospital and Medical Center, Omaha	69.4	13	10	34	1	6	23	3.0	Yes	1.0%
41	Nicklaus Children's Hospital, Miami	68.7	12	11	36	5	6	27	3.1	Yes	4.0%
42	Yale-New Haven/Connecticut Children's Medical Cen., New Haven	68.5	17	8	35	3	4	20	2.5	Yes	1.8%
43	Arnold Palmer Children's Hospital, Orlando, Fla.	67.2	15	12	33	4	4	15	3.6	Yes	0.7%
44	University of Virginia Children's Hospital, Charlottesville	67.1	12	9	35	2	4	17	2.8	A Nurse	1.3%
45	SSM Health Cardinal Glennon Children's Hospital-St. Louis U.	66.2	14	10	35	2	6	16	2.9	No	0.9%
46	Cook Children's Medical Center, Fort Worth	63.3	14	10	31	3	7	24	2.6	Yes	0.5%
47	North Carolina Children's Hospital at UNC, Chapel Hill	63.0	13	3	35	3	4	18	3.9	Yes	0.6%
48	University of Iowa Children's Hospital, Iowa City	61.8	9	10	36	3	4	23	3.0	Yes	0.5%
49	American Family Children's Hospital, Madison, Wis.	61.2	15	9	29	3	4	13	4.7	Yes	0.7%
49	Ochsner Hospital for Children, New Orleans	61.2	14	5	25	5	4	19	3.0	Yes	0.5%
49	Spectrum Hlth. Helen DeVos Children's Hosp., Grand Rapids, Mich.	61.2	16	9	32	3	4	17	2.8	Yes	0.3%

Terms are explained on Page 158.

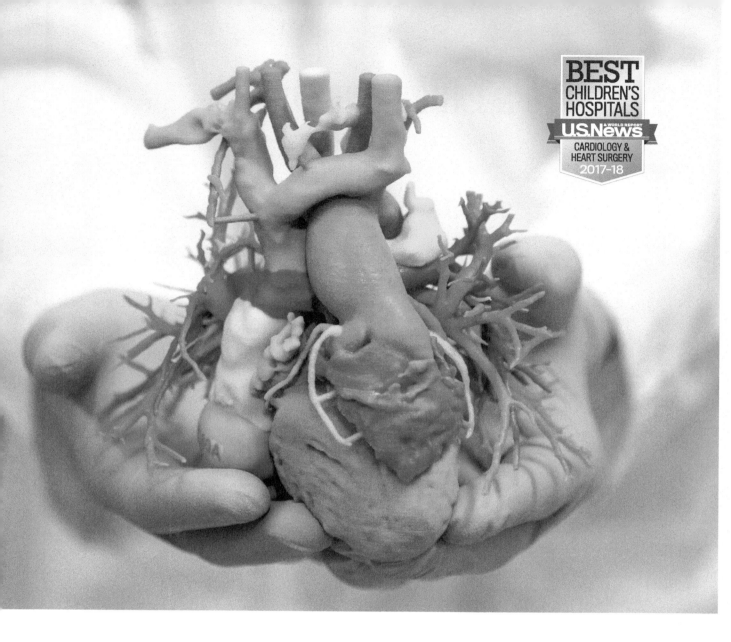

Leading with the heart.

Phoenix Children's Hospital is home to one of the nation's largest and highest-rated pediatric cardiology and congenital heart surgery programs, and the Southwest's only dedicated pediatric heart transplant program. The Phoenix Children's Heart Center uses advanced technology such as integrated 3D multimodality imaging and modeling. It is one of only six programs in the country to receive the Society of Thoracic Surgeons' highest three-star rating, and was once again recognized for excellence in Cardiology and Heart Surgery as a Best Children's Hospital by the experts at *U.S. News & World Report*.

Phoenix Children's delivers family-centered, multidisciplinary care and exceptional outcomes for a wide range of congenital heart conditions, from simple to complex for the children and families of the Southwest.

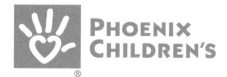

PHOENIX CHILDREN'S

heart.PhoenixChildrens.org

DIABETES & ENDOCRINOLOGY

Rank	Hospital	U.S. News score	Diabetes manage-ment score (42=best)	Hypothyroid manage-ment score (3=best)	Infection prevention score, overall (32=best)	Patient volume score (30=best)	Procedure volume score (26=best)	Nurse-patient ratio (higher is better)	A Nurse Magnet hospital	No. of best practices (108=best)	% of specialists recom-mending hospital
1	Children's Hospital of Philadelphia	100.0	35	3	30	30	26	3.5	Yes	106	62.3%
2	Boston Children's Hospital	99.0	33	3	30	29	26	4.5	Yes	105	63.1%
3	Children's Hospital of Pittsburgh of UPMC	94.2	36	3	30	30	26	3.4	Yes	104	28.9%
4	Yale-New Haven Children's Hospital, New Haven, Conn.	91.9	39	3	30	30	26	2.5	Yes	107	20.1%
5	Children's Hospital Los Angeles	91.1	36	3	28	30	20	3.3	Yes	102	25.4%
6	Texas Children's Hospital, Houston	91.0	33	3	31	29	25	3.7	Yes	102	20.6%
7	Cincinnati Children's Hospital Medical Center	90.3	29	3	28	30	21	4.4	Yes	104	34.2%
8	Children's Hospital Colorado, Aurora	89.0	29	3	29	30	23	3.3	Yes	99	36.5%
9	NY-Presby. Morgan Stanley-Komansky Children's Hospital, N.Y.	87.4	40	3	32	28	25	2.8	No	108	11.0%
10	UCSF Benioff Children's Hospitals, San Francisco and Oakland	86.6	31	3	29	30	20	3.6	Yes	94	18.7%
11	Seattle Children's Hospital	84.8	31	3	28	29	26	2.8	Yes	104	14.9%
12	Johns Hopkins Children's Center, Baltimore	83.7	30	3	32	26	22	3.4	Yes	107	17.3%
13	Nationwide Children's Hospital, Columbus, Ohio	82.6	28	3	30	30	25	3.2	Yes	100	10.8%
14	Riley Hospital for Children at IU Health, Indianapolis	80.8	30	3	24	28	21	4.1	Yes	98	11.7%
15	Rady Children's Hospital, San Diego	80.6	32	3	30	30	26	3.1	Yes	102	3.0%
16	Children's National Medical Center, Washington, D.C.	80.5	28	3	32	30	23	3.2	Yes	104	4.1%
16	Mount Sinai Kravis Children's Hospital, New York	80.5	33	3	32	28	25	3.9	Yes	104	2.6%
18	Children's Medical Center Dallas	78.9	31	3	24	29	25	3.0	Yes	88	9.6%
18	Lucile Packard Children's Hospital Stanford, Palo Alto, Calif.	78.9	29	3	28	29	22	3.9	No	85	16.8%
20	Mayo Clinic Children's Center, Rochester, Minn.	78.2	31	3	31	25	21	3.8	Yes	95	5.7%
21	Arnold Palmer Children's Hospital, Orlando, Fla.	76.9	39	3	27	27	22	3.6	Yes	105	0.5%
22	Ann and Robert H. Lurie Children's Hospital of Chicago	76.7	29	3	30	29	23	3.2	Yes	96	5.6%
23	UF Health Shands Children's Hospital, Gainesville, Fla.	76.6	27	3	25	25	20	2.6	Yes	99	10.6%
24	Monroe Carell Jr. Children's Hospital at Vanderbilt, Nashville, Tenn.	76.3	27	3	27	30	23	3.1	Yes	94	4.9%
25	Holtz Children's Hosp. at UM-Jackson Memorial Med. Cen., Miami	75.1	38	3	24	28	26	3.3	No	107	2.2%
25	MassGeneral Hospital for Children, Boston	75.1	29	3	22	24	21	4.0	Yes	98	7.3%
27	Rainbow Babies and Children's Hospital, Cleveland	75.0	24	3	30	28	22	3.0	Yes	107	5.2%
28	North Carolina Children's Hospital at UNC, Chapel Hill	74.4	27	3	30	28	23	3.9	Yes	103	2.0%
29	NYU Winthrop Hospital Children's Medical Center, Mineola, N.Y.	74.2	34	3	30	24	13	2.1	Yes	107	0.9%
30	Children's Healthcare of Atlanta	73.8	27	3	28	30	26	4.1	No	95	3.4%
30	Nemours Alfred I. duPont Hosp. for Children, Wilmington, Del.	73.8	31	3	30	25	17	4.3	Yes	88	0.7%
32	St. Louis Children's Hospital-Washington University	73.7	25	3	29	29	21	3.4	Yes	92	4.2%
33	Children's Mercy Kansas City, Mo.	73.1	22	3	28	30	24	4.3	Yes	97	3.9%
34	University of Virginia Children's Hospital, Charlottesville	72.9	32	3	27	21	11	2.8	Yes	91	2.3%
35	Duke Children's Hospital and Health Center, Durham, N.C.	72.8	26	3	26	29	22	3.2	Yes	97	3.4%
36	Cohen Children's Center, New Hyde Park, N.Y.	72.7	25	3	32	27	25	3.3	Yes	106	1.5%
37	University of Michigan C.S. Mott Children's Hospital, Ann Arbor	72.4	26	3	27	27	18	3.7	Yes	96	2.7%
38	Nicklaus Children's Hospital, Miami	72.0	30	3	27	30	20	3.1	Yes	99	2.0%
39	Children's Hospital of Wisconsin, Milwaukee	71.9	30	3	23	26	18	4.5	Yes	91	2.1%
40	Doernbecher Children's Hospital, Portland, Ore.	71.4	27	3	27	28	19	3.7	Yes	86	3.6%
41	Univ. of California Davis Children's Hospital, Sacramento	71.2	28	3	31	21	15	5.7	Yes	103	0.6%
42	Children's Hospital at Montefiore, New York	71.0	23	3	32	25	21	3.5	No	106	1.3%
43	CHOC Children's Hospital, Orange, Calif.	70.8	28	3	29	30	20	2.9	Yes	93	2.2%
44	UCLA Mattel Children's Hospital, Los Angeles	70.5	23	3	27	20	23	3.7	Yes	104	4.8%
45	Primary Children's Hospital, Salt Lake City	69.4	31	3	29	27	19	3.9	No	86	0.2%
46	Valley Children's Healthcare and Hospital, Madera, Calif.	69.3	37	3	28	27	9	2.8	Yes	90	0.2%
47	American Family Children's Hospital, Madison, Wis.	69.2	28	3	22	26	13	4.7	Yes	99	2.1%
48	University of Minnesota Masonic Children's Hospital, Minneapolis	68.7	28	3	23	28	19	2.5	No	100	2.8%
49	Children's Hospital of Alabama at UAB, Birmingham	68.2	30	3	24	30	22	3.0	No	95	1.4%
50	Cleveland Clinic Children's Hospital	67.9	22	3	31	29	19	3.5	Yes	87	2.4%

Terms are explained on Page 158.

AMAZING

IS GETTING A HEART AS STRONG AS YOUR SPIRIT.

Jenna was born with only the right half of her heart. A mere six days later, pediatric cardiac surgeons at NewYork-Presbyterian performed the first in a series of three intricate surgeries to keep her alive. At age four, Jenna returned, this time to get a brand new heart. Just a few months after the transplant, this feisty little girl prepared to start kindergarten.

See Jenna's story
at **nyp.org/kids**

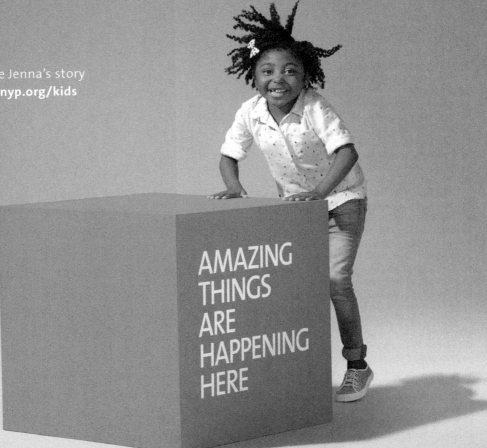

AMAZING
THINGS
ARE
HAPPENING
HERE

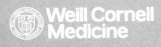 Weill Cornell Medicine

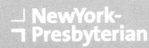 NewYork-Presbyterian

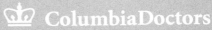 ColumbiaDoctors

GASTROENTEROLOGY & GI SURGERY

Rank	Hospital	U.S. News score	Selected treatments success score (9=best)	Liver transplant survival score (6=best)	Infection prevention score, overall (38=best)	Infection prevention score, ICU (5=best)	Patient volume score (24=best)	Surgery volume score (16=best)	Nonsurgical procedure volume score (24=best)	Nurse-patient ratio (higher is better)	A Nurse Magnet hospital	% of specialists recommending hospital
1	Boston Children's Hospital	100.0	8	6	37	1	24	16	24	4.5	Yes	65.4%
2	Children's Hospital of Philadelphia	96.3	8	5	36	1	23	16	24	3.5	Yes	62.4%
3	Cincinnati Children's Hospital Medical Center	92.8	8	4	35	1	24	14	21	4.4	Yes	63.7%
4	Texas Children's Hospital, Houston	91.6	7	4	38	3	24	16	23	3.7	Yes	38.1%
5	Children's Hospital of Pittsburgh of UPMC	89.1	9	5	35	1	24	16	15	3.4	Yes	22.1%
6	Children's Hospital Colorado, Aurora	88.4	7	4	35	4	22	14	23	3.3	Yes	34.1%
7	Ann and Robert H. Lurie Children's Hospital of Chicago	87.5	7	6	38	2	22	14	18	3.2	Yes	19.3%
7	Children's Hospital Los Angeles	87.5	8	6	36	3	21	14	23	3.3	Yes	14.1%
9	Johns Hopkins Children's Center, Baltimore	86.2	9	4	38	3	23	14	17	3.4	Yes	9.9%
10	NY-Presby. Morgan Stanley-Komansky Children's Hospital, N.Y.	85.6	9	5	38	4	22	16	22	2.8	No	7.3%
11	Children's Healthcare of Atlanta	85.2	8	6	37	3	24	15	24	4.1	No	8.3%
12	Children's National Medical Center, Washington, D.C.	84.6	7	6	38	4	23	16	20	3.2	Yes	3.8%
12	Nationwide Children's Hospital, Columbus, Ohio	84.6	9	NA	37	3	21	15	16	3.2	Yes	46.0%
14	Nemours Alfred I. duPont Hosp. for Children, Wilmington, Del.	83.0	9	6	37	3	16	10	9	4.3	Yes	1.2%
15	St. Louis Children's Hospital-Washington University	81.6	9	5	38	3	17	12	14	3.4	Yes	5.3%
16	Children's Hospital of Wisconsin, Milwaukee	81.5	7	5	30	5	17	11	20	4.5	Yes	6.2%
17	UCSF Benioff Children's Hospitals, San Francisco and Oakland	81.1	6	6	35	3	22	12	13	3.6	Yes	9.0%
18	University of Michigan C.S. Mott Children's Hospital, Ann Arbor	80.7	8	6	33	4	23	14	17	3.7	Yes	3.7%
19	Children's Medical Center Dallas	80.6	8	5	31	2	23	14	22	3.0	Yes	8.0%
20	Seattle Children's Hospital	79.6	6	6	32	1	20	13	18	2.8	Yes	21.7%
21	Monroe Carell Jr. Children's Hosp. at Vanderbilt, Nashville, Tenn.	78.1	9	3	35	3	23	14	19	3.1	Yes	2.8%
21	Riley Hospital for Children at IU Health, Indianapolis	78.1	8	6	30	2	22	12	20	4.1	Yes	4.4%
23	Mount Sinai Kravis Children's Hospital, New York	75.7	8	3	38	4	16	9	14	3.9	Yes	3.8%
24	MassGeneral Hospital for Children, Boston	74.4	6	6	30	4	16	7	14	4.0	Yes	4.2%
25	Children's Mercy Kansas City, Mo.	74.1	8	5	35	1	24	14	17	4.3	Yes	4.2%
26	Lucile Packard Children's Hospital Stanford, Palo Alto, Calif.	73.3	6	6	35	1	22	15	15	3.9	No	13.5%
27	North Carolina Children's Hospital at UNC, Chapel Hill	72.5	6	6	36	3	19	1	15	3.9	Yes	1.3%
28	Cleveland Clinic Children's Hospital	71.7	6	5	38	0	20	14	22	3.5	Yes	5.0%
29	Primary Children's Hospital, Salt Lake City	71.4	7	5	34	3	22	14	17	3.9	No	2.0%
30	Children's Hospital at Montefiore, New York	70.9	6	6	38	3	14	12	13	3.5	No	2.0%
31	UCLA Mattel Children's Hospital, Los Angeles	69.5	6	3	33	3	18	11	14	3.7	Yes	8.2%
32	Le Bonheur Children's Hospital, Memphis, Tenn.	69.4	8	3	35	3	13	13	11	3.2	Yes	1.0%
32	Yale-New Haven Children's Hospital, New Haven, Conn.	69.4	6	6	34	3	13	10	7	2.5	Yes	2.7%
34	Rady Children's Hospital, San Diego	69.3	5	6	36	2	21	14	16	3.1	Yes	2.9%
35	Levine Children's Hospital, Charlotte, N.C.	68.0	7	3	31	4	16	13	15	3.1	Yes	0.6%
36	Children's Hospital of Michigan, Detroit	67.9	9	3	32	3	19	10	11	2.9	No	0.3%
37	Children's Hospital of Alabama at UAB, Birmingham	67.7	9	3	27	3	20	14	13	3.0	No	1.8%
38	Holtz Children's Hosp. at UM-Jackson Memorial Med. Cen., Miami	66.8	5	6	30	5	19	11	14	3.3	No	0.8%
39	Cohen Children's Center, New Hyde Park, N.Y.	66.7	8	NA	38	4	13	10	17	3.3	Yes	1.8%
39	U. of Minnesota Masonic Children's Hospital, Minneapolis	66.7	6	6	30	3	19	12	9	2.5	No	0.3%
41	Duke Children's Hospital and Health Center, Durham, N.C.	64.8	6	5	33	3	15	10	9	3.2	Yes	2.0%
42	Phoenix Children's Hospital	64.4	5	5	34	3	22	12	19	2.8	No	1.7%
43	Rainbow Babies and Children's Hospital, Cleveland	63.8	9	NA	36	2	19	8	12	3.0	Yes	2.2%
44	SSM Health Cardinal Glennon Children's Hospital-St. Louis U.	63.6	6	6	35	2	11	10	9	2.9	No	0.4%
45	American Family Children's Hospital, Madison, Wis.	63.0	6	6	27	3	9	9	7	4.7	Yes	0.3%
46	Nicklaus Children's Hospital, Miami	62.1	8	NA	36	5	14	13	8	3.1	Yes	2.3%
47	MUSC Health-Children's Hospital, Charleston, S.C.	61.6	5	3	30	4	16	11	21	2.8	Yes	1.2%
48	Mayo Clinic Children's Center, Rochester, Minn.	61.5	4	4	35	1	17	11	17	3.8	Yes	2.4%
49	Connecticut Children's Medical Center, Hartford	61.3	9	NA	34	2	18	13	9	2.7	No	1.9%
50	Valley Children's Healthcare and Hospital, Madera, Calif.	58.9	8	NA	34	3	11	13	17	2.8	Yes	0.8%

NA=not applicable; service not provided by hospital. Terms are explained on Page 158.

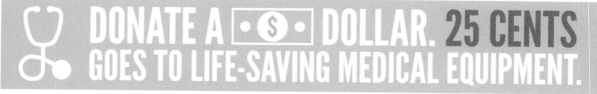

DONATE A ·$· DOLLAR. 25 CENTS GOES TO LIFE-SAVING MEDICAL EQUIPMENT.

Here, these are
TWINS

Despite being four years younger and two feet shorter than her brother, Ella has something nearly identical: her stem cells. So when she needed a bone marrow transplant, Cale was a perfect match. Soon, their family grew to include everyone at our Center for Cancer and Blood Disorders' Bone Marrow Transplant Program, led by Michael Verneris, MD, one of the world's foremost researchers in the field. Ella overcame myelodysplastic syndrome, and together, we created bonds that will last a lifetime. A very long lifetime.

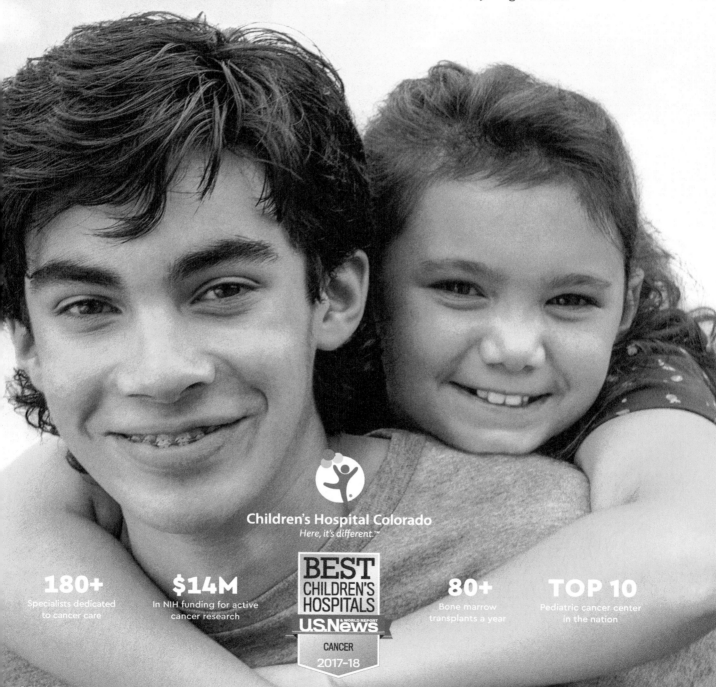

Children's Hospital Colorado
Here, it's different.™

BEST CHILDREN'S HOSPITALS
U.S. News & WORLD REPORT
CANCER
2017–18

180+
Specialists dedicated to cancer care

$14M
In NIH funding for active cancer research

80+
Bone marrow transplants a year

TOP 10
Pediatric cancer center in the nation

NEONATOLOGY

Rank	Hospital	U.S. News score	Leaves NICU on breast milk score (3=best)	Readmissions prevention score (3=best)	Infection prevention score, overall (32=best)	Infection prevention score, NICU (5=best)	Patient volume score (30=best)	Nurse-patient ratio (higher is better)	A Nurse Magnet hospital	No. of best practices (93=best)	% of specialists recommending hospital
1	Children's National Medical Center, Washington, D.C.	100.0	3	3	32	5	30	3.1	Yes	90	11.7%
2	Boston Children's Hospital	97.6	3	3	31	2	24	3.7	Yes	93	46.6%
2	Children's Hospital of Philadelphia	97.6	3	3	30	2	30	3.9	Yes	88	48.3%
4	Johns Hopkins Children's Center, Baltimore	90.0	2	3	31	4	28	3.5	Yes	86	13.5%
5	Rady Children's Hospital, San Diego	89.7	3	3	31	4	22	2.9	Yes	88	5.3%
6	Children's Hospital Los Angeles	89.1	3	2	29	4	26	3.7	Yes	90	12.5%
7	Rainbow Babies and Children's Hospital, Cleveland	89.0	3	3	30	3	18	3.7	Yes	90	19.7%
8	Children's Hospital of Pittsburgh of UPMC	88.5	3	3	30	4	23	3.2	Yes	91	8.3%
9	Monroe Carell Jr. Children's Hospital at Vanderbilt, Nashville, Tenn.	88.3	3	3	29	5	26	2.7	Yes	88	5.6%
10	UCSF Benioff Children's Hospitals, San Francisco and Oakland	87.8	3	3	31	2	26	3.4	Yes	89	11.9%
11	Texas Children's Hospital, Houston	87.6	3	3	32	2	28	2.7	Yes	92	21.9%
12	Nicklaus Children's Hospital, Miami	85.7	3	3	30	5	15	2.8	Yes	87	3.6%
13	Cincinnati Children's Hospital Medical Center	84.8	2	2	31	2	28	3.7	Yes	90	31.0%
14	Seattle Children's Hospital	84.3	3	2	27	3	25	3.4	Yes	80	13.0%
15	Children's Healthcare of Atlanta	83.8	3	3	31	4	27	3.1	No	91	3.9%
16	Univ. of California Davis Children's Hospital, Sacramento	83.7	3	3	32	4	22	3.4	Yes	90	0.6%
17	Ann & Robert H. Lurie Children's Hosp.-Prentice Women's Hosp., Chicago	83.3	3	2	31	4	21	2.3	Yes	86	7.9%
18	St. Louis Children's Hospital-Washington University	83.1	3	3	32	3	27	3.0	Yes	87	8.0%
19	Cohen Children's Center, New Hyde Park, N.Y.	82.8	3	3	28	5	23	2.7	Yes	92	1.1%
20	University of Iowa Children's Hospital, Iowa City	82.1	3	3	28	4	19	2.8	Yes	79	5.9%
21	Nationwide Children's Hospital, Columbus, Ohio	81.1	2	2	31	4	27	2.5	Yes	87	16.2%
22	University of Michigan C.S. Mott Children's Hospital, Ann Arbor	79.9	3	2	25	5	21	2.6	Yes	81	5.1%
23	Lucile Packard Children's Hospital Stanford, Palo Alto, Calif.	79.1	3	2	30	2	21	3.9	No	86	21.1%
24	Children's Mercy Kansas City, Mo.	78.2	2	3	30	3	26	4.1	Yes	89	7.2%
25	Children's Hospital Colorado, Aurora	78.1	3	2	29	1	27	3.6	Yes	90	15.4%
26	NY-Presby. Morgan Stanley-Komansky Children's Hospital, N.Y.	77.8	3	2	32	3	27	2.5	No	86	14.6%
27	University of Rochester-Golisano Children's Hospital, N.Y.	76.3	3	2	31	4	12	3.2	Yes	89	1.8%
28	Duke Children's Hospital and Health Center, Durham, N.C.	76.0	2	2	29	4	23	2.5	Yes	87	6.8%
29	Yale-New Haven Children's Hospital, New Haven, Conn.	75.3	2	3	28	4	17	2.4	Yes	85	2.4%
30	University of Virginia Children's Hospital, Charlottesville	75.0	2	2	28	5	19	2.4	Yes	87	1.6%
31	Children's Hospital of Wisconsin, Milwaukee	74.9	3	2	24	4	24	2.8	Yes	85	1.7%
32	Le Bonheur Children's Hospital, Memphis, Tenn.	74.7	2	2	29	4	22	2.9	Yes	91	0.9%
33	University of Minnesota Masonic Children's Hospital, Minneapolis	74.4	3	3	22	4	19	3.0	No	87	2.2%
34	CHOC Children's Hospital, Orange, Calif.	73.6	3	2	30	3	22	3.0	Yes	91	2.4%
35	Akron Children's Hospital, Ohio	72.9	2	3	28	5	17	3.2	Yes	89	1.2%
36	Doernbecher Children's Hospital, Portland, Ore.	71.8	3	3	29	3	20	2.5	Yes	85	0.6%
37	Mayo Clinic Children's Center, Rochester, Minn.	71.7	3	3	32	2	16	6.2	Yes	84	1.8%
38	Arkansas Children's Hospital, Little Rock	71.3	2	2	26	4	27	2.4	Yes	83	1.8%
39	Primary Children's Hospital, Salt Lake City	70.8	2	2	30	3	30	2.9	No	88	3.1%
40	Cleveland Clinic Children's Hospital	70.6	2	2	28	5	10	2.8	Yes	84	2.1%
41	Nemours Alfred I. duPont Hosp. for Children, Wilmington, Del.	69.7	3	2	31	2	19	2.7	Yes	92	1.3%
42	Children's Medical Center Dallas-Parkland Memorial Hospital	69.1	2	2	25	4	24	2.5	Yes	87	4.3%
43	UCLA Mattel Children's Hospital, Los Angeles	68.6	3	2	27	3	14	4.2	Yes	86	3.9%
44	Inova Children's Hospital, Falls Church, Va.	68.3	3	3	28	5	16	2.3	No	79	2.0%
45	Riley Hospital for Children at IU Health, Indianapolis	67.9	3	3	26	1	26	2.8	Yes	84	3.7%
46	Penn State Children's Hospital, Hershey, Pa.	67.2	2	2	28	3	14	3.0	Yes	82	1.1%
47	North Carolina Children's Hospital at UNC, Chapel Hill	66.2	2	2	30	3	18	2.7	Yes	86	2.2%
48	UF Health Shands Children's Hospital, Gainesville, Fla.	66.0	2	3	24	3	14	3.0	Yes	83	1.6%
49	Children's Hospital of Illinois, Peoria	65.9	2	3	31	4	13	3.9	Yes	81	0.1%
50	Children's Hospital at Montefiore, New York	65.6	3	3	32	2	11	2.7	No	91	1.3%

Terms are explained on Page 158.

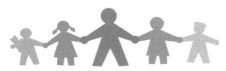

UC**SF** Benioff Children's Hospitals
Oakland | San Francisco

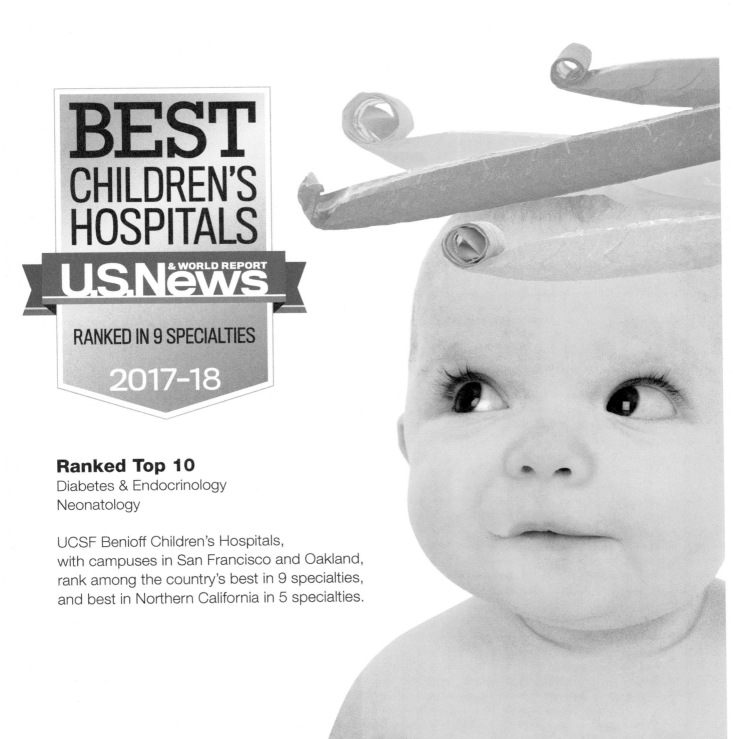

BEST CHILDREN'S HOSPITALS

U.S.News **& WORLD REPORT**

RANKED IN 9 SPECIALTIES

2017-18

Ranked Top 10
Diabetes & Endocrinology
Neonatology

UCSF Benioff Children's Hospitals,
with campuses in San Francisco and Oakland,
rank among the country's best in 9 specialties,
and best in Northern California in 5 specialties.

NEPHROLOGY

Rank	Hospital	U.S. News score	Kidney transplant survival score (24=best)	Biopsy complications prevention score (6=best)	Dialysis management score (12=best)	Infection prevention score, overall (55=best)	Infection prevention score, ICU (5=best)	Infection prevention score, dialysis (9=best)	Patient volume score (24=best)	Nurse-patient ratio (higher is better)	A Nurse Magnet hospital	% of specialists recommending hospital
1	Boston Children's Hospital	100.0	24	6	12	54	1	9	23	4.5	Yes	60.6%
2	Children's Hospital of Philadelphia	97.9	24	6	12	53	1	8	20	3.5	Yes	50.6%
3	Cincinnati Children's Hospital Medical Center	97.4	24	6	11	52	1	9	23	4.4	Yes	62.0%
4	Texas Children's Hospital, Houston	97.0	23	6	12	55	3	8	22	3.7	Yes	35.9%
5	Seattle Children's Hospital	93.5	24	6	12	50	1	6	24	2.8	Yes	51.4%
6	Children's Healthcare of Atlanta	92.5	24	6	12	54	3	9	24	4.1	No	23.7%
7	Children's Mercy Kansas City, Mo.	91.6	24	6	12	53	1	9	23	4.3	Yes	25.7%
8	Lucile Packard Children's Hospital Stanford, Palo Alto, Calif.	90.5	24	6	12	53	1	9	22	3.9	No	34.2%
9	Nationwide Children's Hospital, Columbus, Ohio	90.4	22	5	12	54	3	8	20	3.2	Yes	22.9%
10	Children's National Medical Center, Washington, D.C.	88.8	24	6	12	55	4	7	20	3.2	Yes	6.8%
11	Johns Hopkins Children's Center, Baltimore	88.6	23	6	12	55	3	7	10	3.4	Yes	16.4%
12	UCLA Mattel Children's Hospital, Los Angeles	88.1	20	6	11	49	3	9	19	3.7	Yes	20.9%
13	Ann and Robert H. Lurie Children's Hospital of Chicago	86.0	20	6	12	54	2	7	23	3.2	Yes	12.4%
14	UCSF Benioff Children's Hospitals, San Francisco and Oakland	84.1	21	6	12	53	3	8	17	3.6	Yes	6.2%
15	Children's Hospital of Wisconsin, Milwaukee	83.2	24	6	11	47	5	7	18	4.5	Yes	2.4%
16	University of Michigan C.S. Mott Children's Hospital, Ann Arbor	82.0	23	3	12	50	4	7	20	3.7	Yes	11.6%
17	Children's Medical Center Dallas	81.9	23	6	11	46	2	8	20	3.0	Yes	7.9%
18	Children's Hospital Los Angeles	80.6	23	6	10	53	3	7	18	3.3	Yes	5.4%
18	St. Louis Children's Hospital-Washington University	80.6	24	6	12	55	3	6	13	3.4	Yes	4.6%
20	Children's Hospital of Pittsburgh of UPMC	80.0	24	6	12	52	1	4	16	3.4	Yes	10.5%
21	University of Iowa Children's Hospital, Iowa City	79.9	24	6	10	53	3	7	13	3.0	Yes	7.8%
22	Levine Children's Hospital, Charlotte, N.C.	79.6	22	6	11	49	4	7	20	3.1	Yes	2.3%
23	Univ. of California Davis Children's Hospital, Sacramento	79.2	22	6	11	54	4	9	10	5.7	Yes	1.0%
24	Children's Hospital at Montefiore, New York	78.6	23	6	11	55	3	3	14	3.5	No	8.2%
25	Doernbecher Children's Hospital, Portland, Ore.	78.3	23	6	12	50	1	9	19	3.7	Yes	1.2%
25	Rady Children's Hospital, San Diego	78.3	24	6	10	54	2	8	20	3.1	Yes	5.3%
27	NY-Presby. Morgan Stanley-Komansky Children's Hospital, N.Y.	78.1	23	6	10	55	4	9	15	2.8	No	1.8%
28	MUSC Health-Children's Hospital, Charleston, S.C.	77.6	23	6	12	52	4	8	15	2.8	Yes	0.6%
29	Riley Hospital for Children at IU Health, Indianapolis	77.5	24	6	12	47	2	8	15	4.1	Yes	3.9%
30	Duke Children's Hospital and Health Center, Durham, N.C.	76.9	24	6	11	52	3	8	19	3.2	Yes	3.5%
31	Holtz Children's Hosp. at UM-Jackson Memorial Med. Cen., Miami	76.5	24	6	11	44	5	7	16	3.3	No	2.5%
31	Monroe Carell Jr. Children's Hosp. at Vanderbilt, Nashville, Tenn.	76.5	22	5	8	52	3	9	17	3.1	Yes	2.1%
31	U. of Minn. Masonic Children's Hosp.-Children's Minn., Minneapolis	76.5	23	6	12	47	3	7	18	2.5	No	5.2%
34	Children's Hospital Colorado, Aurora	76.3	23	5	8	51	4	7	13	3.3	Yes	3.6%
35	Le Bonheur Children's Hospital, Memphis, Tenn.	76.2	22	6	8	51	3	8	18	3.2	Yes	5.2%
36	Spectrum Hlth. Helen DeVos Children's Hosp., Grand Rapids, Mich.	75.9	24	6	11	50	3	9	16	2.8	Yes	0.4%
37	North Carolina Children's Hospital at UNC, Chapel Hill	75.3	24	6	9	51	3	7	14	3.9	Yes	0.8%
38	Nemours Alfred I. duPont Hosp. for Children, Wilmington, Del.	75.1	24	6	8	50	3	5	16	4.3	Yes	1.9%
39	Mount Sinai Kravis Children's Hospital, New York	74.2	23	4	10	55	4	7	9	3.9	Yes	3.1%
40	Phoenix Children's Hospital	73.7	23	6	11	50	3	9	19	2.8	No	1.4%
41	Children's Hospital of Michigan, Detroit	73.1	17	6	12	51	3	7	19	2.9	No	2.0%
42	Rainbow Babies and Children's Hospital, Cleveland	73.0	20	6	12	53	2	6	19	3.0	Yes	1.9%
43	Children's Hospital of Alabama at UAB, Birmingham	72.6	22	6	8	47	3	6	23	3.0	No	3.4%
43	University of Rochester-Golisano Children's Hospital, N.Y.	72.6	24	6	12	49	2	7	10	3.0	Yes	1.3%
45	Children's Hospital of Richmond at VCU, Va.	71.7	19	6	12	42	2	9	13	2.0	Yes	0.9%
45	Cohen Children's Center, New Hyde Park, N.Y.	71.7	NR	6	12	55	4	9	16	3.3	Yes	0.7%
47	Primary Children's Hospital, Salt Lake City	71.1	22	6	9	52	3	4	20	3.9	No	1.9%
48	SSM Health Cardinal Glennon Children's Hospital-St. Louis U.	71.0	24	6	11	49	2	8	15	2.9	No	0.9%
49	American Family Children's Hospital, Madison, Wis.	70.9	24	6	12	45	3	6	12	4.7	Yes	0.3%
50	Connecticut Children's Medical Center, Hartford	70.3	22	6	11	51	2	7	21	2.7	No	0.6%

NR=data not reported or unavailable. Terms are explained on Page 158.

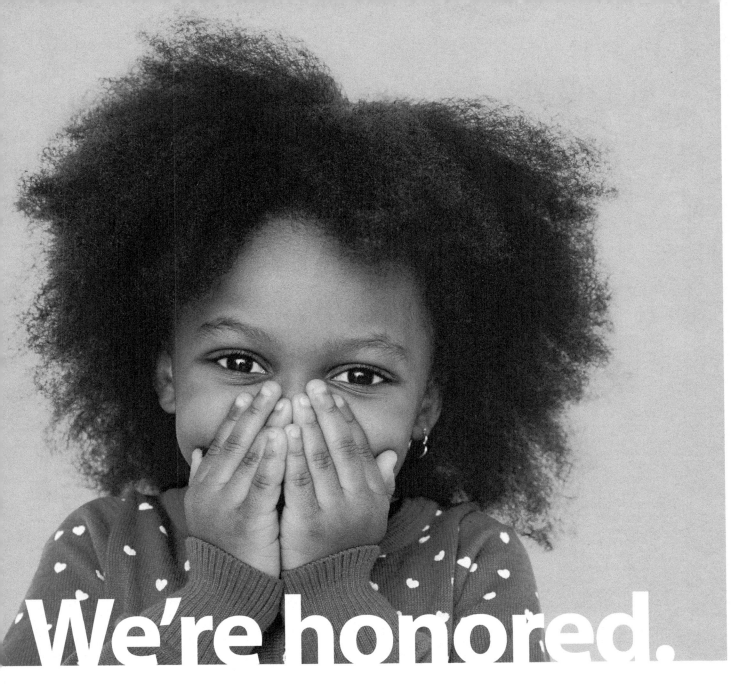

We're honored.

Proud to be ranked #9 on the Honor Roll of America's Best Children's Hospitals by *U.S. News & World Report.* And to be part of this elite list eight years in a row. We're honored by this consistent recognition, but our biggest privilege is caring for your child. To learn more, visit CHP.edu/USNews.

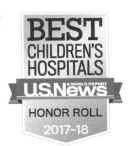

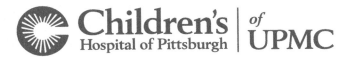

NEUROLOGY & NEUROSURGERY

Rank	Hospital	U.S. News score	Surgical survival score (12=best)	Surgical complications prevention score (22=best)	Epilepsy management score (8=best)	Infection prevention score, overall (36=best)	Surgery volume score (42=best)	Nurse-patient ratio (higher is better)	A Nurse Magnet hospital	% of specialists recommending hospital
1	Boston Children's Hospital	100.0	11	20	8	34	42	4.5	Yes	66.1%
2	Children's Hospital of Philadelphia	95.9	12	18	8	34	35	3.5	Yes	54.2%
3	Cincinnati Children's Hospital Medical Center	95.0	12	20	8	34	39	4.4	Yes	31.4%
4	Texas Children's Hospital, Houston	94.0	12	18	8	36	39	3.7	Yes	36.2%
5	Johns Hopkins Children's Center, Baltimore	92.2	12	21	8	36	32	3.4	Yes	28.7%
6	Nationwide Children's Hospital, Columbus, Ohio	90.5	12	22	8	35	34	3.2	Yes	15.9%
7	St. Louis Children's Hospital-Washington University	89.1	12	19	8	36	30	3.4	Yes	25.8%
8	Ann and Robert H. Lurie Children's Hospital of Chicago	88.9	12	20	8	35	39	3.2	Yes	19.3%
9	Children's National Medical Center, Washington, D.C.	88.7	12	22	6	36	38	3.2	Yes	17.5%
10	Children's Hospital Los Angeles	87.3	12	22	8	34	38	3.3	Yes	11.1%
11	Nicklaus Children's Hospital, Miami	86.1	12	20	8	34	35	3.1	Yes	13.8%
12	Children's Hospital of Pittsburgh of UPMC	85.9	12	19	8	34	36	3.4	Yes	12.1%
13	Children's Hospital Colorado, Aurora	83.9	11	17	7	33	40	3.3	Yes	20.6%
14	Rady Children's Hospital, San Diego	82.0	12	22	8	35	42	3.1	Yes	2.7%
15	Seattle Children's Hospital	81.0	11	16	7	33	38	2.8	Yes	24.7%
16	Cleveland Clinic Children's Hospital	80.4	12	18	6	36	28	3.5	Yes	15.7%
16	Rainbow Babies and Children's Hospital, Cleveland	80.4	12	21	8	34	19	3.0	Yes	7.6%
18	Children's Medical Center Dallas	79.3	12	21	8	29	38	3.0	Yes	4.1%
18	Le Bonheur Children's Hospital, Memphis, Tenn.	79.3	12	18	7	33	28	3.2	Yes	7.6%
20	Mayo Clinic Children's Center, Rochester, Minn.	78.4	12	16	8	35	26	3.8	Yes	7.0%
21	University of Michigan C.S. Mott Children's Hospital, Ann Arbor	78.2	12	21	8	31	28	3.7	Yes	5.8%
22	Primary Children's Hospital, Salt Lake City	77.9	12	18	7	34	35	3.9	No	8.7%
23	Cohen Children's Center, New Hyde Park, N.Y.	76.6	12	22	6	36	32	3.3	Yes	1.9%
24	Children's Hospital of Wisconsin, Milwaukee	76.4	12	18	8	28	30	4.5	Yes	3.0%
25	NY-Presby. Morgan Stanley-Komansky Children's Hospital, N.Y.	76.0	12	19	8	35	31	2.8	No	9.0%
26	Monroe Carell Jr. Children's Hospital at Vanderbilt, Nashville, Tenn.	75.7	12	15	8	33	36	3.1	Yes	2.6%
27	CHOC Children's Hospital, Orange, Calif.	75.0	11	21	7	33	33	2.9	Yes	3.1%
27	Mount Sinai Kravis Children's Hospital, New York	75.0	12	20	8	35	20	3.9	Yes	0.2%
29	UCSF Benioff Children's Hospitals, San Francisco and Oakland	74.7	11	7	7	35	34	3.6	Yes	17.2%
30	Children's Hospital of Alabama at UAB, Birmingham	73.8	12	20	8	25	36	3.0	No	7.8%
31	Children's Mercy Kansas City, Mo.	72.5	12	19	6	33	28	4.3	Yes	2.2%
32	UCLA Mattel Children's Hospital, Los Angeles	72.1	12	21	4	30	25	3.7	Yes	9.1%
33	Duke Children's Hospital and Health Center, Durham, N.C.	72.0	12	15	8	33	34	3.2	Yes	3.4%
34	Children's Healthcare of Atlanta	71.6	12	15	6	34	40	4.1	No	2.9%
35	Levine Children's Hospital, Charlotte, N.C.	71.1	12	20	6	30	26	3.1	Yes	0.5%
36	Lucile Packard Children's Hospital Stanford, Palo Alto, Calif.	70.5	10	17	6	34	28	3.9	No	10.3%
37	Riley Hospital for Children at IU Health, Indianapolis	68.4	12	15	6	29	29	4.1	Yes	2.8%
38	Yale-New Haven Children's Hospital, New Haven, Conn.	67.9	12	20	4	34	18	2.5	Yes	2.3%
39	Phoenix Children's Hospital	67.8	9	16	8	34	32	2.8	No	4.4%
40	Cook Children's Medical Center, Fort Worth	67.5	12	18	7	28	25	2.6	Yes	2.0%
41	Doernbecher Children's Hospital, Portland, Ore.	67.0	11	17	5	32	25	3.7	Yes	1.8%
42	University of Chicago Comer Children's Hospital	65.9	12	22	6	28	22	3.3	No	1.1%
43	Johns Hopkins All Children's Hospital, St. Petersburg, Fla.	65.6	12	20	5	32	31	3.2	No	0.9%
44	University of Rochester-Golisano Children's Hospital, N.Y.	64.8	12	15	4	32	16	3.0	Yes	3.4%
45	Joseph M. Sanzari Children's Hospital, Hackensack, N.J.	64.1	12	18	8	25	21	2.8	Yes	1.4%
45	MUSC Health-Children's Hospital, Charleston, S.C.	64.1	10	16	7	33	21	2.8	Yes	0.0%
47	Children's Hospital of Michigan, Detroit	63.9	11	12	8	32	28	2.9	No	1.3%
48	North Carolina Children's Hospital at UNC, Chapel Hill	63.7	12	13	4	33	20	3.9	Yes	0.6%
49	UF Health Shands Children's Hospital, Gainesville, Fla.	63.2	11	15	8	29	17	2.6	Yes	0.5%
50	Children's Memorial Hermann Hospital, Houston	62.1	12	11	8	31	26	2.8	Yes	0.7%

Terms are explained on Page 158.

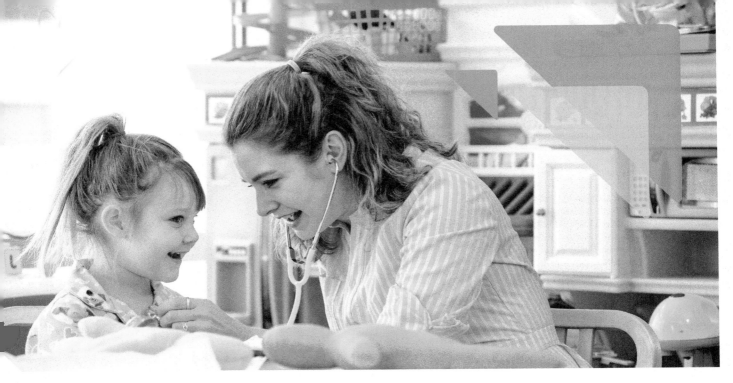

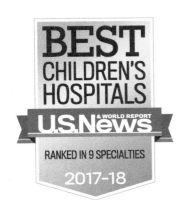

BEST
CHILDREN'S
HOSPITALS
U.S.News & WORLD REPORT

RANKED IN 9 SPECIALTIES

2017-18

We see another year of rankings.
Our patients see it as really good care.

We've once again been ranked among the nation's top hospitals on this year's *U.S. News & World Report*'s Best Children's Hospitals list. Our center was recognized for superior pediatric care in nine different specialties: **Cancer, Diabetes/Endocrinology, Gastroenterology/Gastrointestinal Surgery, Neonatology, Nephrology, Neurology/Neurosurgery, Orthopaedics, Pulmonology and Urology.**

Cohen Children's offer the region's only freestanding kids' emergency department, exceptional outpatient care and a wide range of specialty pediatric practices—in New York and beyond.

To find a pediatric specialist, call **(631) 414-5373** or visit **Northwell.edu/cohenchildrens.**

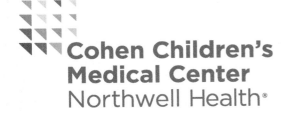

Cohen Children's
Medical Center
Northwell Health®

21966 7-17

ORTHOPEDICS

Rank	Hospital	U.S. News score	Fracture repair score (6=best)	Surgical complications prevention score (12=best)	Infection prevention score, overall (33=best)	Patient volume score (21=best)	Procedure volume score (23=best)	Nurse-patient ratio (higher is better)	A Nurse Magnet hospital	No. of best practices (66=best)	% of specialists recommending hospital
1	Boston Children's Hospital	100.0	6	12	32	19	23	4.5	Yes	66	67.1%
2	Children's Hospital of Philadelphia	98.4	6	12	31	21	23	3.5	Yes	65	58.6%
3	Rady Children's Hospital, San Diego	93.6	6	12	32	17	16	3.1	Yes	65	50.1%
4	Cincinnati Children's Hospital Medical Center	93.3	6	12	31	17	20	4.4	Yes	66	31.8%
5	Children's Medical Cen. Dallas-Texas Scottish Rite Hosp. for Children	93.0	6	12	26	20	22	3.0	Yes	61	54.3%
6	Children's Hospital Los Angeles	90.9	6	12	31	19	22	3.3	Yes	65	25.3%
7	Nemours Alfred I. duPont Hosp. for Children, Wilmington, Del.	86.1	5	11	32	21	18	4.3	Yes	65	22.6%
8	Nationwide Children's Hospital, Columbus, Ohio	84.6	6	12	32	19	21	3.2	Yes	63	6.4%
9	Children's National Medical Center, Washington, D.C.	84.0	6	12	33	19	16	3.2	Yes	66	4.7%
10	Johns Hopkins Children's Center, Baltimore	83.9	6	12	33	13	20	3.4	Yes	66	7.5%
11	Ann and Robert H. Lurie Children's Hospital of Chicago	82.2	6	12	33	10	14	3.2	Yes	63	8.7%
12	Rainbow Babies and Children's Hospital, Cleveland	81.6	6	12	31	15	20	3.0	Yes	64	7.0%
13	Monroe Carell Jr. Children's Hospital at Vanderbilt, Nashville, Tenn.	81.4	6	12	30	19	19	3.1	Yes	61	4.5%
14	University of Michigan C.S. Mott Children's Hospital, Ann Arbor	78.8	6	12	28	10	16	3.7	Yes	59	3.7%
15	UCLA Mattel Children's Hospital, Los Angeles	78.6	6	12	28	15	14	3.7	Yes	60	2.9%
16	Texas Children's Hospital, Houston	78.5	6	8	33	17	14	3.7	Yes	63	8.7%
17	Children's Healthcare of Atlanta	78.4	4	12	32	20	20	4.1	No	63	14.4%
18	North Carolina Children's Hospital at UNC, Chapel Hill	78.2	6	12	31	11	15	3.9	Yes	64	0.2%
18	UC Davis Childrens Hospital/Shriners Hospitals N. Calif., Sacramento	78.2	5	12	33	16	17	5.7	Yes	66	4.4%
20	Seattle Children's Hospital	77.4	6	9	30	17	19	2.8	Yes	53	13.3%
21	Children's Hospital of Wisconsin, Milwaukee	76.7	6	12	26	14	18	4.5	Yes	58	1.2%
22	UCSF Benioff Children's Hospitals, San Francisco and Oakland	76.5	5	12	32	15	20	3.6	Yes	56	2.5%
23	Children's Hospital at Montefiore, New York	75.8	6	12	33	14	13	3.5	No	65	0.5%
23	Primary Children's Hosp.-Shriners Hosps. for Children, Salt Lake City	75.8	6	10	32	16	20	3.9	No	58	6.7%
25	St. Louis Children's Hospital-Washington University/Shriners Hospital	75.5	4	11	33	17	21	3.4	Yes	57	13.0%
26	Le Bonheur Children's Hospital, Memphis, Tenn.	75.2	6	9	30	16	15	3.2	Yes	59	5.9%
27	Mayo Clinic Children's Center, Rochester, Minn.	75.0	5	12	33	10	14	3.8	Yes	61	2.9%
28	Children's Mercy Kansas City, Mo.	74.7	6	8	31	21	20	4.3	Yes	65	3.2%
28	Hospital for Special Surgery, New York	74.7	6	12	24	15	15	5.6	Yes	58	3.4%
30	Riley Hospital for Children at IU Health, Indianapolis	74.0	6	10	26	17	18	4.1	Yes	63	1.7%
31	Nicklaus Children's Hospital, Miami	73.8	5	12	31	10	14	3.1	Yes	56	4.0%
32	Joe DiMaggio Children's Hospital at Memorial, Hollywood, Fla.	73.0	6	12	30	16	21	3.3	No	65	1.3%
33	Arnold Palmer Children's Hospital, Orlando, Fla.	72.6	6	12	28	7	11	3.6	Yes	60	3.5%
33	Children's Hospital of Pittsburgh of UPMC	72.6	6	8	31	17	16	3.4	Yes	58	2.0%
35	Cohen Children's Center, New Hyde Park, N.Y.	72.4	5	11	33	12	13	3.3	Yes	66	0.4%
36	Valley Children's Healthcare and Hospital, Madera, Calif.	72.3	6	12	31	16	12	2.8	Yes	61	0.4%
37	Levine Children's Hospital, Charlotte, N.C.	71.7	6	12	27	16	14	3.1	Yes	55	0.8%
38	CHOC Children's Hospital, Orange, Calif.	71.6	6	10	31	11	16	2.9	Yes	65	1.6%
38	NY-Presby. Morgan Stanley-Komansky Children's Hospital, N.Y.	71.6	5	12	33	9	12	2.8	No	51	8.4%
40	Johns Hopkins All Children's Hospital, St. Petersburg, Fla.	71.3	6	11	30	18	13	3.2	No	63	2.5%
41	Cleveland Clinic Children's Hospital	70.7	5	12	33	10	7	3.5	Yes	56	2.4%
41	University of Virginia Children's Hospital, Charlottesville	70.7	6	11	30	7	11	2.8	Yes	61	0.2%
43	Lucile Packard Children's Hospital Stanford, Palo Alto, Calif.	70.0	4	12	31	16	18	3.9	No	59	3.6%
44	Children's Hospital of Alabama at UAB, Birmingham	69.3	6	12	25	13	16	3.0	No	57	1.3%
44	Cook Children's Medical Center, Fort Worth	69.3	6	12	26	17	12	2.6	Yes	58	0.1%
46	Penn State Children's Hospital, Hershey, Pa.	68.1	6	12	28	7	5	3.1	Yes	43	0.4%
47	Dell Children's Medical Center of Central Texas, Austin	66.8	6	12	23	12	9	2.7	Yes	56	0.6%
48	Spectrum Hlth. Helen DeVos Children's Hosp., Grand Rapids, Mich.	66.7	6	9	28	9	11	2.8	Yes	58	0.8%
49	Children's Hospital of Michigan, Detroit	66.6	6	9	30	13	16	2.9	No	64	0.8%
49	Duke Children's Hospital and Health Center, Durham, N.C.	66.6	5	12	30	8	10	3.2	Yes	52	0.5%

Terms are explained on Page 158.

 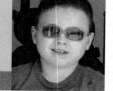

Our Partners
PUT THE MONEY
WHERE THE MIRACLES ARE.

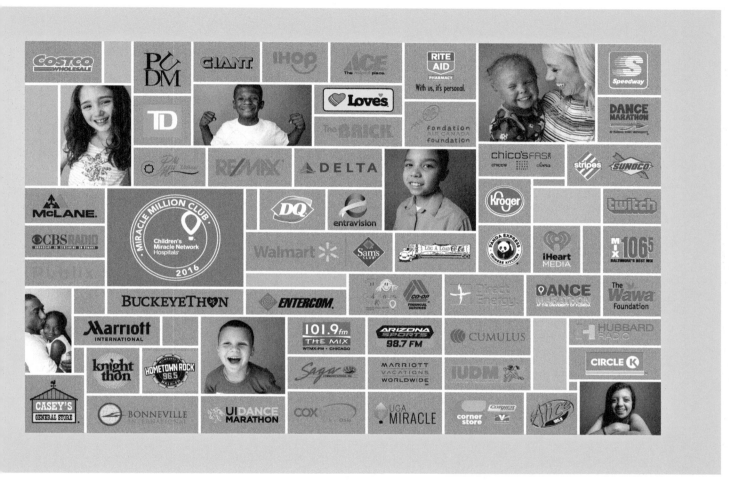

Thanks to all of our partners, we raised more than
$378 million last year for children's hospitals.

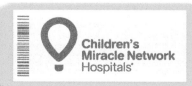

CMNHospitals.org

PULMONOLOGY

Rank	Hospital	U.S. News score	Asthma inpatient care score (5=best)	Lung transplant survival score (6=best)	Cystic fibrosis management score (16=best)	Infection prevention score, overall (45=best)	Infection prevention score, ICU (5=best)	Patient volume score (19=best)	Nurse-patient ratio (higher is better)	A Nurse Magnet hospital	% of specialists recommending hospital
1	Children's Hospital of Philadelphia	100.0	4	4	12	42	1	18	3.5	Yes	62.6%
2	Texas Children's Hospital, Houston	99.5	3	4	13	44	3	18	3.7	Yes	45.0%
3	Boston Children's Hospital	99.1	5	3	8	44	1	18	4.5	Yes	55.9%
4	Cincinnati Children's Hospital Medical Center	98.3	4	2	15	41	1	16	4.4	Yes	61.7%
5	Children's Hospital of Pittsburgh of UPMC	96.7	5	4	13	43	1	18	3.4	Yes	27.7%
6	Nationwide Children's Hospital, Columbus, Ohio	95.2	4	4	13	44	3	19	3.2	Yes	20.2%
7	Children's Hospital Colorado, Aurora	92.8	5	NA	11	42	4	14	3.3	Yes	48.0%
8	St. Louis Children's Hospital-Washington University	91.8	5	2	13	43	3	15	3.4	Yes	21.7%
9	North Carolina Children's Hospital at UNC, Chapel Hill	88.1	4	3	11	41	3	11	3.9	Yes	18.9%
10	Johns Hopkins Children's Center, Baltimore	87.8	4	NA	12	45	3	14	3.4	Yes	24.5%
11	Lucile Packard Children's Hospital Stanford, Palo Alto, Calif.	86.7	5	4	10	43	1	16	3.9	No	15.3%
12	Seattle Children's Hospital	85.6	5	NA	10	41	1	14	2.8	Yes	38.7%
13	Monroe Carell Jr. Children's Hosp. at Vanderbilt, Nashville, Tenn.	84.7	5	NA	15	41	3	12	3.1	Yes	7.6%
14	NY-Presby. Morgan Stanley-Komansky Children's Hospital, N.Y.	84.0	4	6	10	45	4	14	2.8	No	4.9%
14	Riley Hospital for Children at IU Health, Indianapolis	84.0	4	3	10	36	2	17	4.1	Yes	16.1%
16	Children's National Medical Center, Washington, D.C.	83.8	5	NA	10	45	4	13	3.2	Yes	6.0%
17	Children's Hospital of Wisconsin, Milwaukee	83.4	5	NA	14	38	5	14	4.5	Yes	2.9%
18	Children's Hospital Los Angeles	83.0	4	NA	14	43	3	15	3.3	Yes	13.9%
19	Rainbow Babies and Children's Hospital, Cleveland	81.6	5	NR	10	42	2	11	3.0	Yes	17.1%
20	Ann and Robert H. Lurie Children's Hospital of Chicago	79.3	4	NA	13	43	2	11	3.2	Yes	10.6%
21	University of Michigan C.S. Mott Children's Hospital, Ann Arbor	76.0	4	NA	12	40	4	13	3.7	Yes	3.7%
22	Le Bonheur Children's Hospital, Memphis, Tenn.	75.2	5	NA	12	36	3	10	3.2	Yes	4.3%
23	Duke Children's Hospital and Health Center, Durham, N.C.	74.9	5	3	9	41	3	9	3.2	Yes	1.1%
24	Nicklaus Children's Hospital, Miami	74.5	4	NA	12	43	5	12	3.1	Yes	1.7%
25	Cohen Children's Center, New Hyde Park, N.Y.	74.2	5	NA	10	44	4	11	3.3	Yes	0.7%
26	Rady Children's Hospital, San Diego	73.0	5	NA	12	42	2	13	3.1	Yes	4.1%
27	UCSF Benioff Children's Hospitals, San Francisco and Oakland	72.6	4	NA	10	40	3	11	3.6	No	3.8%
28	Children's Healthcare of Atlanta	72.3	5	NA	10	41	3	17	4.1	No	1.8%
29	Children's Hospital of Alabama at UAB, Birmingham	72.1	5	NA	11	35	3	16	3.0	No	7.4%
30	NYU Winthrop Hospital Children's Medical Center, Mineola, N.Y.	72.0	5	NA	15	43	3	8	2.1	Yes	0.5%
31	Nemours Alfred I. duPont Hosp. for Children, Wilmington, Del.	71.8	4	NA	11	44	3	10	4.3	Yes	0.5%
32	Mount Sinai Kravis Children's Hospital, New York	71.1	3	NA	14	45	4	7	3.9	Yes	0.1%
33	UF Health Shands Children's Hospital, Gainesville, Fla.	70.7	5	4	11	38	2	9	2.6	Yes	0.4%
34	Children's Hospitals and Clinics of Minnesota, Minneapolis	70.0	5	NA	12	36	4	12	3.3	No	1.6%
35	Cleveland Clinic Children's Hospital	69.8	5	NA	9	45	0	13	3.5	Yes	2.7%
36	Arnold Palmer Children's Hospital, Orlando, Fla.	69.6	4	NA	13	40	4	9	3.6	Yes	0.6%
37	CHOC Children's Hospital, Orange, Calif.	69.1	5	NA	12	43	2	11	2.9	Yes	1.6%
38	Mayo Clinic Children's Center, Rochester, Minn.	68.8	4	NA	12	44	1	6	3.8	Yes	1.7%
39	Yale-New Haven Children's Hospital, New Haven, Conn.	68.6	5	NA	12	43	3	9	2.5	Yes	2.5%
40	MassGeneral Hospital for Children, Boston	68.4	4	NA	7	32	4	7	4.0	Yes	2.5%
41	Spectrum Hlth. Helen DeVos Children's Hosp., Grand Rapids, Mich.	67.7	5	NA	11	35	3	9	2.8	Yes	0.7%
42	American Family Children's Hospital, Madison, Wis.	67.5	4	NA	10	31	3	10	4.7	Yes	1.2%
43	UCLA Mattel Children's Hospital, Los Angeles	67.4	4	NA	10	40	3	8	3.7	Yes	3.2%
43	University of Minnesota Masonic Children's Hospital, Minneapolis	67.4	4	3	12	34	3	9	2.5	No	0.7%
45	University of Iowa Children's Hospital, Iowa City	66.4	4	NA	11	43	3	11	3.0	Yes	1.6%
46	Children's Mercy Kansas City, Mo.	66.3	4	NA	10	41	1	12	4.3	Yes	2.2%
47	Arkansas Children's Hospital, Little Rock	66.1	4	NA	13	34	4	9	3.2	Yes	1.6%
48	Children's Hospital of Michigan, Detroit	66.0	5	NA	6	42	3	12	2.9	No	0.2%
49	Primary Children's Hospital, Salt Lake City	65.3	5	NA	11	41	3	12	3.9	No	0.1%
50	Doernbecher Children's Hospital, Portland, Ore.	65.1	5	NA	11	40	1	9	3.7	Yes	0.9%

NA=not applicable; service not provided by hospital. NR=data not reported or unavailable. Terms are explained on Page 158.

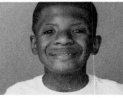

UROLOGY

Rank	Hospital	U.S. News score	Surgical complications prevention score (18=best)	Testicular torsion care score (2=best)	Infection prevention score, overall (28=best)	Patient volume score (33=best)	Surgery volume score (23=best)	Minimally invasive volume score (12=best)	Nurse-patient ratio (higher is better)	A Nurse Magnet hospital	% of specialists recommending hospital
1	Boston Children's Hospital	100.0	17	2	26	30	20	12	4.5	Yes	73.6%
2	Children's Hospital of Philadelphia	94.9	14	2	25	31	20	11	3.5	Yes	76.2%
3	Cincinnati Children's Hospital Medical Center	93.0	15	2	25	30	20	12	4.4	Yes	43.0%
4	Ann and Robert H. Lurie Children's Hospital of Chicago	90.7	15	2	27	29	18	12	3.2	Yes	40.1%
5	Riley Hospital for Children at IU Health, Indianapolis	88.7	14	2	20	32	23	11	4.1	Yes	52.4%
6	Texas Children's Hospital, Houston	86.7	12	2	27	29	21	12	3.7	Yes	37.2%
7	Johns Hopkins Children's Center, Baltimore	86.4	15	2	27	26	19	11	3.4	Yes	23.7%
7	Monroe Carell Jr. Children's Hosp. at Vanderbilt, Nashville, Tenn.	86.4	13	2	24	31	22	11	3.1	Yes	39.0%
9	Cohen Children's Center, New Hyde Park, N.Y.	84.7	18	2	27	28	20	12	3.3	Yes	5.8%
10	Nationwide Children's Hospital, Columbus, Ohio	83.5	15	2	26	29	19	11	3.2	Yes	17.1%
11	Seattle Children's Hospital	81.1	17	1	24	22	20	9	2.8	Yes	35.7%
12	Children's Hospital of Pittsburgh of UPMC	80.5	14	2	25	25	22	12	3.4	Yes	10.4%
13	Children's Hospital Colorado, Aurora	79.5	15	2	25	24	19	8	3.3	Yes	9.5%
14	Children's Medical Center Dallas	79.3	16	2	20	27	17	11	3.0	Yes	11.7%
14	St. Louis Children's Hospital-Washington University	79.3	17	2	27	21	18	8	3.4	Yes	4.5%
16	Children's Hospital Los Angeles	79.0	14	2	25	24	19	12	3.3	Yes	11.3%
17	Nicklaus Children's Hospital, Miami	75.1	16	2	25	14	18	11	3.1	Yes	4.1%
18	CHOC Children's Hospital, Orange, Calif.	74.7	16	2	25	23	16	7	2.9	Yes	4.1%
19	Le Bonheur Children's Hospital, Memphis, Tenn.	74.4	14	2	24	25	16	9	3.2	Yes	3.6%
20	Children's Mercy Kansas City, Mo.	74.0	15	2	25	23	16	6	4.3	Yes	1.2%
21	Children's National Medical Center, Washington, D.C.	73.7	8	2	27	26	18	11	3.2	Yes	17.8%
22	Rady Children's Hospital, San Diego	73.5	12	2	26	25	17	7	3.1	Yes	8.6%
23	American Family Children's Hospital, Madison, Wis.	73.0	16	2	19	24	16	7	4.7	Yes	2.6%
24	Cleveland Clinic Children's Hospital	72.6	15	2	27	12	13	9	3.5	Yes	0.6%
25	Children's Hospital of Michigan, Detroit	72.3	17	2	24	20	13	5	2.9	No	3.4%
26	Children's Healthcare of Atlanta	71.4	12	2	26	28	16	12	4.1	No	9.4%
26	UC Davis Children's Hospital/Shriners Hospitals N. Calif., Sacramento	71.4	15	2	27	20	13	6	5.7	Yes	1.0%
28	University of Michigan C.S. Mott Children's Hospital, Ann Arbor	71.1	14	2	22	21	19	8	3.7	Yes	3.2%
29	Children's Hospital of Illinois, Peoria	70.0	17	2	26	14	13	7	3.2	Yes	0.8%
30	Akron Children's Hospital, Ohio	69.7	15	2	23	24	12	8	3.4	Yes	1.9%
30	Mount Sinai Kravis Children's Hospital, New York	69.7	15	2	27	12	13	5	3.9	Yes	0.7%
32	Lucile Packard Children's Hospital Stanford, Palo Alto, Calif.	69.5	13	2	25	27	13	5	3.9	No	5.0%
33	Spectrum Hlth. Helen DeVos Children's Hosp., Grand Rapids, Mich.	69.4	16	2	22	18	15	7	2.8	Yes	0.6%
34	Mayo Clinic Children's Center, Rochester, Minn.	69.3	12	2	27	25	13	7	3.8	Yes	4.1%
35	Primary Children's Hospital, Salt Lake City	69.0	11	2	26	28	22	9	3.9	No	9.1%
36	University of Iowa Children's Hospital, Iowa City	68.4	14	2	25	24	19	6	3.0	Yes	3.0%
37	MUSC Health-Children's Hospital, Charleston, S.C.	67.8	15	2	24	15	11	7	2.8	Yes	1.0%
38	Children's Hospital of Wisconsin, Milwaukee	66.2	11	2	20	22	19	10	4.5	Yes	2.6%
39	Bristol-Myers Squibb Children's Hosp., New Brunswick, N.J.	66.1	16	2	19	19	13	7	2.3	Yes	0.5%
40	UCLA Mattel Children's Hospital, Los Angeles	65.8	12	2	22	11	12	4	3.7	Yes	4.8%
41	Children's Hospital at Montefiore, New York	65.4	15	2	27	11	9	5	3.5	No	0.4%
42	Nemours Alfred I. duPont Hosp. for Children, Wilmington, Del.	65.3	9	2	26	19	13	10	4.3	Yes	1.9%
43	NY-Presby. Morgan Stanley-Komansky Children's Hospital, N.Y.	65.1	12	2	27	18	15	8	2.8	Yes	3.7%
44	Duke Children's Hospital and Health Center, Durham, N.C.	63.2	11	2	24	22	13	6	3.2	Yes	3.1%
45	Arnold Palmer Children's Hospital, Orlando, Fla.	62.5	15	2	22	10	12	8	3.6	Yes	0.4%
45	Yale-New Haven/Connecticut Children's Medical Centers, New Haven	62.5	13	1	25	24	13	11	2.5	Yes	6.3%
47	NYU Winthrop Hospital Children's Medical Center, Mineola, N.Y.	62.1	18	2	25	5	8	2	2.1	Yes	0.7%
48	Arkansas Children's Hospital, Little Rock	61.7	11	2	22	18	10	10	3.2	Yes	1.1%
48	Joe DiMaggio Children's Hospital at Memorial, Hollywood, Fla.	61.7	15	2	24	11	11	6	3.3	No	1.2%
50	Phoenix Children's Hospital	61.1	10	2	25	29	17	6	2.8	No	2.8%
50	Rainbow Babies and Children's Hospital, Cleveland	61.1	17	1	25	12	10	4	3.0	Yes	1.5%

Terms are explained on Page 158.

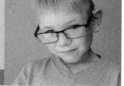

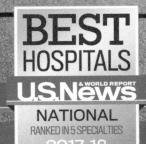

Keck Medical Center of USC recognized as a top 10 California hospital —
once again

CHAPTER 6

BEST REGIONAL HOSPITALS

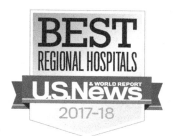

BEST REGIONAL HOSPITALS
U.S.News & WORLD REPORT
2017-18

Great care can be found close to home. Whether you seek expertise for highly specialized complex conditions or more commonplace treatment like joint replacement surgery, most states boast at least one facility, and many states have many, that we recognize as a Best Regional Hospital.

STAR POWER NEAR HOME

How we identified and ranked the top hospitals state by state

By Ben Harder and Avery Comarow

I f you're like most people facing hospitalization, you would much prefer to stay close to home. You'll feel more comfortable, and lower stress can lead to faster recovery. Your family can visit without racking up hotel bills. And a battle with your health insurer over coverage at an out-of-network facility might be avoidable.

Since 2011, our Best Regional Hospitals listings have showcased hundreds of facilities around the U.S. that offer high-quality care across a range of clinical services. These services include both complex, highly specialized care for the sickest patients – the focus of the Best Hospitals rankings (Page 96) – and safe, effective treatment for those whose medical needs are more commonplace, such as patients seeking hip or knee replacement surgery for age-related arthritis. These state-by-state rankings, which can be found in their entirety at usnews.com/bestregionalhospitals, offer readers in most parts of the country a number of high-quality choices that are apt to be convenient and in-network.

These evaluations include ratings of how well hospitals handle nine relatively common procedures and conditions in addition to their assessments in 12 specialties. The nine areas of care are heart bypass surgery, aortic valve surgery, abdominal aortic aneurysm repair, heart failure, hip replacement, knee replacement, colon cancer surgery, lung cancer surgery and chronic obstructive pulmonary disease. Hospitals are assigned a rating of "high performing," "average" or "below average" in each area in which they treated enough patients to be evaluated.

Recognition as a 2017-18 Best Regional Hospital means a hospital was nationally ranked in at least one of the 12 Best Hospitals specialties that use objective data* or that it earned at least three "high performing" ratings across the nine procedures and conditions and the 12 specialties. In the specialties, high performing signifies a score below those of the 50 top hospitals but within the high-

Duke is one of 48 hospitals earning top honors in routine care.

est 10 percent of hospitals that we evaluated. (An FAQ at usnews.com/best-hospitals offers more details.)

This year 535 hospitals merited Best Regional Hospitals status. They appear ranked by state on the following pages. In each state with at least two Best Regional Hospitals that met certain criteria, hospitals are numerically ordered according to the following rules:

1. The higher rank went to the hospital with the better status in the Best Hospitals Honor Roll ranking, if any.

2. Next, the higher rank went to the hospital that earned more points according to the following three rules: (a) A hospital received two points for each of the 12 specialties in which it was ranked among the top 50. (b) A hospital received one point for each specialty, procedure or condition in which it was rated high performing. (c) A hospital lost one point for each procedure or condition in which it was rated below average.

Based on the same rules, hospitals in major metropolitan areas also received rankings that compare them to other top hospitals in the same metropolis. Our website displays these rankings for 47 metro areas with at least 1 million residents. The website also lists top hospitals in some 200 U.S. News-de-

---

*Cancer; cardiology & heart surgery; diabetes & endocrinology; ear, nose & throat; gastroenterology & GI surgery; geriatrics; gynecology; nephrology; neurology & neurosurgery; orthopedics; pulmonology; and urology.

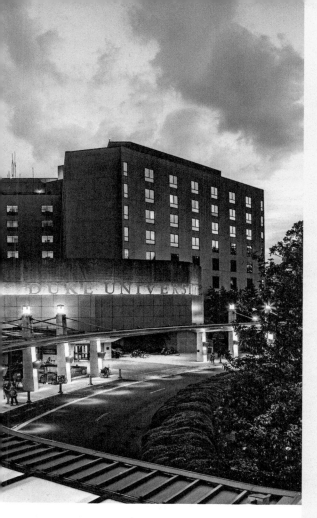

fined regions, such as Southern Indiana and Texas Hill Country, to help consumers outside the biggest urban centers searching for high-quality care.

How a hospital performed in four specialties – ophthalmology, psychiatry, rehabilitation and rheumatology – is not a factor in the regional rankings. That these specialties are important is undeniable. But objective data on which to compare hospitals' performance are either not available or do not meet our rigorous analytical standards.

Consequently, some hospitals that excel in one or more of those specialties may not appear among the Best Regional Hospitals. Specialty hospitals such as dedicated cancer centers and surgical hospitals also were not considered in the regional rankings. Specialty hospitals have indisputable but narrow value; such a hospital might only do surgery, say, or only treat heart patients. Our goal with the state and metro area rankings is to identify general medical-surgical hospitals that offer both high-quality care and breadth of care, so only hospitals that deliver a wide range of clinical services for adult patients were considered for Best Regional Hospitals status.

Children's hospitals are excluded from consideration in the regional rankings because so few metro areas have more than one or two. There are fewer than 200 in the entire country. ●

TOPS AT ROUTINE CARE

U.S. News evaluated more than 4,500 hospitals for their handling of nine surgical procedures and chronic conditions: colon cancer surgery, lung cancer surgery, COPD, heart failure, heart bypass surgery, aortic valve surgery, abdominal aortic aneurysm repair, knee replacement and hip replacement. Of that total, 1,214 earned at least one top rating of "high performing." But only these 48 standouts, just over 1 percent of the hospitals evaluated, got the top rating in all nine:

- **Abbott Northwestern Hospital,** Minneapolis
- **Aurora St. Luke's Medical Center,** Milwaukee
- **Baptist Health Lexington,** Ky.
- **Barnes-Jewish Hospital,** St. Louis
- **Baystate Medical Center,** Springfield, Mass.
- **Beaumont Hospital-Royal Oak,** Mich.
- **Carilion Roanoke Memorial Hospital,** Roanoke, Va.
- **Carolinas Medical Center,** Charlotte, N.C.
- **Cedars-Sinai Medical Center,** Los Angeles
- **CHI Memorial Hospital,** Chattanooga, Tenn.
- **Christ Hospital,** Cincinnati
- **Christiana Care Hospitals,** Newark, Del.
- **Duke University Hospital,** Durham, N.C.
- **Eisenhower Medical Center,** Rancho Mirage, Calif.
- **Emory St. Joseph's Hospital,** Atlanta
- **Emory University Hospital,** Atlanta
- **Florida Hospital,** Orlando
- **Hoag Memorial Hospital Presbyterian,** Newport Beach, Calif.
- **Houston Methodist Hospital**
- **John Muir Medical Center, Concord,** Calif.
- **Lancaster General Hospital,** Lancaster, Pa.
- **Lehigh Valley Hospital,** Allentown, Pa.
- **Maine Medical Center,** Portland
- **Massachusetts General Hospital,** Boston

- **Mayo Clinic,** Rochester, Minn.
- **Mayo Clinic Jacksonville,** Fla.
- **Mayo Clinic Phoenix**
- **Missouri Baptist Medical Center,** St. Louis
- **Morristown Medical Center,** Morristown, N.J.
- **Moses H. Cone Memorial Hospital,** Greensboro, N.C.
- **Munson Medical Center,** Traverse City, Mich.
- **Northwestern Memorial Hospital,** Chicago
- **OHSU Hospital,** Portland, Ore.
- **Orlando Regional Medical Center**
- **Providence St. Vincent Medical Center,** Portland, Ore.
- **Rush University Medical Center,** Chicago
- **Sanford USD Medical Center,** Sioux Falls, S.D.
- **Sarasota Memorial Health-Sarasota Hospital,** Sarasota, Fla.
- **Scripps La Jolla Hospitals,** La Jolla, Calif.
- **Spectrum Health-Butterworth-Blodgett Hospitals,** Grand Rapids, Mich.
- **St. Cloud Hospital,** St. Cloud, Minn.
- **St. Joseph Hospital Health Center,** Syracuse, N.Y.
- **St. Luke's Regional Medical Center,** Boise, Idaho
- **Stanford Health Care-Stanford Hospital,** Stanford, Calif.
- **Thomas Jefferson University Hospitals,** Philadelphia
- **UNC Rex Hospital,** Raleigh, N.C.
- **University of Tennessee Medical Center,** Knoxville
- **Vanderbilt University Medical Center,** Nashville

	COMPLEX SPECIALTY CARE	COMMON PROCEDURES & CONDITIONS
COMPLEX SPECIALTY CARE	● Nationally ranked ● High performing	
COMMON PROCEDURES & CONDITIONS	○ High performing ○ Average ● Below average	

Column headers (Complex Specialty Care): Cancer · Cardiology & Heart Surgery · Diabetes & Endocrinology · Ear, Nose & Throat · Gastroenterology & GI Surgery · Geriatrics · Gynecology · Nephrology · Neurology & Neurosurgery · Orthopedics · Pulmonology · Urology

Column headers (Common Procedures & Conditions): Colon Cancer Surgery · Lung Cancer Surgery · Heart Bypass Surgery · Heart Failure · Heart Valve Surgery · Abdominal Aortic Aneurysm · Hip Replacement · Knee Replacement · COPD

State Rank Hospital	Can	Cardio	Diab	ENT	Gastro	Geri	Gyn	Neph	Neuro	Ortho	Pulm	Urol	Colon	Lung	Bypass	HtFail	Valve	AAA	Hip	Knee	COPD
ALABAMA																					
1 University of Alabama at Birmingham Hospital	●	●	●	●	●	●	●	●	●	●	●	●	●	●	●	●	●	●	●	●	●
2 Huntsville Hospital, Huntsville	–	–	–	–	–	–	–	–	–	–	–	–	●	●	●	●	●	●	●	●	●
ARIZONA																					
1 Mayo Clinic Phoenix	●	●	●	●	●	–	●	●	●	●	●	●	●	●	●	●	●	●	●	●	●
2 Banner University Medical Center Phoenix	–	●	●	–	●	●	●	●	●	–	●	●	●	●	●	●	●	●	●	●	●
2 Banner University Medical Center Tucson	●	–	●	●	●	●	●	–	●	●	●	●	●	●	●	●	●	●	●	●	●
4 Banner Estrella Medical Center, Phoenix	–	●	●	–	–	–	●	–	–	–	●	●	●	●	●	●	●	–	–	●	●
5 Flagstaff Medical Center, Flagstaff	–	–	●	–	●	–	–	–	●	●	●	–	●	●	●	●	●	●	●	●	●
5 St. Joseph's Hospital and Medical Center, Phoenix	–	–	–	–	–	●	●	–	●	●	●	–	●	●	●	●	●	●	●	●	●
7 Banner Boswell Medical Center, Sun City	–	–	–	–	–	–	–	–	–	–	–	–	●	●	●	●	●	●	●	●	●
8 HonorHealth Scottsdale Shea Medical Center, Scottsdale	–	–	–	–	–	–	–	–	–	–	–	–	●	●	●	●	●	●	●	●	●
9 Chandler Regional Medical Center, Chandler	–	–	–	–	–	–	–	●	–	–	●	–	●	●	●	●	●	●	●	●	●
9 HonorHealth Scottsdale Osborn Medical Center, Scottsdale	–	–	–	–	–	–	–	–	–	–	–	–	●	●	●	●	●	–	●	●	●
9 HonorHealth Scottsdale Thompson Peak Medical Center, Scottsdale	–	–	–	–	–	–	–	–	–	–	–	–	●	●	–	●	–	–	●	●	●
12 Carondelet St. Joseph's Hospital, Tucson	–	–	–	–	–	–	–	–	–	–	–	–	●	●	●	●	●	●	●	●	●
12 HonorHealth Deer Valley Medical Center, Phoenix	–	–	–	–	–	–	–	–	–	–	–	–	●	●	●	●	●	●	●	●	●
12 TMC Healthcare-Tucson	–	–	–	–	–	–	–	–	–	–	–	–	●	●	●	●	●	●	●	●	●
ARKANSAS																					
1 CHI St. Vincent Infirmary, Little Rock	–	–	–	–	–	–	–	–	–	–	–	–	●	●	●	●	●	●	●	●	●
2 Baptist Health Medical Center-Little Rock	–	–	–	–	–	–	–	–	–	–	–	–	●	●	●	●	●	●	●	●	●
CALIFORNIA																					
1 UCSF Medical Center, San Francisco	●	●	●	●	●	●	●	●	●	●	●	●	●	●	●	●	●	●	●	●	●
2 Ronald Reagan UCLA Medical Center, Los Angeles[1]	●	●	●	●	●	●	●	●	●	●	●	●	●	●	●	●	●	●	●	●	●
3 Stanford Health Care-Stanford Hospital, Stanford	●	●	●	●	●	●	●	●	●	●	●	●	●	●	●	●	●	●	●	●	●
4 Cedars-Sinai Medical Center, Los Angeles	●	●	●	●	●	●	●	●	●	●	●	●	●	●	●	●	●	●	●	●	●
5 University of California, Davis Medical Center, Sacramento	●	●	●	●	●	●	●	●	●	●	●	●	●	●	●	●	●	●	●	●	●
6 Scripps La Jolla Hospitals, La Jolla	●	●	–	●	●	●	●	●	●	●	●	●	●	●	●	●	●	●	●	●	●
7 UC San Diego Medical Center[2]	●	●	–	●	●	●	●	●	●	●	●	●	●	●	●	●	●	●	●	●	●
8 Hoag Memorial Hospital Presbyterian, Newport Beach	–	–	–	●	●	–	●	–	●	●	●	●	●	●	●	●	●	●	●	●	●
9 Huntington Memorial Hospital, Pasadena	–	●	●	●	●	–	●	●	●	●	●	–	●	●	●	●	●	–	●	●	●
10 Keck Hospital of USC, Los Angeles[3]	●	●	●	–	●	●	●	–	●	●	–	●	●	●	●	●	●	●	●	●	●
11 John Muir Medical Center, Walnut Creek	–	–	–	●	●	●	●	–	●	●	●	–	●	●	●	●	●	●	●	●	●
11 UC Irvine Medical Center, Orange	●	–	–	●	●	●	●	●	●	●	●	–	●	●	●	●	●	●	●	●	●
13 John Muir Medical Center, Concord	–	–	–	●	●	●	–	●	●	●	–	●	●	●	●	●	●	●	●	●	●
13 Long Beach Memorial Medical Center, Long Beach	–	–	–	●	●	–	●	●	●	–	●	●	●	●	●	●	●	●	●	●	●
15 Sharp Memorial Hospital, San Diego	–	–	–	–	●	–	●	–	–	–	●	–	●	●	●	●	●	●	●	●	●
16 Eisenhower Medical Center, Rancho Mirage	–	–	–	–	●	–	–	–	–	–	–	–	●	●	●	●	●	●	●	●	●
16 Providence Little Company of Mary Medical Center Torrance	–	●	–	–	●	–	●	–	●	–	●	–	●	●	●	●	–	●	●	●	●
18 El Camino Hospital, Mountain View	–	–	–	–	–	–	–	●	–	●	–	–	●	●	●	●	●	●	●	●	●
18 St. Joseph Hospital, Orange	–	–	–	–	–	–	–	●	–	●	–	–	●	●	●	●	●	●	●	●	●
18 St. Jude Medical Center, Fullerton	–	●	–	–	–	–	–	●	–	●	–	–	●	●	●	●	●	●	●	●	●
18 Sutter Medical Center, Sacramento	–	–	–	–	–	–	–	●	–	●	–	–	●	●	●	●	●	●	●	●	●
22 Kaiser Permanente Los Angeles Medical Center	–	–	–	●	●	–	●	●	●	–	●	–	●	●	●	–	●	●	●	●	●
22 Providence Holy Cross Medical Center, Mission Hills	–	–	–	–	●	●	–	–	–	●	●	–	●	●	●	●	●	●	●	●	●

In complex care specialties, (-) indicates hospital is not nationally ranked or high performing.
In procedures and conditions, (-) indicates care not offered or hospital has too few Medicare patients to be rated.

A footnote indicates that another hospital's results are included, that the hospital has a different name in one or more areas of care, or both.
[1] Santa Monica-UCLA Medical Center and Orthopedic Hospital. [2] UC San Diego Health-Moores Cancer Center; UC San Diego Health-Sulpizio Cardiovascular Center.
[3] USC Norris Cancer Hospital-Keck Medical Center of USC.

More @ usnews.com/bestregionalhospitals

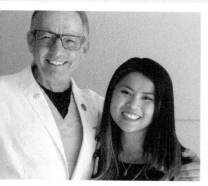
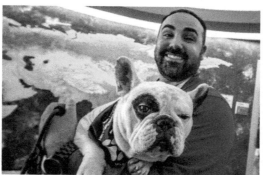
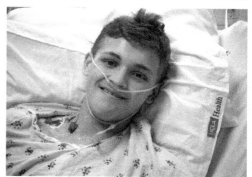
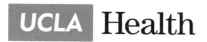
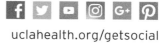

COMPLEX SPECIALTY CARE   COMMON PROCEDURES & CONDITIONS

COMPLEX SPECIALTY CARE
- ● Nationally ranked
- ● High performing

COMMON PROCEDURES & CONDITIONS
- ● High performing
- ○ Average
- ● Below average

State Rank	Hospital	Cancer	Cardiology & Heart Surgery	Diabetes & Endocrinology	Ear, Nose & Throat	Gastroenterology & GI Surgery	Geriatrics	Gynecology	Nephrology	Neurology & Neurosurgery	Orthopedics	Pulmonology	Urology	Colon Cancer Surgery	Lung Cancer Surgery	Heart Bypass Surgery	Heart Failure	Heart Valve Surgery	Abdominal Aortic Aneurysm	Hip Replacement	Knee Replacement	COPD
CALIFORNIA (CONTINUED)																						
24	Kaiser Permanente Anaheim Medical Center, Anaheim	–	–	–	–	–	–	–	–	●	–	–	●	●	–	●	–	–	●	●	●	
24	Orange Coast Memorial Medical Center, Fountain Valley	–	–	–	–	●	–	●	–	●	–	–	●	●	●	●	●	●	–	●	●	●
26	Kaiser Permanente San Francisco Medical Center	–	●	–	–	–	–	●	–	●	–	●	–	●	●	●	●	●	●	●	●	●
26	Torrance Memorial Medical Center, Torrance	–	–	–	–	–	–	–	–	–	–	●	–	●	●	●	●	●	●	●	●	●
28	Glendale Adventist Medical Center, Los Angeles	–	–	–	–	●	–	●	–	●	●	–	●	●	●	●	●	–	●	●	●	●
28	Mission Hospitals, Mission Viejo and Laguna Beach, Mission Viejo	–	–	–	–	–	–	–	–	●	–	●	–	●	●	●	●	●	●	●	●	●
28	Oroville Hospital, Oroville	–	–	–	●	●	–	●	–	–	●	–	●	●	–	●	●	–	●	–	●	●
28	Sharp Grossmont Hospital, La Mesa	–	–	–	–	–	–	–	–	–	–	●	–	●	●	●	●	●	●	●	●	●
32	California Pacific Medical Center, San Francisco	–	–	–	–	–	–	–	–	●	–	●	–	●	●	●	●	●	●	●	●	●
32	Kaiser Permanente Downey Medical Center, Downey	–	–	–	–	–	–	–	–	●	–	–	●	●	●	●	–	●	–	●	●	●
32	Kaiser Permanente Oakland Medical Center, Oakland	–	–	–	–	–	–	–	–	–	–	–	●	●	●	●	●	–	–	●	●	●
32	Kaiser Permanente Roseville Medical Center, Roseville	–	–	–	–	–	–	–	–	–	–	–	●	●	●	●	●	●	–	●	●	●
32	Kaiser Permanente Santa Clara Medical Center, Santa Clara	–	–	–	–	–	–	–	–	–	–	–	●	●	●	●	●	●	–	●	●	●
32	Kaiser Permanente South Bay Medical Center, Harbor City	●	–	–	–	–	–	–	–	–	–	–	●	●	–	●	●	–	–	●	●	●
32	Memorial Medical Center, Modesto	–	–	–	–	–	–	●	–	–	–	–	●	●	●	●	●	●	●	●	●	●
32	Mercy General Hospital, Sacramento	–	–	–	–	–	–	–	–	–	–	●	–	●	●	●	●	●	●	●	●	●
32	NorthBay Medical Center, Fairfield	–	–	–	–	–	–	–	–	–	–	●	–	●	●	●	●	–	●	●	●	●
32	Providence Tarzana Medical Center, Tarzana	–	–	●	–	●	–	–	–	–	–	–	●	●	●	●	●	●	●	●	●	●
32	Scripps Mercy Hospital, San Diego	–	–	–	–	–	–	●	–	–	–	–	●	●	●	●	●	●	●	●	●	●
32	Washington Hospital, Fremont	–	–	–	–	–	–	–	–	–	–	–	●	●	●	●	●	●	–	●	●	●
44	Alta Bates Summit Medical Center, Oakland	–	–	–	–	–	–	–	–	–	–	–	●	●	–	●	●	–	●	●	●	●
44	Kaiser Permanente Antioch Medical Center, Antioch	–	–	–	–	–	–	–	–	–	–	–	–	–	–	●	●	–	–	●	●	●
44	Kaiser Permanente Fontana and Ontario Medical Centers, Fontana	–	–	–	–	–	–	–	–	–	–	–	●	●	●	●	●	●	–	●	●	●
44	Loma Linda University Medical Center, Loma Linda	–	–	–	–	–	–	–	–	●	–	–	●	●	●	●	●	●	–	●	●	●
44	Providence St. John's Health Center, Santa Monica	–	–	–	–	–	–	–	–	–	–	–	●	●	●	●	●	●	–	●	●	●
44	Sequoia Hospital, Redwood City	–	–	–	–	–	–	–	–	–	–	–	●	●	●	●	●	●	●	●	●	●
44	St. Helena Hospital Napa Valley, St. Helena	–	–	–	–	–	–	–	–	–	–	–	●	●	●	●	●	●	–	●	●	●
44	St. Vincent Medical Center, Los Angeles	–	–	–	–	–	–	–	–	–	–	–	●	●	●	●	●	–	●	●	●	●
52	Los Robles Hospital and Medical Center, Thousand Oaks	–	–	–	–	–	–	–	–	–	–	–	●	●	●	●	●	●	●	●	●	●
53	Centinela Hospital Medical Center, Inglewood	–	–	–	–	●	–	–	–	–	–	–	●	●	●	●	●	●	–	●	●	●
COLORADO																						
1	University of Colorado Hospital, Aurora[4]	●	●	●	–	●	●	●	●	●	●	●	●	●	●	●	●	●	●	●	●	●
2	Porter Adventist Hospital, Denver	–	–	–	●	●	●	–	●	–	●	●	●	●	●	●	●	●	●	●	●	●
3	Rose Medical Center, Denver	–	–	–	–	●	●	●	–	●	–	●	–	●	●	●	●	●	●	●	●	●
4	Medical Center of Aurora	–	–	●	–	●	–	–	●	–	●	●	●	●	●	●	●	–	●	●	●	●
5	Medical Center of the Rockies, Loveland	–	–	–	–	●	–	–	–	●	–	●	●	●	●	●	●	●	●	●	●	●
5	Parker Adventist Hospital, Parker	–	–	–	–	●	–	–	–	●	●	–	●	●	–	●	●	–	●	●	●	●
5	Sky Ridge Medical Center, Lone Tree	–	–	–	–	–	●	–	●	–	●	–	●	●	●	●	●	●	●	●	●	●
8	Penrose-St. Francis Health Services, Colorado Springs	–	–	–	–	–	–	–	–	–	–	–	●	●	●	●	●	●	–	●	●	●
8	Poudre Valley Hospital, Fort Collins	–	–	–	–	–	–	–	–	–	–	–	●	●	●	●	●	–	–	●	●	●
10	Lutheran Medical Center, Wheat Ridge	–	–	–	–	–	–	–	–	–	–	–	●	●	●	●	●	●	●	●	●	●
10	Presbyterian-St. Luke's Medical Center, Denver	●	–	–	–	–	–	–	–	●	–	–	●	●	●	●	●	●	●	●	●	●
10	St. Mary's Medical Center, Grand Junction	–	–	–	–	–	–	–	–	–	–	●	–	●	●	●	●	●	●	●	●	●

In complex care specialties, (-) indicates hospital is not nationally ranked or high performing.
In procedures and conditions, (-) indicates care not offered or hospital has too few Medicare patients to be rated.

A footnote indicates that another hospital's results are included, that the hospital has a different name in one or more areas of care, or both.
[4]National Jewish Health, Denver-University of Colorado Hospital, Aurora.

More @ usnews.com/bestregionalhospitals

For Our Community

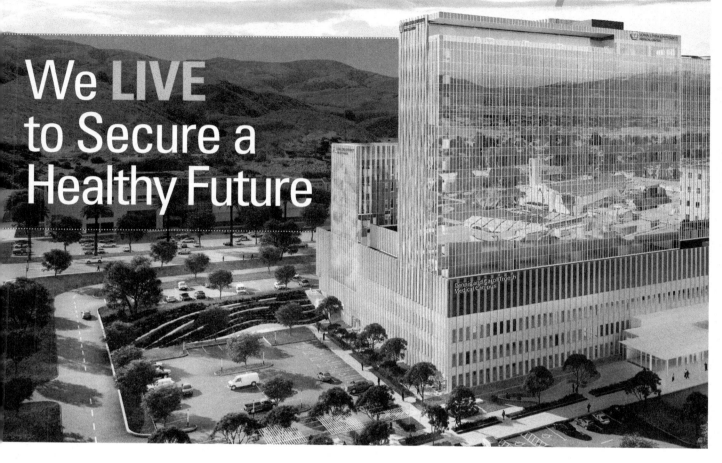

We **LIVE** to Secure a Healthy Future

From our humble beginnings over a century ago, Loma Linda University Health has developed into a world-class leader in health and education. Today, our determination to deliver unsurpassed service and care is only rivaled by our desire to grow and meet the needs of our communities. That is why we have embarked on an ambitious and transformative campaign that will bring into the region new state-of-the-art hospitals designed to enhance the health and healing process, as well as restore lives and families.

Providing world class care for our community is why we **LIVE TO SECURE A HEALTHY FUTURE.**

Find out more about Loma Linda University Health's Vision 2020.
Visit **lluhvision2020.org**

MANY STRENGTHS. ONE MISSION.

A Seventh-day Adventist Organization

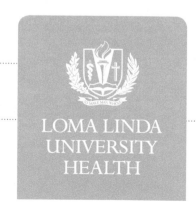

LOMA LINDA
UNIVERSITY
HEALTH

	COMPLEX SPECIALTY CARE	COMMON PROCEDURES & CONDITIONS

COMPLEX SPECIALTY CARE
- ● Nationally ranked
- ● High performing

COMMON PROCEDURES & CONDITIONS
- ● High performing
- ● Average
- ● Below average

State Rank Hospital	CANCER	CARDIOLOGY & HEART SURGERY	DIABETES & ENDOCRINOLOGY	EAR, NOSE & THROAT	GASTROENTEROLOGY & GI SURGERY	GERIATRICS	GYNECOLOGY	NEPHROLOGY	NEUROLOGY & NEUROSURGERY	ORTHOPEDICS	PULMONOLOGY	UROLOGY	COLON CANCER SURGERY	LUNG CANCER SURGERY	HEART BYPASS SURGERY	HEART FAILURE	HEART VALVE SURGERY	ABDOMINAL AORTIC ANEURYSM	HIP REPLACEMENT	KNEE REPLACEMENT	COPD
CONNECTICUT																					
1 Yale-New Haven Hospital, New Haven	●	–	●	●	●	●	–	●	●	●	●	●	●	●	●	●	●	●	●	●	●
2 Hartford Hospital, Hartford	–	–	●	–	●	●	–	●	–	●	●	–	●	●	●	●	●	●	●	●	●
3 Greenwich Hospital, Greenwich	–	–	–	–	●	●	–	–	–	–	–	–	●	●	–	●	–	–	●	●	●
3 St. Francis Hospital and Medical Center, Hartford	–	–	–	–	●	●	–	●	–	●	●	–	●	●	●	●	●	●	●	●	●
5 Danbury Hospital, Danbury	–	–	–	–	●	–	–	–	–	–	–	–	●	●	●	●	●	●	●	●	●
5 Middlesex Hospital, Middletown	–	–	–	–	–	–	–	–	–	–	–	–	●	●	●	●	●	●	●	●	●
5 Stamford Hospital, Stamford	–	–	–	–	–	–	–	–	–	–	–	●	●	●	●	●	●	●	●	●	●
DELAWARE																					
1 Christiana Care Hospitals, Newark	–	–	●	–	●	●	–	●	●	●	●	●	●	●	●	●	●	●	●	●	●
2 Bayhealth Kent General Hospital, Dover	–	–	–	–	–	–	–	–	–	–	–	–	●	●	●	●	●	●	●	●	●
FLORIDA																					
1 Mayo Clinic Jacksonville	●	●	–	●	●	●	–	●	●	●	●	●	●	●	●	●	●	●	●	●	●
2 Tampa General Hospital	–	●	–	●	●	–	●	●	●	●	●	●	●	●	●	●	●	●	●	●	●
3 UF Health Shands Hospital, Gainesville	●	–	●	●	●	●	●	●	●	●	●	●	●	●	●	●	●	●	●	●	●
4 Florida Hospital, Orlando	–	–	–	●	●	●	–	●	–	–	–	–	●	●	●	●	●	●	●	●	●
4 Orlando Regional Medical Center	–	–	●	–	●	–	–	●	–	●	–	–	●	●	●	●	●	●	●	●	●
6 Baptist Hospital of Miami[5]	–	–	–	●	●	–	–	●	●	●	–	–	●	●	●	●	●	●	●	●	●
7 Baptist Medical Center Jacksonville	–	–	–	●	●	–	–	●	–	●	–	–	●	●	●	●	●	●	●	●	●
8 Cleveland Clinic Florida, Weston	●	–	–	●	●	–	●	–	●	–	–	–	●	●	●	●	●	●	●	●	●
8 Sarasota Memorial Health-Sarasota Hospital, Sarasota	–	–	–	–	●	–	–	–	–	●	–	–	●	●	●	●	●	●	●	●	●
10 Holy Cross Hospital, Fort Lauderdale	–	–	–	–	–	–	–	–	–	–	–	–	●	●	●	●	●	●	●	●	●
10 Morton Plant Hospital, Clearwater	–	–	–	–	–	–	–	–	–	–	–	–	●	●	●	●	●	●	●	●	●
12 NCH Downtown Naples Hospital, Naples	–	–	–	–	–	–	–	–	–	–	–	–	●	●	●	●	●	●	●	●	●
12 University of Miami Hospital	–	–	–	●	–	–	–	–	●	–	–	–	●	●	●	●	●	●	●	●	●
14 Lee Memorial Hospital, Fort Myers	–	–	–	–	–	–	–	–	–	–	–	–	●	●	●	●	●	●	●	●	●
14 Memorial Regional Hospital, Hollywood	–	–	–	–	–	–	–	–	–	–	–	–	●	●	●	●	●	●	●	●	●
16 Boca Raton Regional Hospital, Boca Raton	–	–	–	–	–	–	–	–	–	–	–	–	●	●	●	●	●	●	●	●	●
16 Flagler Hospital, St. Augustine	–	–	–	–	–	–	–	–	–	–	–	–	●	●	●	●	●	●	●	●	●
16 Munroe Regional Medical Center, Ocala	–	–	–	–	–	–	–	–	–	–	–	–	●	●	●	●	●	●	●	●	●
16 South Miami Hospital	–	–	–	–	–	–	–	–	–	–	–	–	●	●	●	●	●	●	●	●	●
16 St. Joseph's Hospital, Tampa	–	–	–	–	–	–	–	–	–	–	–	–	●	●	●	●	●	●	●	●	●
16 West Kendall Baptist Hospital, Miami	–	–	–	●	–	–	–	–	–	–	–	–	●	●	–	●	–	–	●	●	●
16 Winter Haven Hospital, Winter Haven	–	–	–	–	–	–	–	–	–	–	–	–	●	●	–	●	–	●	●	●	●
23 Baptist Medical Center Beaches, Jacksonville Beach	–	–	–	–	–	–	–	–	–	–	–	–	●	●	–	●	–	●	●	●	●
23 Bethesda Hospital East, Boynton Beach	–	–	–	–	–	–	–	–	–	–	–	–	●	●	●	●	●	●	●	●	●
23 Florida Hospital Waterman, Tavares	–	–	–	–	–	–	–	–	–	–	–	–	●	●	●	●	●	●	●	●	●
23 Health First Holmes Regional Medical Center, Melbourne	–	–	–	–	–	–	–	–	–	–	–	–	●	●	●	●	●	●	●	●	●
23 Heart of Florida Regional Medical Center, Davenport	–	–	–	–	–	–	–	–	–	–	–	–	●	●	–	●	–	●	●	●	●
23 Homestead Hospital, Homestead	–	–	–	–	–	–	–	–	–	–	–	–	●	●	–	●	–	●	●	●	●
23 Lakeland Regional Health, Lakeland	–	–	–	–	–	–	–	–	–	–	–	–	●	●	–	●	–	●	●	●	●
23 Mease Countryside Hospital, Safety Harbor	–	–	–	–	–	–	–	–	–	–	–	–	●	●	–	●	–	●	●	●	●
23 Mount Sinai Medical Center, Miami Beach	–	–	–	–	●	–	–	–	–	–	–	–	●	●	●	●	●	●	●	●	●
23 UF Health Jacksonville	–	–	●	–	●	–	●	–	–	–	–	–	●	●	●	●	●	●	●	●	●
33 Memorial Hospital West, Pembroke Pines	–	–	–	–	–	–	–	–	–	–	–	–	●	●	–	●	–	●	●	●	●
33 North Florida Regional Medical Center, Gainesville	–	–	–	–	–	–	–	–	–	–	–	–	●	●	●	●	●	●	●	●	●
35 Martin Medical Center, Stuart	–	–	–	–	–	–	–	–	–	–	–	–	●	●	●	●	●	●	●	●	●

In complex care specialties, (-) indicates hospital is not nationally ranked or high performing.
In procedures and conditions, (-) indicates care not offered or hospital has too few Medicare patients to be rated.
A footnote indicates that another hospital's results are included, that the hospital has a different name in one or more areas of care, or both.
[5] Miami Cancer Institute, Baptist Hospital of Miami; Baptist Health Neuroscience Center; Miami Cardiac & Vascular Institute; Miami Orthopedics & Sports Medicine Institute.

More @ usnews.com/bestregionalhospitals

CHOSEN AGAIN
#1 HOSPITAL IN ORLANDO

Florida Hospital is recognized by *U.S. News & World* Report as one of Florida's best hospitals in 14 types of care.

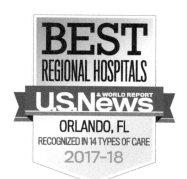

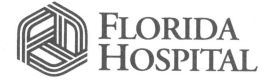

FloridaHospital.com/USNews

COMPLEX SPECIALTY CARE
- ● Nationally ranked
- ● High performing

COMMON PROCEDURES & CONDITIONS
- ● High performing
- ● Average
- ● Below average

COMPLEX SPECIALTY CARE — **COMMON PROCEDURES & CONDITIONS**

State Rank / Hospital	Cancer	Cardiology & Heart Surgery	Diabetes & Endocrinology	Ear, Nose & Throat	Gastroenterology & GI Surgery	Geriatrics	Gynecology	Nephrology	Neurology & Neurosurgery	Orthopedics	Pulmonology	Urology	Colon Cancer Surgery	Lung Cancer Surgery	Heart Bypass Surgery	Heart Failure	Heart Valve Surgery	Abdominal Aortic Aneurysm	Hip Replacement	Knee Replacement	COPD
GEORGIA																					
1 Emory University Hospital, Atlanta[6]	●	●	–	–	●	●	–	●	●	●	–	●	●	●	●	●	●	●	●	●	●
2 Emory St. Joseph's Hospital, Atlanta	–	–	–	–	●	–	–	–	–	–	–	–	●	●	●	●	●	●	●	●	●
3 Navicent Health Medical Center, Macon	–	–	–	–	–	–	–	–	–	–	–	–	●	●	●	●	●	●	●	●	●
3 Northeast Georgia Medical Center, Gainesville	–	–	–	–	–	–	–	–	–	–	–	–	●	●	●	●	●	●	●	●	●
3 University Hospital, Augusta	–	–	–	–	–	–	–	–	–	–	–	–	●	●	●	●	●	●	●	●	●
3 WellStar Kennestone Hospital, Marietta	–	–	–	–	–	–	–	–	–	–	–	–	●	●	●	●	●	●	●	●	●
7 Gwinnett Medical Center, Lawrenceville	–	–	–	–	–	–	–	–	–	–	–	–	●	●	●	●	●	●	●	●	●
7 Memorial University Medical Center, Savannah	–	–	●	–	–	–	–	–	–	–	–	–	●	●	●	●	●	●	●	●	●
7 St. Joseph's Hospital, Savannah	–	–	–	–	–	–	–	–	–	–	–	–	●	●	●	●	●	●	●	●	●
10 Piedmont Atlanta Hospital, Atlanta	–	–	–	–	–	–	–	–	–	–	–	–	●	●	●	●	●	●	●	●	●
11 Candler Hospital, Savannah	–	–	–	–	–	–	–	–	–	–	–	–	●	●	●	●	–	●	–	–	●
11 Emory University Hospital Midtown, Atlanta	–	–	–	–	–	–	–	–	–	–	–	–	●	●	●	●	●	●	●	●	●
13 Athens Regional Medical Center, Athens	–	–	–	–	–	–	–	–	–	–	–	–	●	●	●	●	●	●	● (below avg)	●	●
HAWAII																					
– Queen's Medical Center, Honolulu	●	–	●	●	●	–	●	●	●	●	–	●	●	●	●	●	●	●	●	●	●
IDAHO																					
1 St. Luke's Regional Medical Center, Boise	–	–	●	–	–	–	–	–	–	–	●	–	●	●	●	●	●	●	●	●	●
2 Kootenai Health-Coeur D'Alene	–	–	–	–	–	–	–	–	–	–	–	–	●	●	●	●	●	●	●	●	●
ILLINOIS																					
1 Northwestern Memorial Hospital, Chicago	●	●	●	–	●	●	●	●	●	●	●	●	●	●	●	●	●	●	●	●	●
2 Rush University Medical Center, Chicago	●	●	●	●	●	●	●	●	●	●	●	●	●	●	●	●	●	●	●	●	●
3 Loyola University Medical Center, Maywood	●	●	–	–	●	●	–	●	●	●	–	●	●	●	●	●	●	●	●	●	●
4 Advocate Christ Medical Center, Oak Lawn	–	●	●	–	●	●	–	●	●	●	–	●	●	●	●	●	●	●	●	●	●
5 NorthShore University Health-Evanston Hospital, Evanston	–	–	–	–	●	●	–	●	●	●	–	●	●	●	●	●	●	●	●	●	●
5 Northwestern Medicine Central DuPage Hospital, Winfield	–	–	–	–	●	–	●	–	●	●	–	●	●	●	●	●	●	●	●	●	●
5 OSF St. Francis Medical Center, Peoria	–	–	–	–	●	●	–	●	●	●	–	●	●	●	●	●	●	●	●	●	●
8 Advocate Lutheran General Hospital, Park Ridge	●	–	–	–	●	●	–	–	●	●	–	●	●	●	●	●	●	●	●	●	●
8 University of Chicago Medical Center	●	–	–	–	●	●	–	●	●	●	–	●	●	●	●	●	●	●	●	●	●
10 Advocate Good Samaritan Hospital, Downers Grove	–	–	–	–	●	●	–	●	●	●	–	●	●	●	●	●	●	●	●	●	●
11 Amita Health Elk Grove Village	–	–	–	–	●	●	–	●	●	●	–	●	●	●	●	●	●	●	●	●	●
12 Advocate Sherman Hospital, Elgin	–	–	–	–	●	●	–	–	–	–	–	–	●	●	●	●	●	●	●	●	●
13 Edward Hospital, Naperville[7]	–	–	–	–	●	●	–	●	●	●	–	●	●	●	●	●	●	●	●	●	●
13 Memorial Medical Center, Springfield	–	–	–	–	–	–	–	●	●	●	–	●	●	●	●	●	●	●	●	●	●
13 Presence St. Joseph Medical Center, Joliet	–	–	–	–	–	–	–	●	●	●	–	●	●	●	●	●	●	●	●	●	●
16 Amita Health Adventist Medical Center-Hinsdale	–	–	–	–	●	●	–	●	●	●	–	●	●	●	●	●	–	●	●	●	●
16 Riverside Medical Center, Kankakee	–	–	–	–	●	●	–	●	●	●	–	●	●	●	●	●	●	●	●	●	●
18 Advocate Illinois Masonic Medical Center, Chicago	–	–	–	–	–	–	–	●	●	–	●	–	●	●	●	●	●	●	●	●	●
18 Carle Foundation Hospital, Urbana	–	–	–	–	●	●	–	●	●	●	–	–	●	●	●	●	●	●	●	●	●
18 Elmhurst Memorial Hospital, Elmhurst	–	–	–	–	●	●	–	●	●	●	–	–	●	●	●	●	●	●	●	●	●
18 Northwest Community Hospital, Arlington Heights	–	–	–	–	–	●	–	–	–	–	–	–	●	●	●	●	●	●	●	●	●
18 UnityPoint Health-Peoria	–	–	–	–	–	–	–	–	–	–	–	–	●	●	●	●	●	●	●	●	●
23 Advocate Good Shepherd Hospital, Barrington	–	–	–	–	–	–	–	–	–	–	–	–	●	●	●	●	●	●	●	●	●
23 Centegra Hospital-McHenry	–	–	–	–	–	–	–	–	●	–	–	–	●	●	●	●	●	●	●	●	●
23 Northwestern Lake Forest Hospital, Lake Forest	–	–	–	–	–	–	●	–	●	–	●	–	●	●	●	–	●	–	–	●	●
23 OSF St. Anthony Medical Center, Rockford	–	–	–	–	–	–	–	–	–	–	–	–	●	●	●	●	●	●	●	●	●

In complex care specialties, (-) indicates hospital is not nationally ranked or high performing.
In procedures and conditions, (-) indicates care not offered or hospital has too few Medicare patients to be rated.

A footnote indicates that another hospital's results are included, that the hospital has a different name in one or more areas of care, or both.
[6]Emory Wesley Woods Geriatric Hospital. [7]Edward Cancer Center, Edward Heart Hospital.

More @ usnews.com/bestregionalhospitals

COMPLEX SPECIALTY CARE
- ● Nationally ranked
- ● High performing

COMMON PROCEDURES & CONDITIONS
- ● High performing
- ○ Average
- ● Below average

State Rank / Hospital	Cancer	Cardiology & Heart Surgery	Diabetes & Endocrinology	Ear, Nose & Throat	Gastroenterology & GI Surgery	Geriatrics	Gynecology	Nephrology	Neurology & Neurosurgery	Orthopedics	Pulmonology	Urology	Colon Cancer Surgery	Lung Cancer Surgery	Heart Bypass Surgery	Heart Failure	Heart Valve Surgery	Abdominal Aortic Aneurysm	Hip Replacement	Knee Replacement	COPD
ILLINOIS (CONTINUED)																					
23 OSF St. Joseph Medical Center, Bloomington	–	–	–	–	–	–	–	–	–	–	○	○	○	○	○	○	○	○	○	○	○
23 Palos Community Hospital, Palos Heights	–	–	–	–	–	–	–	–	–	–	○	○	○	○	○	○	○	○	○	○	○
23 Swedish American Hospital, Rockford	–	–	–	–	–	–	–	–	–	–	○	○	○	○	○	○	○	○	○	○	○
30 St. John's Hospital, Springfield	–	–	–	–	–	–	–	–	–	–	○	○	○	○	○	○	○	○	○	○	○
INDIANA																					
1 Indiana University Health University Hospital, Indianapolis	●	●	●	–	●	●	–	●	●	●	●	●	○	○	○	○	○	○	○	○	○
2 Indiana University Health North Hospital, Carmel	–	–	–	–	–	–	–	–	–	–	–	–	○	○	–	○	–	–	○	○	○
3 Indiana University Health West Hospital, Avon	–	–	–	–	●	●	–	●	–	●	–	○	○	○	○	○	○	○	○	○	○
3 St. Mary's Medical Center of Evansville	–	–	–	–	–	–	–	–	–	●	–	○	○	○	○	○	○	○	○	○	○
5 Indiana University Health Bloomington Hospital, Bloomington	–	–	–	–	–	–	–	–	–	–	●	○	○	○	○	○	○	○	○	○	○
6 Deaconess Hospital, Evansville	–	–	–	–	–	–	–	–	–	–	●	○	○	○	–	○	○	○	○	○	○
6 Hendricks Regional Health, Danville	–	–	–	–	–	–	–	–	–	–	●	○	○	○	–	○	○	○	○	○	○
6 Indiana University Health Arnett Hospital, Lafayette	–	–	–	–	–	–	–	–	–	–	●	○	○	○	○	○	○	○	○	○	○
6 Indiana University Health Ball Memorial Hospital, Muncie	–	–	–	–	–	–	–	–	–	–	●	○	○	○	○	○	○	○	○	○	○
10 Parkview Regional Medical Center, Fort Wayne	–	–	–	–	–	–	–	–	–	–	●	○	○	○	○	○	○	○	○	○	○
10 St. Vincent Indianapolis Hospital	–	–	–	–	–	–	–	–	–	–	●	○	○	○	○	○	○	○	○	○	○
12 Community Hospital, Munster	–	–	–	–	–	–	–	–	–	–	●	○	○	●	○	○	○	○	○	○	○
12 Franciscan St. Francis Health-Indianapolis	–	–	–	–	–	–	–	–	–	–	●	○	○	○	○	○	●	○	○	○	○
IOWA																					
1 University of Iowa Hospitals and Clinics, Iowa City	●	–	–	●	●	●	–	●	●	●	●	●	○	○	○	○	○	○	○	○	○
2 UnityPoint Health-St. Luke's Hospital, Cedar Rapids	–	–	–	–	–	–	–	–	–	–	●	○	○	○	○	○	○	○	○	○	○
3 Mercy Medical Center-Des Moines	–	–	–	–	–	–	–	–	–	–	●	○	○	○	○	○	○	○	○	○	○
4 UnityPoint Health-Iowa Methodist Medical Center, Des Moines	–	–	–	–	–	–	–	–	–	–	●	○	○	○	○	○	○	○	○	○	○
5 Genesis Medical Center-Davenport	–	–	–	–	–	–	–	–	–	–	●	○	○	○	○	○	○	○	○	○	○
5 Mercy Medical Center-Dubuque	–	–	–	–	–	–	–	–	–	–	●	○	○	○	○	○	○	○	○	○	○
KANSAS																					
1 University of Kansas Hospital, Kansas City	●	●	●	–	●	●	–	●	●	●	●	●	○	○	○	○	○	○	○	○	○
2 Stormont Vail Hospital, Topeka	–	–	–	–	–	–	–	–	–	–	●	○	○	○	○	○	○	○	○	○	○
KENTUCKY																					
1 University of Kentucky Albert B. Chandler Hospital, Lexington	●	–	●	–	●	●	–	●	●	●	●	●	○	○	○	○	○	○	○	○	○
2 St. Elizabeth Healthcare Edgewood-Covington Hospitals, Edgewood	–	–	–	–	–	–	–	●	–	–	●	○	○	○	○	○	○	○	○	○	○
3 Baptist Health Lexington	–	–	–	–	–	–	–	–	–	–	●	○	○	○	○	○	○	○	○	○	○
4 Norton Hospital, Louisville	–	–	–	–	–	–	–	–	–	–	●	○	○	○	○	○	○	○	○	○	○
5 Baptist Health Louisville	–	–	–	–	–	–	–	–	–	–	●	○	○	○	○	○	○	○	○	○	○
6 Jewish Hospital, Louisville	–	–	–	–	–	–	–	–	–	–	●	○	○	○	○	○	○	○	○	○	○
7 Owensboro Health Regional Hospital, Owensboro	–	–	–	–	–	–	–	–	–	–	○	○	○	●	○	●	–	○	○	○	○
LOUISIANA																					
1 Ochsner Medical Center, New Orleans	●	–	●	●	●	●	–	●	●	●	●	●	○	○	○	○	○	○	○	○	○
2 Our Lady of the Lake Regional Medical Center, Baton Rouge	–	–	–	●	–	–	–	–	–	–	●	○	○	○	○	○	○	○	○	○	○
3 Willis-Knighton Medical Center, Shreveport	–	–	–	–	–	–	–	–	–	–	●	○	○	○	○	○	○	○	○	○	○
4 East Jefferson General Hospital, Metairie	–	–	–	–	–	–	–	–	–	–	●	○	○	○	○	○	○	○	○	○	○
MAINE																					
– Maine Medical Center, Portland	–	–	–	–	–	–	–	–	–	–	●	○	○	○	○	○	○	○	○	○	○
MARYLAND																					
1 Johns Hopkins Hospital, Baltimore	●	●	●	●	●	●	●	●	●	●	●	●	○	○	○	○	○	○	○	○	○
2 University of Maryland Medical Center, Baltimore	●	–	●	–	–	–	●	–	●	●	●	●	○	○	○	○	○	○	○	○	○

In complex care specialties, (-) indicates hospital is not nationally ranked or high performing.
In procedures and conditions, (-) indicates care not offered or hospital has too few Medicare patients to be rated.

Legend

COMPLEX SPECIALTY CARE
- ● Nationally ranked
- ● High performing

COMMON PROCEDURES & CONDITIONS
- ● High performing
- ● Average
- ● Below average

	COMPLEX SPECIALTY CARE												COMMON PROCEDURES & CONDITIONS								
State Rank — Hospital	Cancer	Cardiology & Heart Surgery	Diabetes & Endocrinology	Ear, Nose & Throat	Gastroenterology & GI Surgery	Geriatrics	Gynecology	Nephrology	Neurology & Neurosurgery	Orthopedics	Pulmonology	Urology	Colon Cancer Surgery	Lung Cancer Surgery	Heart Bypass Surgery	Heart Failure	Heart Valve Surgery	Abdominal Aortic Aneurysm	Hip Replacement	Knee Replacement	COPD
MARYLAND (CONTINUED)																					
3 Mercy Medical Center, Baltimore	–	–	–	–	–	–	–	●	–	–	●	–	●	●	–	●	–	●	●	●	●
3 Sinai Hospital of Baltimore	–	–	–	–	●	–	–	●	–	●	–	–	●	●	●	●	–	●	●	●	●
5 Anne Arundel Medical Center, Annapolis	–	–	–	–	–	–	–	–	–	–	–	–	●	●	●	●	●	●	●	●	●
5 MedStar Union Memorial Hospital, Baltimore	–	–	–	●	–	–	–	–	–	–	–	–	●	●	●	●	●	●	●	●	●
5 University of Maryland St. Joseph Medical Center, Towson	–	–	–	–	–	–	–	–	–	–	–	–	●	●	●	●	●	●	●	●	●
8 University of Maryland Shore Medical Center at Easton	–	–	–	–	–	–	–	–	–	–	–	–	●	–	●	●	–	●	●	●	●
9 MedStar Franklin Square Medical Center, Baltimore	–	–	–	–	–	–	–	–	–	–	–	–	●	●	●	●	●	●	●	●	●
9 MedStar Harbor Hospital, Baltimore	–	–	–	–	–	–	–	–	–	–	–	–	●	●	●	●	●	●	●	●	●
11 Holy Cross Hospital, Silver Spring	–	–	–	–	–	–	–	–	–	–	–	–	●	●	●	●	●	●	●	●	●
11 Johns Hopkins Bayview Medical Center, Baltimore	–	–	–	–	–	–	–	●	–	–	–	–	●	●	●	●	●	●	●	●	●
11 MedStar Good Samaritan Hospital, Baltimore	–	–	–	–	–	–	–	–	–	–	–	–	●	●	●	●	●	●	●	●	●
11 Peninsula Regional Medical Center, Salisbury	–	–	–	–	–	–	–	–	–	–	–	–	●	●	●	●	●	●	●	●	●
11 Suburban Hospital, Bethesda	–	–	–	–	–	–	–	–	–	–	–	–	●	●	●	●	●	●	●	●	●
11 U. of Maryland Baltimore Washington Medical Center, Glen Burnie	–	–	–	–	–	–	–	–	–	–	–	–	●	●	●	●	●	●	●	●	●
17 MedStar Southern Maryland Hospital Center, Clinton	–	–	–	–	–	–	–	–	–	–	●	–	●	●	–	●	–	●	●	●	●
MASSACHUSETTS																					
1 Massachusetts General Hospital, Boston[8]	●	●	●	●	●	●	●	●	●	●	●	●	●	●	●	●	●	●	●	●	●
2 Brigham and Women's Hospital, Boston[9]	●	●	●	–	●	●	●	●	●	●	●	●	●	●	●	●	●	●	●	●	●
3 Baystate Medical Center, Springfield	–	–	–	–	●	–	–	●	●	–	–	–	●	●	●	●	●	●	●	●	●
4 Beth Israel Deaconess Medical Center, Boston	●	–	●	–	●	●	–	●	●	●	●	●	●	●	●	●	●	●	●	●	●
5 UMass Memorial Medical Center, Worcester	–	–	–	–	●	–	–	●	●	–	●	–	●	●	●	●	●	●	●	●	●
6 Tufts Medical Center, Boston	–	●	–	–	●	–	–	●	–	–	–	–	●	●	●	●	●	●	●	●	●
7 South Shore Hospital, South Weymouth	–	–	–	–	●	–	–	–	–	–	–	–	●	●	–	●	–	●	●	●	●
8 Lahey Hospital and Medical Center, Burlington	–	–	–	–	●	–	–	–	–	–	–	–	●	●	●	●	●	●	●	●	●
9 Southcoast Charlton Memorial Hospital, Fall River	–	–	–	–	–	–	–	–	–	–	–	–	●	●	●	●	●	●	●	●	●
10 Boston Medical Center	–	–	–	–	●	–	●	●	●	–	–	–	●	●	●	●	●	●	●	●	●
MICHIGAN																					
1 University of Michigan Hospitals and Health Centers, Ann Arbor	●	●	●	●	●	●	●	●	●	●	●	●	●	●	●	●	●	●	●	●	●
2 Beaumont Hospital-Royal Oak	–	●	●	–	●	●	●	●	●	●	●	●	●	●	●	●	●	●	●	●	●
3 Spectrum Health-Butterworth and Blodgett Campuses, Grand Rapids	–	–	●	–	●	–	●	–	●	●	●	●	●	●	●	●	●	●	●	●	●
4 DMC Harper University Hospital, Detroit	–	–	●	–	●	–	–	●	●	–	●	●	●	●	●	●	●	●	●	●	●
4 Munson Medical Center, Traverse City	–	●	–	–	●	–	–	–	–	–	–	–	●	●	●	●	●	●	●	●	●
6 Beaumont Hospital-Troy	–	●	–	–	●	–	–	–	–	–	–	–	●	●	●	●	●	●	●	●	●
7 St. Joseph Mercy Ann Arbor Hospital, Ypsilanti	–	–	–	●	–	–	–	–	–	–	–	–	●	●	●	●	●	●	●	●	●
8 Bronson Methodist Hospital, Kalamazoo	–	–	–	–	–	–	–	–	–	–	–	–	●	●	●	●	●	●	●	●	●
8 Henry Ford Hospital, Detroit	–	–	●	–	●	–	–	–	●	–	●	●	●	●	●	●	●	●	●	●	●
10 McLaren Northern Michigan Hospital, Petoskey	–	–	–	–	●	–	–	–	–	–	●	–	●	●	●	●	●	●	●	●	●
10 Mercy Health St. Mary's Campus, Grand Rapids	–	–	–	–	●	–	–	–	–	–	–	–	●	●	●	●	●	●	●	●	●
12 MidMichigan Medical Center-Midland	–	–	–	–	–	–	–	●	–	–	●	–	●	●	–	●	–	●	●	●	●
13 Providence-Providence Park Hospital, Southfield Campus	–	–	–	–	–	–	–	–	–	–	–	–	●	●	●	●	●	●	●	●	●
13 St. John Hospital and Medical Center, Detroit	–	–	–	–	–	–	–	–	–	–	–	–	●	●	●	●	●	●	●	●	●
15 Beaumont Hospital-Dearborn	–	–	–	–	–	–	–	●	–	–	–	–	●	●	●	●	●	●	●	●	●
15 Beaumont Hospital-Grosse Pointe	–	–	–	–	●	–	–	–	–	–	–	–	●	●	●	●	–	●	●	●	●
15 Sparrow Hospital, Lansing	–	–	–	–	–	–	–	–	●	–	●	–	●	●	●	●	●	●	●	●	●

In complex care specialties, (-) indicates hospital is not nationally ranked or high performing.
In procedures and conditions, (-) indicates care not offered or hospital has too few Medicare patients to be rated.

A footnote indicates that another hospital's results are included, that the hospital has a different name in one or more areas of care, or both.
[8]Massachusetts Eye and Ear Infirmary, Massachusetts General Hospital. [9]Dana-Farber/Brigham and Women's Cancer Center.

▶ More @ usnews.com/bestregionalhospitals

COMPLEX SPECIALTY CARE   **COMMON PROCEDURES & CONDITIONS**

State Rank / Hospital	Cancer	Cardiology & Heart Surgery	Diabetes & Endocrinology	Ear, Nose & Throat	Gastroenterology & GI Surgery	Geriatrics	Gynecology	Nephrology	Neurology & Neurosurgery	Orthopedics	Pulmonology	Urology	Colon Cancer Surgery	Lung Cancer Surgery	Heart Bypass Surgery	Heart Failure	Heart Valve Surgery	Abdominal Aortic Aneurysm	Hip Replacement	Knee Replacement	COPD
MICHIGAN (CONTINUED)																					
15 St. Joseph Mercy Oakland, Pontiac	–	–	–	–	–	–	–	–	–	–	–	–	●	●	●	●	●	–	●	●	●
19 DMC Huron Valley-Sinai Hospital, Commerce Township	–	–	–	–	–	–	–	–	–	–	–	–	●	●	●	●	●	–	●	●	●
19 McLaren Greater Lansing Hospital, Lansing	–	–	–	–	–	–	–	–	–	–	–	–	●	●	–	●	–	●	●	●	●
21 St. John Macomb-Oakland Hospital, Warren	–	–	–	–	–	–	–	–	–	–	–	–	●	●	●	●	●	●	●	●	●
22 DMC-Sinai-Grace Hospital, Detroit	–	–	–	–	–	–	–	●	–	–	–	–	●	●	●	–	–	●	●	●	●
MINNESOTA																					
1 Mayo Clinic, Rochester	●	●	●	●	●	●	●	●	●	●	●	●	●	●	●	●	●	●	●	●	●
2 Abbott Northwestern Hospital, Minneapolis[10]	–	●	●	●	●	●	●	●	●	●	●	●	●	●	●	●	●	●	●	●	●
3 St. Cloud Hospital, St. Cloud	–	●	●	–	●	●	●	–	●	●	●	–	●	●	●	●	●	●	●	●	●
4 U. of Minnesota Medical Center, West Bank Campus, Minneapolis	●	–	–	●	●	–	●	●	●	●	●	●	●	●	●	●	●	●	●	●	●
5 Mercy Hospital, Coon Rapids	–	–	–	–	●	–	–	–	–	●	–	–	●	●	●	●	●	●	●	●	●
6 Essentia Health-St. Mary's Medical Center, Duluth	–	–	●	–	–	–	–	–	●	–	●	–	●	●	●	●	●	●	●	●	●
6 Fairview Southdale Hospital, Edina	–	–	–	–	–	–	–	–	●	●	–	–	●	●	●	●	●	●	●	●	●
8 Park Nicollet Methodist Hospital, St. Louis Park	–	–	–	–	–	–	–	–	–	–	–	–	●	●	●	●	●	●	●	●	●
8 United Hospital, St. Paul	–	●	–	–	–	–	–	–	–	–	–	–	●	●	●	●	●	●	●	●	●
10 North Memorial Medical Center, Robbinsdale	–	–	–	–	–	–	–	–	–	–	–	–	●	●	●	●	●	●	●	●	●
10 Regions Hospital, St. Paul	–	–	–	–	–	–	–	–	–	–	–	–	●	●	●	●	●	●	●	●	●
12 Maple Grove Hospital, Maple Grove	–	–	–	–	–	–	–	–	–	–	–	–	●	●	●	●	●	●	●	●	●
12 Mayo Clinic Mankato	–	–	–	–	–	–	–	–	●	–	●	–	–	–	–	–	–	●	●	●	●
MISSISSIPPI																					
– Mississippi Baptist Medical Center, Jackson	–	–	–	–	–	–	–	–	–	–	–	–	●	●	●	●	●	●	●	●	●
MISSOURI																					
1 Barnes-Jewish Hospital, St. Louis	●	●	●	●	●	●	●	●	●	●	●	●	●	●	●	●	●	●	●	●	●
2 St. Luke's Hospital of Kansas City	–	●	●	–	●	●	●	–	●	●	●	–	●	●	●	●	●	●	●	●	●
3 Missouri Baptist Medical Center, St. Louis	–	–	●	–	●	●	●	–	●	●	–	–	●	●	●	●	●	●	●	●	●
4 Boone Hospital Center, Columbia	–	–	–	–	●	●	–	–	●	–	–	–	●	●	●	●	●	●	●	●	●
5 Mercy Hospital Springfield	–	–	–	–	–	–	–	–	–	–	–	–	●	●	●	●	●	●	●	●	●
5 Mercy Hospital St. Louis	–	–	–	–	–	–	–	–	–	–	–	–	●	●	●	●	●	●	●	●	●
7 Barnes-Jewish West County Hospital, St. Louis	–	–	–	–	●	–	–	–	●	●	●	–	●	●	●	●	●	●	●	●	●
7 St. Luke's Hospital, Chesterfield	–	–	–	–	–	–	–	–	●	●	●	–	–	–	●	–	●	●	●	●	●
9 CoxHealth Springfield	–	–	–	–	–	–	–	–	–	–	–	–	●	●	●	●	●	●	●	●	●
10 Cox Medical Center Branson	–	–	–	–	–	–	–	–	–	–	–	–	●	●	●	●	●	●	●	●	●
11 SSM DePaul Health Center, Bridgeton	–	–	–	–	–	–	–	–	–	–	–	–	–	●	●	–	–	●	●	●	●
									●	–	–		●	●	●	●	●	●	●	●	●
MONTANA																					
1 Billings Clinic, Billings	–	–	●	–	–	–	●	–	●	–	●	–	●	●	●	●	●	●	●	●	●
2 St. Patrick Hospital, Missoula	–	–	–	–	–	–	–	–	●	●	●	–	●	●	●	●	●	●	●	●	●
NEBRASKA																					
1 Nebraska Medicine-Nebraska Medical Center, Omaha	●	–	–	●	●	●	●	●	–	●	●	●	●	●	●	●	●	●	●	●	●
2 Bryan Medical Center, Lincoln	–	–	–	–	–	–	–	–	–	●	–	–	●	●	●	●	●	●	●	●	●
2 Nebraska Methodist Hospital, Omaha	–	–	–	–	–	–	–	–	–	–	–	–	●	●	●	●	●	●	●	●	●
4 CHI Health St Elizabeth, Lincoln	–	–	–	–	–	–	–	–	–	–	–	–	●	●	●	●	●	●	●	●	●
5 CHI Health Bergan Mercy, Omaha	–	–	–	–	–	–	–	–	–	–	–	–	●	●	●	●	–	●	●	●	●
5 CHI Health Good Samaritan, Kearney	–	–	–	–	–	–	–	–	–	–	–	–	●	●	●	●	●	●	●	●	●

In complex care specialties, (-) indicates hospital is not nationally ranked or high performing.
In procedures and conditions, (-) indicates care not offered or hospital has too few Medicare patients to be rated.

A footnote indicates that another hospital's results are included, that the hospital has a different name in one or more areas of care, or both.
[10] Minneapolis Heart Institute at Abbott Northwestern Hospital.

	COMPLEX SPECIALTY CARE												COMMON PROCEDURES & CONDITIONS								
State Rank Hospital	CANCER	CARDIOLOGY & HEART SURGERY	DIABETES & ENDOCRINOLOGY	EAR, NOSE & THROAT	GASTROENTEROLOGY & GI SURGERY	GERIATRICS	GYNECOLOGY	NEPHROLOGY	NEUROLOGY & NEUROSURGERY	ORTHOPEDICS	PULMONOLOGY	UROLOGY	COLON CANCER SURGERY	LUNG CANCER SURGERY	HEART BYPASS SURGERY	HEART FAILURE	HEART VALVE SURGERY	ABDOMINAL AORTIC ANEURYSM	HIP REPLACEMENT	KNEE REPLACEMENT	COPD
NEW HAMPSHIRE																					
1 Dartmouth-Hitchcock Medical Center, Lebanon	●	–	–	–	–	–	●	–	–	–	–	●	●	●	●	●	●	●	●	●	●
2 St. Joseph Hospital, Nashua	–	–	–	–	–	–	–	–	●	●	–	●	–	–	●	–	–	●	●	●	
3 Exeter Hospital, Exeter	–	–	–	–	–	–	–	–	–	–	–	●	●	–	●	–	–	●	●	●	
NEW JERSEY																					
1 Hackensack University Medical Center, Hackensack	●	–	●	–	●	–	●	●	●	●	–	●	●	●	●	●	●	●	●	●	●
2 Morristown Medical Center, Morristown	–	●	–	–	●	●	●	●	●	●	–	●	●	●	●	●	●	●	●	●	●
3 Robert Wood Johnson University Hospital, New Brunswick	●	–	–	●	●	–	●	●	–	–	–	●	●	●	●	●	●	●	●	●	●
4 Jersey Shore University Medical Center, Neptune	–	–	–	–	–	–	–	–	–	–	–	●	●	●	●	●	●	●	●	●	●
5 AtlantiCare Regional Medical Center, Atlantic City	–	–	–	–	–	–	–	●	–	–	–	●	●	●	●	●	●	●	●	●	●
5 Valley Hospital, Ridgewood	–	–	–	–	–	–	–	–	–	–	–	●	●	●	●	●	●	●	●	●	●
7 Virtua Voorhees, Voorhees Township	–	–	–	–	–	–	–	–	–	–	–	●	●	●	●	–	●	–	●	●	●
8 Ocean Medical Center, Brick Township	–	–	–	–	–	–	–	–	–	–	–	●	●	●	●	–	●	–	●	●	●
8 Overlook Medical Center, Summit	–	–	●	–	–	–	–	–	●	–	–	●	●	–	●	–	–	–	●	●	●
8 Riverview Medical Center, Red Bank	–	–	–	–	–	–	–	–	–	–	–	●	●	–	●	–	–	–	●	●	●
8 Robert Wood Johnson University Hospital Somerset, Somerville	–	–	●	–	–	–	–	–	–	–	–	●	●	–	●	–	–	–	●	●	●
8 University Medical Center of Princeton at Plainsboro	–	–	–	–	–	–	–	–	–	–	–	●	●	–	●	–	–	–	●	●	●
13 Capital Health Medical Center-Hopewell, Pennington	–	–	–	–	–	–	–	●	–	–	–	●	●	–	●	–	–	–	●	●	●
13 Capital Health Regional Medical Center, Trenton	–	–	–	–	–	–	●	–	–	–	–	●	●	–	●	–	–	–	●	●	●
13 Community Medical Center, Toms River	–	–	–	–	–	–	–	–	–	–	–	●	●	–	●	–	–	–	●	●	●
13 Englewood Hospital and Medical Center, Englewood	–	–	–	–	–	–	–	–	–	–	–	●	●	–	●	–	–	–	●	●	●
13 Hunterdon Medical Center, Flemington	–	–	–	–	–	–	–	–	–	–	–	●	●	–	●	–	–	–	●	●	●
13 Inspira Medical Center-Elmer	–	–	–	–	–	–	–	–	–	–	–	●	●	–	●	–	–	–	●	●	●
13 Inspira Medical Center-Vineland	–	–	–	–	–	–	–	–	–	–	–	●	●	–	●	–	●	●	●	●	●
13 Kennedy Health System, Cherry Hill	–	–	–	–	–	–	–	–	–	–	–	●	●	–	●	–	–	–	●	●	●
13 St. Barnabas Medical Center, Livingston	–	–	–	–	–	–	–	–	–	–	–	●	●	–	●	–	–	–	●	●	●
13 St. Joseph's Healthcare System, Paterson	–	–	–	–	–	–	–	–	–	–	–	●	●	–	●	–	–	–	●	●	●
13 St. Peter's University Hospital, New Brunswick	–	–	–	–	–	–	–	–	–	–	–	●	●	–	●	–	–	●	●	●	●
24 Holy Name Medical Center, Teaneck	–	–	–	–	–	–	●	–	–	–	–	●	●	–	●	–	–	●	●	●	●
NEW MEXICO																					
– Presbyterian Hospital, Albuquerque	–	–	–	–	–	–	–	–	–	–	–	●	●	●	●	●	●	●	●	●	●
NEW YORK																					
1 New York-Presbyterian Hospital	●	●	●	●	●	●	●	●	●	●	●	●	●	●	●	●	●	●	●	●	●
2 Mount Sinai Hospital, New York	●	●	●	–	●	●	●	●	●	●	●	●	●	●	●	●	●	●	●	●	●
3 NYU Langone Medical Center, New York[11]	●	●	●	–	●	●	–	●	●	●	●	●	●	●	●	●	●	●	●	●	●
4 Strong Memorial Hospital of the University of Rochester	–	●	●	–	●	●	–	●	●	●	●	●	●	●	●	●	●	–	●	●	●
5 St. Francis Hospital, Roslyn	–	●	–	–	–	–	–	–	–	–	–	●	●	●	●	●	●	●	●	●	●
6 NYU Winthrop Hospital, Mineola	–	–	●	–	●	–	–	●	●	–	●	●	●	●	●	●	●	●	●	●	●
6 Rochester General Hospital, Rochester	–	–	–	–	●	–	–	●	–	●	–	●	●	●	●	●	●	●	●	●	●
8 Montefiore Medical Center, Bronx	●	–	●	–	●	–	–	●	–	–	–	●	●	●	●	●	●	●	●	●	●
9 Lenox Hill Hospital, New York[12]	●	–	–	●	●	–	–	●	–	●	–	●	●	●	●	●	●	●	●	●	●
9 St. Joseph's Hospital Health Center, Syracuse	–	–	–	–	–	–	–	–	–	–	–	●	●	●	●	●	●	●	●	●	●
11 Buffalo General Medical Center	–	–	–	–	–	–	–	–	–	–	–	●	●	●	●	●	●	●	●	●	●
12 St. Peter's Hospital, Albany	–	–	–	–	–	–	–	–	–	–	–	●	●	●	●	●	●	●	●	●	●
13 Albany Medical Center, Albany	–	–	–	–	–	–	●	–	–	–	–	●	●	●	●	●	●	●	●	●	●

COMPLEX SPECIALTY CARE
- ● Nationally ranked
- ● High performing

COMMON PROCEDURES & CONDITIONS
- ● High performing
- ● Average
- ● Below average

In complex care specialties, (-) indicates hospital is not nationally ranked or high performing.
In procedures and conditions, (-) indicates care not offered or hospital has too few Medicare patients to be rated.

A footnote indicates that another hospital's results are included, that the hospital has a different name in one or more areas of care, or both.
[11]Hospital for Joint Diseases, NYU Langone Medical Center. [12]Lenox Hill Hospital-Manhattan Eye, Ear and Throat Institute.

● More @ usnews.com/bestregionalhospitals

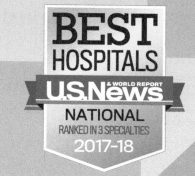
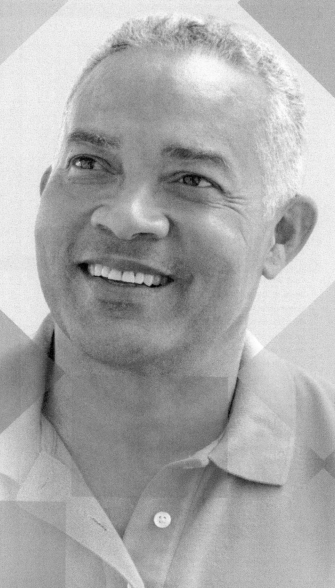
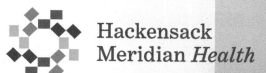

COMPLEX SPECIALTY CARE
- ● Nationally ranked
- ● High performing

COMMON PROCEDURES & CONDITIONS
- ● High performing
- ● Average
- ● Below average

State Rank / Hospital	Cancer	Cardiology & Heart Surgery	Diabetes & Endocrinology	Ear, Nose & Throat	Gastroenterology & GI Surgery	Geriatrics	Gynecology	Nephrology	Neurology & Neurosurgery	Orthopedics	Pulmonology	Urology	Colon Cancer Surgery	Lung Cancer Surgery	Heart Bypass Surgery	Heart Failure	Heart Valve Surgery	Abdominal Aortic Aneurysm	Hip Replacement	Knee Replacement	COPD
NEW YORK (CONTINUED)																					
13 North Shore University Hospital, Manhasset	–	–	–	–	–	●	–	–	●	–	–	–	●	●	●	●	●	●	●	●	●
13 Stony Brook University Hospital, Stony Brook	–	–	–	–	●	●	–	●	●	–	●	●	●	●	●	●	●	●	●	●	●
16 Long Island Jewish Medical Center, New Hyde Park	–	–	–	–	–	–	●	–	●	–	–	●	●	●	●	–	●	–	●	●	●
17 Huntington Hospital, Huntington	–	–	–	–	–	–	–	–	●	–	–	–	●	●	●	●	●	–	●	●	●
18 Northern Westchester Hospital, Mount Kisco	–	–	–	–	–	–	●	–	–	–	–	–	●	–	●	●	●	–	●	●	●
18 South Nassau Communities Hospital, Oceanside	–	–	–	–	–	–	–	–	–	●	–	–	●	●	●	●	●	●	●	●	●
18 Staten Island University Hospital, Staten Island	–	–	●	–	–	–	–	–	–	–	–	–	●	●	●	●	●	●	●	●	●
21 Glens Falls Hospital, Glens Falls	–	–	–	–	–	–	–	–	–	–	–	–	●	–	●	●	●	–	●	●	●
21 Highland Hospital, Rochester	–	–	–	–	–	–	–	–	–	–	–	–	●	–	●	●	●	–	●	●	●
21 John T. Mather Memorial Hospital, Port Jefferson	–	–	–	–	–	–	–	–	–	–	–	–	●	–	●	●	●	–	●	●	●
21 Mount Sinai Beth Israel, New York	–	–	–	–	–	–	–	–	–	–	–	–	●	●	●	●	●	●	●	●	●
21 Mount Sinai St. Luke's-Roosevelt, New York	–	–	–	–	–	●	–	–	–	–	–	–	●	●	●	●	●	–	●	●	●
21 Orange Regional Medical Center, Middletown	–	–	–	–	–	–	–	–	–	–	–	–	●	–	●	●	●	–	●	●	●
21 Our Lady of Lourdes Memorial Hospital, Binghamton	–	–	–	–	–	–	–	–	–	–	–	–	●	●	●	●	●	●	●	●	●
28 Maimonides Medical Center, Brooklyn	–	–	–	–	–	–	–	–	–	–	–	–	●	●	●	●	●	●	●	●	●
28 NewYork-Presbyterian Brooklyn Methodist Hospital, Brooklyn	–	–	–	–	–	–	–	●	–	–	–	–	●	●	●	●	●	–	●	●	●
30 New York-Presbyterian/Queens, Flushing	–	–	–	–	–	–	–	–	–	–	–	–	●	●	●	●	●	●	●	●	●
NORTH CAROLINA																					
1 Duke University Hospital, Durham	●	●	●	–	●	●	●	●	●	●	●	●	●	●	●	●	●	●	●	●	●
2 Wake Forest Baptist Medical Center, Winston-Salem	●	–	●	●	–	●	●	●	●	●	●	●	●	●	●	●	●	●	●	●	●
3 University of North Carolina Hospitals, Chapel Hill	●	–	–	●	●	●	●	●	●	–	●	●	●	●	●	●	●	●	●	●	●
4 Carolinas Medical Center, Charlotte	●	–	●	●	●	–	●	●	●	–	●	●	●	●	●	●	●	●	●	●	●
5 Vidant Medical Center, Greenville	–	●	–	●	–	–	●	●	●	–	●	●	●	●	●	●	●	●	●	●	●
6 Moses H. Cone Memorial Hospital, Greensboro	–	–	–	–	●	–	–	–	–	–	●	–	●	●	●	●	●	●	●	●	●
7 Mission Hospital, Asheville	–	–	–	–	–	–	–	●	●	–	–	–	●	●	●	●	●	●	●	●	●
8 UNC Rex Hospital, Raleigh	–	–	–	–	–	–	–	–	–	–	–	–	●	●	●	●	●	●	●	●	●
9 Novant Health Forsyth Medical Center, Winston-Salem	–	–	–	–	–	–	–	–	–	–	–	–	●	●	●	●	●	●	●	●	●
9 Novant Health Presbyterian Medical Center, Charlotte	–	–	–	–	–	–	–	–	●	–	●	–	●	●	●	●	●	●	●	●	●
11 FirstHealth Moore Regional Hospital, Pinehurst	–	–	–	–	–	–	–	–	–	–	–	–	●	●	●	●	●	●	●	●	●
11 WakeMed Health and Hospitals, Raleigh Campus	–	–	–	–	–	–	–	–	–	–	–	–	●	●	●	●	●	●	●	●	●
13 Cape Fear Valley Medical Center, Fayetteville	–	–	–	–	–	–	–	–	–	–	–	–	●	●	●	●	–	–	●	●	●
13 Duke Raleigh Hospital, Raleigh	–	–	–	–	–	–	–	–	–	–	–	–	●	●	●	–	–	–	●	●	●
13 Duke Regional Hospital, Durham	–	–	–	–	–	–	–	–	●	–	–	–	●	–	●	●	–	–	●	●	●
13 New Hanover Regional Medical Center, Wilmington	–	–	–	–	–	–	–	–	–	–	–	–	●	●	●	●	●	●	●	●	●
17 High Point Regional Hospital, High Point	–	–	–	–	–	–	–	–	–	–	–	–	●	●	●	●	–	●	●	●	●
18 Southeastern Health, Lumberton	–	–	–	–	–	–	–	–	–	–	–	–	●	●	●	●	–	●	●	●	●
NORTH DAKOTA																					
1 CHI St. Alexius Health, Bismarck	–	–	–	–	●	–	–	–	●	●	–	●	●	●	●	●	●	●	●	●	●
2 Sanford Medical Center Bismarck	–	–	–	–	–	–	–	–	–	–	–	●	●	●	●	●	●	–	●	●	●
3 Sanford Medical Center Fargo	–	–	–	–	–	–	–	–	–	–	–	–	●	●	●	●	●	●	●	●	●
OHIO																					
1 Cleveland Clinic	●	●	●	●	●	●	●	●	●	●	●	●	●	●	●	●	●	●	●	●	●
2 University Hospitals Cleveland Medical Center[13]	●	●	●	●	●	●	●	●	●	●	●	●	●	●	●	●	●	●	●	●	●
3 Ohio State University Wexner Medical Center, Columbus[14]	●	●	●	●	●	●	–	●	●	●	●	●	●	●	●	●	●	●	●	●	●
4 Miami Valley Hospital, Dayton	–	●	–	–	●	–	●	●	●	–	●	●	●	●	●	●	●	●	●	●	●

In complex care specialties, (-) indicates hospital is not nationally ranked or high performing.
In procedures and conditions, (-) indicates care not offered or hospital has too few Medicare patients to be rated.

A footnote indicates that another hospital's results are included, that the hospital has a different name in one or more areas of care, or both.
[13]University Hospitals Seidman Cancer Center. [14]Ohio State University James Cancer Hospital.

● More @ usnews.com/bestregionalhospitals

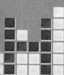
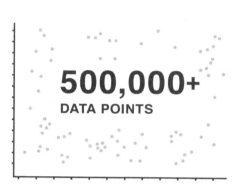
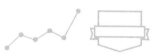
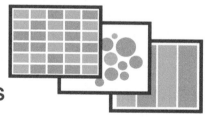
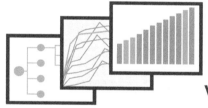
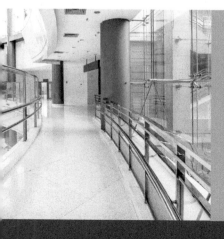

COMPLEX SPECIALTY CARE

COMMON PROCEDURES & CONDITIONS

Legend

COMPLEX SPECIALTY CARE
- ● Nationally ranked
- ● High performing

COMMON PROCEDURES & CONDITIONS
- ● High performing
- ○ Average
- ● Below average

State Rank / Hospital	Cancer	Cardiology & Heart Surgery	Diabetes & Endocrinology	Ear, Nose & Throat	Gastroenterology & GI Surgery	Geriatrics	Gynecology	Nephrology	Neurology & Neurosurgery	Orthopedics	Pulmonology	Urology	Colon Cancer Surgery	Lung Cancer Surgery	Heart Bypass Surgery	Heart Failure	Heart Valve Surgery	Abdominal Aortic Aneurysm	Hip Replacement	Knee Replacement	COPD
OHIO (CONTINUED)																					
5 Christ Hospital, Cincinnati	–	–	●	–	●	●	●	–	●	–	●	●	●	●	●	●	●	●	●	●	●
6 Cleveland Clinic Fairview Hospital, Cleveland	●	●	●	–	●	●	●	●	●	–	●	●	●	●	●	●	●	●	●	●	●
7 Hillcrest Hospital, Cleveland	–	–	●	–	●	●	●	–	●	●	●	●	●	●	●	●	●	●	●	●	●
8 ProMedica Toledo Hospital, Toledo	–	●	●	–	●	●	–	●	●	–	●	●	●	●	●	●	●	●	●	●	●
9 OhioHealth Riverside Methodist Hospital, Columbus	–	–	–	–	–	●	●	●	–	●	●	●	●	●	●	●	●	●	●	●	●
10 Cleveland Clinic Akron General, Akron	–	–	●	–	●	●	●	–	●	●	●	●	●	●	●	●	●	●	●	●	●
11 Good Samaritan Hospital, Cincinnati	–	–	–	–	●	●	●	–	●	–	●	●	●	●	●	●	●	●	●	●	●
12 Aultman Hospital, Canton	–	–	–	–	–	●	●	–	–	●	●	●	●	●	●	●	●	●	●	●	●
13 Bethesda North Hospital, Cincinnati	–	–	–	–	–	●	●	–	●	–	●	●	●	●	●	●	●	●	●	●	●
14 University of Cincinnati Medical Center	–	–	–	●	●	–	●	–	●	–	●	●	●	●	●	●	●	●	●	●	●
15 Summa Health-Akron Campus	–	–	–	–	●	●	●	–	●	–	●	●	●	●	●	●	●	●	●	●	●
16 MetroHealth Medical Center, Cleveland	–	–	–	–	●	●	●	–	●	–	●	●	●	●	●	●	●	–	●	●	●
16 OhioHealth Grant Medical Center, Columbus	–	–	–	–	–	●	●	–	●	–	●	●	●	●	●	●	●	●	●	●	●
18 Good Samaritan Hospital, Dayton	–	–	–	–	–	●	●	–	●	–	●	●	●	●	●	●	●	●	●	●	●
18 Kettering Medical Center, Kettering	–	–	–	–	–	●	●	–	●	–	●	●	●	●	●	●	●	●	●	●	●
18 Mercy Health-St. Elizabeth Youngstown Hospital, Youngstown	–	–	–	–	–	●	●	–	●	–	●	●	●	●	●	●	●	●	●	●	●
18 Mount Carmel East and West Hospitals, Columbus	–	–	–	–	–	●	●	–	●	–	●	●	●	●	●	●	●	●	●	●	●
22 Mercy Health-St. Elizabeth Boardman Hospital, Boardman	–	–	–	–	–	●	●	–	–	–	●	●	●	●	–	●	●	–	●	●	●
22 Southern Ohio Medical Center, Portsmouth	–	–	–	–	–	●	●	–	–	–	●	●	●	●	●	●	●	–	●	●	●
24 Marymount Hospital, Garfield Heights	–	–	–	–	–	–	●	–	–	–	●	●	●	●	●	●	–	●	●	●	●
24 South Pointe Hospital, Warrensville Heights	–	–	–	–	●	–	●	–	●	–	●	●	●	●	●	–	–	●	●	●	●
26 Southwest General Health Center, Middleburg Heights	–	–	–	–	–	–	–	–	–	–	●	●	●	●	●	●	●	●	●	●	●
OKLAHOMA																					
1 St. John Medical Center, Tulsa	–	–	–	–	–	–	–	–	–	–	●	●	●	●	●	●	●	●	●	●	●
2 Integris Baptist Medical Center, Oklahoma City	–	–	–	–	–	–	–	–	–	–	●	●	●	●	●	●	●	●	●	●	●
2 St. Francis Hospital, Tulsa	–	–	–	–	–	–	–	–	–	–	●	●	●	●	●	●	●	●	●	●	●
OREGON																					
1 OHSU Hospital, Portland	●	●	●	●	●	●	●	●	●	–	●	●	●	●	●	●	●	●	●	●	●
2 Providence Portland Medical Center, Portland	–	–	●	●	●	●	–	–	–	–	●	●	●	●	●	●	●	●	●	●	●
2 Providence St. Vincent Medical Center, Portland	–	–	●	–	–	●	–	–	–	–	●	●	●	●	●	●	●	●	●	●	●
4 Salem Hospital, Salem	–	–	–	–	–	–	●	–	–	–	●	●	●	●	●	●	●	●	●	●	●
5 Asante Rogue Regional Medical Center, Medford	–	–	–	–	–	–	●	–	–	–	●	●	●	●	●	●	●	●	●	●	●
6 Kaiser Permanente Sunnyside Medical Center, Clackamas	–	–	–	–	–	–	–	–	–	–	●	●	●	●	●	●	●	●	●	●	●
7 PeaceHealth Sacred Heart Medical Center at RiverBend, Springfield	–	–	–	–	–	–	–	–	–	–	●	●	●	●	●	●	●	●	●	●	●
7 St. Charles Medical Center, Bend	–	–	●	–	–	–	–	–	–	–	●	●	●	●	●	●	●	●	●	●	●
9 Legacy Good Samaritan Hospital and Medical Center, Portland	–	–	●	–	–	–	–	–	●	–	●	●	●	●	●	●	–	●	●	●	●
PENNSYLVANIA																					
1 Hospitals of the U. of Pennsylvania-Penn Presbyterian, Philadelphia	●	●	●	●	●	–	●	●	●	●	●	●	●	●	●	●	●	●	●	●	●
2 UPMC Presbyterian Shadyside, Pittsburgh	●	●	●	●	●	●	●	●	●	●	●	●	●	●	●	●	●	●	●	●	●
3 Thomas Jefferson University Hospitals, Philadelphia[15]	●	●	●	●	●	–	●	●	●	●	●	●	●	●	●	●	●	●	●	●	●
4 Penn State Milton S. Hershey Medical Center, Hershey	●	–	–	–	●	●	●	●	●	–	●	●	●	●	●	●	●	●	●	●	●
5 Lehigh Valley Hospital, Allentown	–	–	–	–	●	●	●	–	●	–	●	●	●	●	●	●	●	●	●	●	●
6 Lancaster General Hospital, Lancaster	–	–	–	–	●	–	●	–	●	–	●	●	●	●	●	●	●	●	●	●	●
7 Lankenau Medical Center, Wynnewood	–	–	–	–	●	–	●	–	●	–	●	●	●	●	●	●	●	●	●	●	●

In complex care specialties, (-) indicates hospital is not nationally ranked or high performing.
In procedures and conditions, (-) indicates care not offered or hospital has too few Medicare patients to be rated.

A footnote indicates that another hospital's results are included, that the hospital has a different name in one or more areas of care, or both.
[15] Rothman Institute at Thomas Jefferson University Hospitals.

▶ **More** @ usnews.com/bestregionalhospitals

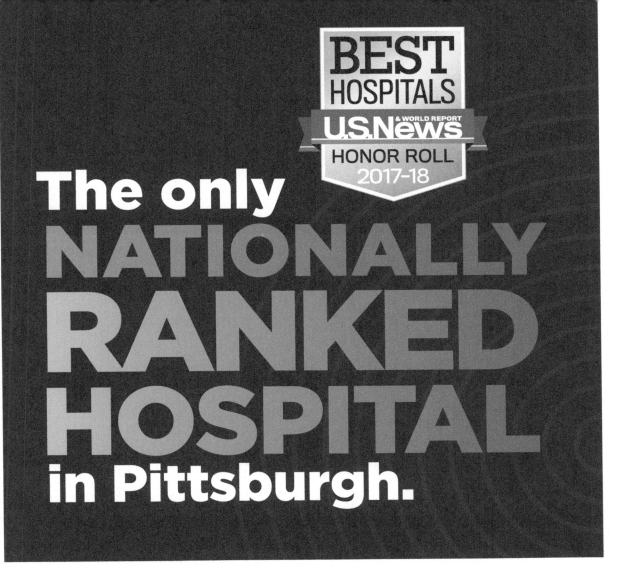

We're proud to once again be named to the *U.S. News & World Report* Honor Roll of America's Best Hospitals, with rankings in 14 specialties. It is an honor to be part of this elite group and to be ranked #1 in Pittsburgh. But the greater honor is to continue to provide the best care to those who rely on us every day. **To learn more, visit UPMC.com/HonorRoll.**

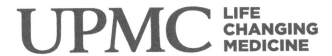

Affiliated with the University of Pittsburgh School of Medicine, UPMC Presbyterian Shadyside is ranked on the *U.S. News & World Report* Best Hospitals Honor Roll.

	COMPLEX SPECIALTY CARE												COMMON PROCEDURES & CONDITIONS								
State Rank Hospital	CANCER	CARDIOLOGY & HEART SURGERY	DIABETES & ENDOCRINOLOGY	EAR, NOSE & THROAT	GASTROENTEROLOGY & GI SURGERY	GERIATRICS	GYNECOLOGY	NEPHROLOGY	NEUROLOGY & NEUROSURGERY	ORTHOPEDICS	PULMONOLOGY	UROLOGY	COLON CANCER SURGERY	LUNG CANCER SURGERY	HEART BYPASS SURGERY	HEART FAILURE	HEART VALVE SURGERY	ABDOMINAL AORTIC ANEURYSM	HIP REPLACEMENT	KNEE REPLACEMENT	COPD
PENNSYLVANIA (CONTINUED)																					
7 **Reading Hospital**, West Reading	–	–	–	●	–	●	–	●	–	–	●	●	●	●	●	●	●	●	●	●	●
9 **Penn Medicine Chester County Hospital**, West Chester	–	–	–	–	●	●	–	●	–	–	●	●	●	–	●	●	●	●	●	●	●
9 **St. Luke's University Hospital-Bethlehem Campus**	–	–	–	–	–	●	●	–	–	–	–	●	●	●	●	●	●	●	●	●	●
9 **UPMC Hamot**, Erie	–	–	●	–	–	–	–	●	–	●	–	●	●	●	●	●	●	●	●	●	●
12 **Bryn Mawr Hospital**, Bryn Mawr	–	–	–	–	●	●	–	–	●	–	–	●	●	●	●	●	●	●	●	●	●
12 **PinnacleHealth Hospitals**, Harrisburg	–	–	–	–	–	–	–	–	–	–	●	●	●	●	●	●	●	●	●	●	●
14 **Pennsylvania Hospital**, Philadelphia	–	–	–	–	–	●	–	–	●	–	–	●	●	●	●	●	●	●	●	●	●
15 **Geisinger Medical Center**, Danville	–	–	–	–	–	–	–	–	–	–	●	●	●	●	●	●	●	●	●	●	●
15 **Paoli Hospital**, Paoli	–	–	–	–	–	–	–	–	–	–	●	●	●	●	●	●	●	●	●	●	●
15 **Riddle Hospital**, Media	–	–	–	–	–	–	–	–	●	–	–	●	–	–	●	–	–	●	●	●	●
18 **Abington Hospital-Jefferson Health**, Abington	–	–	–	–	–	–	–	–	–	–	●	●	●	●	●	●	●	●	●	●	●
18 **Allegheny General Hospital**, Pittsburgh	–	–	–	–	–	–	–	–	–	–	●	●	●	●	●	●	●	●	●	●	●
18 **Hahnemann University Hospital**, Philadelphia	–	–	–	–	●	–	–	–	–	●	–	●	●	●	●	●	●	●	●	●	●
18 **Temple University Hospital**, Philadelphia	●	–	–	–	–	–	●	–	●	–	–	●	●	●	●	●	●	●	●	●	●
18 **UPMC St. Margaret**, Pittsburgh	–	–	–	–	–	–	–	–	–	–	●	●	●	●	●	●	–	●	●	●	●
23 **Doylestown Hospital**, Doylestown	–	–	–	–	–	–	–	–	–	–	●	●	●	●	●	●	●	–	●	●	●
23 **Excela Health Westmoreland Hospital**, Greensburg	–	–	–	–	–	–	–	–	–	–	●	●	●	●	●	●	●	●	●	●	●
23 **Lehigh Valley Hospital-Muhlenberg**, Bethlehem	–	–	–	–	–	–	–	–	–	–	●	●	●	●	●	●	●	–	●	●	●
23 **St. Mary Medical Center**, Langhorne	–	–	–	–	–	–	–	–	–	–	●	●	●	●	●	●	●	●	●	●	●
23 **WellSpan York Hospital**, York	–	–	–	–	–	–	–	–	–	–	●	●	●	●	●	●	●	●	●	●	●
RHODE ISLAND																					
1 **Miriam Hospital**, Providence	–	–	–	–	–	–	–	–	–	–	●	●	●	●	●	●	●	●	●	●	●
2 **Rhode Island Hospital**, Providence	–	–	–	–	–	–	–	–	–	–	●	●	●	●	●	●	●	●	●	●	●
SOUTH CAROLINA																					
1 **MUSC Health-University Medical Center**, Charleston	●	–	–	●	●	●	●	●	●	●	●	●	●	●	●	●	●	●	●	●	●
2 **Spartanburg Medical Center**, Spartanburg	–	–	–	–	–	–	–	–	–	–	●	●	●	●	●	●	●	●	●	●	●
3 **AnMed Health Medical Center**, Anderson	–	–	–	–	–	–	–	–	–	–	●	●	●	●	●	●	●	●	●	●	●
4 **McLeod Regional Medical Center**, Florence	–	–	–	–	–	–	–	–	–	–	●	●	●	●	●	●	●	●	●	●	●
4 **Providence Hospital**, Columbia	–	–	–	–	–	–	–	–	–	–	●	●	●	●	●	●	●	●	●	●	●
6 **Roper St. Francis**, Charleston	–	–	–	–	–	–	–	–	–	–	●	●	●	●	●	●	●	●	●	●	●
7 **Bon Secours St. Francis Hospital**, Charleston	–	–	–	–	–	–	–	–	–	●	–	●	–	–	●	–	–	●	–	●	●
7 **GHS Greer Memorial Hospital**, Greer	–	–	–	–	–	–	–	–	–	–	–	–	–	–	●	–	●	–	●	●	●
7 **Grand Strand Regional Medical Center**, Myrtle Beach	–	–	–	–	–	–	–	–	–	–	●	●	●	●	●	●	●	●	●	●	●
SOUTH DAKOTA																					
1 **Sanford USD Medical Center**, Sioux Falls	●	–	●	–	●	–	●	●	–	●	●	●	●	●	●	●	●	●	●	●	●
2 **Avera McKennan Hospital and University Health Center**, Sioux Falls	●	–	–	–	●	–	–	●	–	●	●	●	–	●	–	–	●	●	●	●	●
3 **Rapid City Regional Hospital**, Rapid City	–	–	–	–	●	–	–	–	●	–	●	●	●	●	●	●	●	●	●	●	●
TENNESSEE																					
1 **Vanderbilt University Medical Center**, Nashville	●	●	●	–	●	●	●	●	●	●	●	●	●	●	●	●	●	●	●	●	●
2 **University of Tennessee Medical Center**, Knoxville	–	–	–	–	–	–	●	–	●	–	●	●	●	●	●	●	●	●	●	●	●
3 **CHI Memorial Hospital**, Chattanooga	–	–	–	–	–	–	–	–	–	–	●	●	●	●	●	●	●	●	●	●	●
4 **Methodist Hospitals of Memphis**	–	–	–	–	–	–	●	–	–	–	–	●	●	●	●	●	●	●	●	●	●
4 **St. Thomas West Hospital**, Nashville	–	–	–	–	–	–	–	–	–	–	–	●	●	●	●	●	●	●	●	●	●
6 **Baptist Memorial Hospital-Memphis**	–	–	–	–	–	–	–	–	–	–	●	●	●	●	●	●	●	●	●	●	●
7 **St. Thomas Midtown Hospital**, Nashville	–	–	–	–	–	–	–	–	–	–	●	●	●	●	●	●	●	●	●	●	●
8 **TriStar Centennial Medical Center**, Nashville	–	–	–	–	–	–	–	–	–	–	●	●	●	●	●	●	●	●	●	●	●

In complex care specialties, (-) indicates hospital is not nationally ranked or high performing.
In procedures and conditions, (-) indicates care not offered or hospital has too few Medicare patients to be rated.

More @ usnews.com/bestregionalhospitals

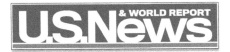
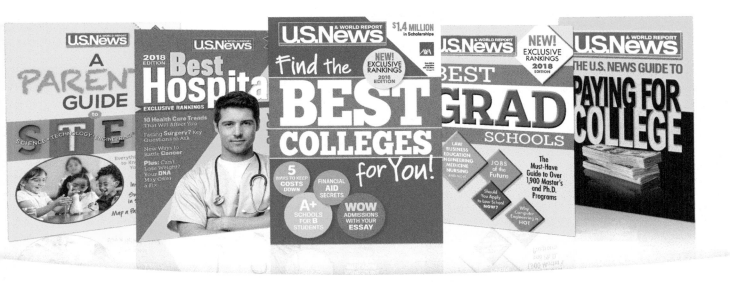
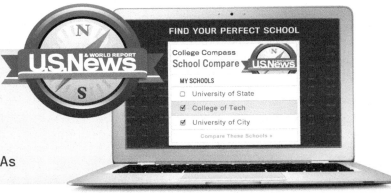

Legend

COMPLEX SPECIALTY CARE
- ● Nationally ranked
- ● High performing

COMMON PROCEDURES & CONDITIONS
- ● High performing
- ● Average
- ● Below average

State Rank	Hospital	CANCER	CARDIOLOGY & HEART SURGERY	DIABETES & ENDOCRINOLOGY	EAR, NOSE & THROAT	GASTROENTEROLOGY & GI SURGERY	GERIATRICS	GYNECOLOGY	NEPHROLOGY	NEUROLOGY & NEUROSURGERY	ORTHOPEDICS	PULMONOLOGY	UROLOGY	COLON CANCER SURGERY	LUNG CANCER SURGERY	HEART BYPASS SURGERY	HEART FAILURE	HEART VALVE SURGERY	ABDOMINAL AORTIC ANEURYSM	HIP REPLACEMENT	KNEE REPLACEMENT	COPD
	TEXAS																					
1	**Houston Methodist Hospital**	●	●	●	–	●	●		●	●	●	●	●	●	●	●	●	●	●	●	●	●
2	**UT Southwestern Medical Center**, Dallas	●	–	●	●	●	●	●	●	●	●	●	●	●	●	●	●	●	●	●	●	●
3	**Baylor University Medical Center**, Dallas[16]	●	●	●	●	●	●	●	●	●	●	–	●	●	●	●	●	●	●	●	●	●
4	**Baylor St. Luke's Medical Center**, Houston[17]	●	●	●	●	●	●	●	●	●	●	●	●	●	●	●	●	●	●	●	●	●
5	**Memorial Hermann-Texas Medical Center**, Houston	–	●	●	–	●	–	●	●	●	●	●	●	●	●	●	●	●	●	●	●	●
6	**Medical City Dallas Hospital**	●	–	–	–	–	–	●	–	–	–	–	–	●	●	●	●	●	●	●	●	●
7	**Memorial Hermann Greater Heights Hospital**, Houston	–	–	–	–	–	–	–	–	–	–	–	–	●	●	●	●	●	●	●	●	●
7	**Scott and White Memorial Hospital**, Temple	–	–	●	●	–	–	–	–	–	–	–	–	●	●	●	●	●	●	●	●	●
7	**Seton Medical Center Austin**	–	–	–	–	–	–	–	–	–	–	–	–	●	●	●	●	●	●	●	●	●
7	**Texas Health Presbyterian Hospital Dallas**	–	–	–	–	–	–	–	–	–	–	–	–	●	●	●	●	●	●	●	●	●
11	**Texas Health Harris Methodist Hospital Fort Worth**	–	–	–	–	–	–	–	–	–	–	–	–	●	●	●	●	●	●	●	●	●
12	**Christus Mother Frances Hospital-Tyler**	–	–	–	–	–	–	–	–	–	–	–	–	●	●	●	●	●	●	●	●	●
12	**Covenant Medical Center**, Lubbock	–	–	–	–	–	–	–	–	–	–	–	–	●	●	●	●	●	●	–	●	●
12	**Houston Methodist Willowbrook Hospital**, Houston	–	–	–	–	●	●	–	–	–	–	–	–	●	●	●	●	●	●	–	●	●
12	**Memorial Hermann Memorial City Medical Center**, Houston	–	–	–	–	–	–	–	–	–	●	–	–	●	●	●	●	●	●	●	●	●
12	**Methodist Hospital**, San Antonio	–	–	–	–	–	–	–	–	–	●	–	–	●	●	●	●	●	●	●	●	●
12	**St. David's Medical Center**, Austin	–	–	–	–	–	–	–	–	–	–	–	–	●	●	●	●	●	●	●	●	●
12	**Texas Health Presbyterian Hospital Plano**	–	–	–	–	–	–	–	–	–	–	–	–	●	●	●	●	●	●	●	●	●
12	**University Hospital**, San Antonio	–	–	–	–	–	●	●	–	–	–	–	–	●	●	●	●	●	●	–	●	●
20	**Baptist Medical Center**, San Antonio	–	–	–	–	–	●	●	–	–	–	–	–	●	●	●	●	●	●	–	●	●
20	**Medical City Fort Worth Hospital**	–	–	–	–	–	–	–	–	–	–	–	–	●	●	●	●	●	●	●	●	●
20	**Texas Health Harris Methodist Hospital Southwest**, Fort Worth	–	–	–	–	–	–	–	–	–	–	–	–	●	●	–	●	–	●	●	●	●
23	**Baylor Medical Center at Irving**	–	–	–	–	–	–	–	–	–	–	–	–	●	●	–	●	–	●	●	●	●
23	**Baylor Regional Medical Center at Plano**	–	–	–	–	–	–	●	–	–	–	–	–	●	●	●	●	●	–	●	●	●
23	**Baylor Scott and White Medical Center-Grapevine**	–	–	–	–	–	–	●	–	–	–	–	–	●	●	–	●	–	●	–	●	●
23	**Christus Southeast Texas Hospital-St. Elizabeth**, Beaumont	–	–	–	–	–	–	–	–	–	–	–	–	●	●	●	●	●	●	●	●	●
23	**Christus Spohn Hospital Corpus Christi-Memorial**, Corpus Christi	–	–	–	–	–	–	–	–	–	–	–	–	●	●	●	●	●	●	●	●	●
23	**Clear Lake Regional Medical Center**, Webster	–	–	●	–	–	–	–	–	–	–	–	–	●	●	●	●	●	●	●	●	●
23	**Denton Regional Medical Center**, Denton	–	–	–	–	–	–	–	–	–	–	–	–	●	●	●	●	●	●	●	●	●
23	**Houston Methodist San Jacinto Hospital**, Baytown	–	–	–	–	●	–	–	–	–	–	–	–	●	●	●	●	●	●	–	●	●
23	**Medical Center of Plano**	–	–	–	–	–	–	–	–	–	–	–	–	●	●	●	●	●	–	●	●	●
23	**Texas Health Arlington Memorial Hospital**, Arlington	–	–	–	–	–	–	–	–	–	–	–	–	●	●	●	●	●	–	●	●	●
33	**University of Texas Medical Branch**, Galveston	–	–	–	–	–	●	–	–	–	–	–	–	●	●	–	●	–	●	●	●	●
34	**Baylor All Saints Medical Center at Fort Worth**	–	–	–	●	–	–	–	–	–	–	–	–	●	●	●	●	●	–	●	●	●
	UTAH																					
1	**University of Utah Health Care-Hospital and Clinics**, Salt Lake City[18]	●	–	–	●	–	–	●	●	●	●	●	●	●	●	●	●	●	●	●	●	●
2	**Intermountain Medical Center**, Murray	–	–	●	–	–	–	–	–	–	●	●	●	●	●	●	●	●	●	●	●	●
	VERMONT																					
–	**Rutland Regional Medical Center**, Rutland	–	–	–	–	–	–	–	–	–	–	–	–	●	●	–	●	–	–	●	●	●
	VIRGINIA																					
1	**University of Virginia Medical Center**, Charlottesville	●	●	●	●	●	●	●	●	●	●	●	●	●	●	●	●	●	●	●	●	●
2	**Sentara Norfolk General Hospital**, Norfolk[19]	–	●	●	–	●	–	●	●	●	●	●	●	●	●	●	●	●	●	●	●	●
3	**Carilion Roanoke Memorial Hospital**, Roanoke	–	–	●	–	–	–	●	●	●	●	●	●	●	●	●	●	●	●	–	–	●
3	**VCU Medical Center**, Richmond	●	–	●	–	–	–	–	●	●	●	●	●	●	●	●	●	●	●	●	●	●

In complex care specialties, (-) indicates hospital is not nationally ranked or high performing.
In procedures and conditions, (-) indicates care not offered or hospital has too few Medicare patients to be rated.

A footnote indicates that another hospital's results are included, that the hospital has a different name in one or more areas of care, or both.
[16]Baylor University Medical Center and Heart and Vascular Hospital. [17]Texas Heart Institute at Baylor St. Luke's Medical Center.
[18]Huntsman Cancer Institute at the University of Utah. [19]Sentara Norfolk General Hospital-Sentara Heart Hospital.

More @ usnews.com/bestregionalhospitals

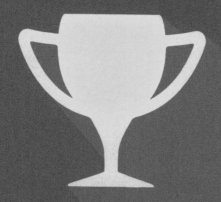

Most nationally ranked hospitals than any other health care system in Texas.

Baylor Scott & White Health is proud to lead our state with four nationally ranked hospitals and two hospitals ranked in the Texas Top Ten, as recognized by *U.S. News & World Report.* For you, these recognitions confirm our commitment to providing quality health care each day.

To find out more about our award-winning care, call 1.844.BSW.DOCS or visit BSWHealth.com/BestHospitals.

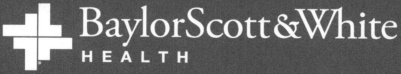

BaylorScott&White
HEALTH

Changing Health Care. **For Life.®**

COMPLEX SPECIALTY CARE
- ● Nationally ranked
- ● High performing

COMMON PROCEDURES & CONDITIONS
- ● High performing
- ● Average
- ● Below average

COMPLEX SPECIALTY CARE · COMMON PROCEDURES & CONDITIONS

State Rank Hospital	Cancer	Cardiology & Heart Surgery	Diabetes & Endocrinology	Ear, Nose & Throat	Gastroenterology & GI Surgery	Geriatrics	Gynecology	Nephrology	Neurology & Neurosurgery	Orthopedics	Pulmonology	Urology	Colon Cancer Surgery	Lung Cancer Surgery	Heart Bypass Surgery	Heart Failure	Heart Valve Surgery	Abdominal Aortic Aneurysm	Hip Replacement	Knee Replacement	COPD
VIRGINIA (CONTINUED)																					
5 Centra Lynchburg General Hospital, Lynchburg	–	–	–	–	●	●	–	●	–	–	●	–	●	●	●	●	●	●	●	●	●
6 Mary Washington Hospital, Fredericksburg	–	–	–	–	–	–	–	–	–	–	●	–	●	●	●	●	–	●	●	●	●
7 Bon Secours Memorial Regional Medical Center, Mechanicsville	–	–	●	–	●	–	–	–	–	–	–	–	●	●	●	●	●	●	●	●	●
7 Inova Fairfax Hospital, Falls Church	–	–	–	–	–	–	–	–	–	–	–	–	●	●	●	●	●	●	●	●	●
9 Bon Secours St. Mary's Hospital, Richmond	–	–	–	–	–	–	–	–	–	–	–	–	●	●	●	●	●	●	●	●	●
9 Sentara Leigh Hospital, Norfolk	–	–	–	–	–	–	●	–	–	–	●	–	●	●	●	●	–	–	●	●	●
9 Sentara Princess Anne Hospital, Virginia Beach	–	–	~	–	–	–	●	–	–	–	●	–	●	●	●	●	–	–	●	●	●
9 Virginia Hospital Center, Arlington	–	–	–	–	–	–	–	–	–	–	–	–	●	●	●	●	–	–	●	●	●
9 Winchester Medical Center, Winchester	–	–	●	–	–	–	–	–	–	–	–	–	●	●	●	●	●	●	●	●	●
14 Inova Fair Oaks Hospital, Fairfax	–	–	–	–	–	–	–	–	–	–	–	–	●	●	●	●	–	–	●	●	●
15 Inova Loudoun Hospital, Leesburg	–	–	–	–	●	–	–	–	–	–	–	–	●	●	●	●	–	–	–	●	●
15 Sentara RMH Medical Center, Harrisonburg	–	–	–	–	–	–	–	–	–	●	●	–	●	●	●	●	–	–	●	●	●
15 Sentara Williamsburg Regional Medical Center, Williamsburg	–	–	●	–	–	–	–	–	–	–	–	–	●	●	●	●	–	–	●	●	●
18 Inova Mount Vernon Hospital, Alexandria	–	–	–	–	–	–	●	–	–	●	–	–	●	●	–	●	–	–	●	●	●
18 Sentara Martha Jefferson Hospital, Charlottesville	–	–	–	–	–	–	–	–	–	–	●	–	●	●	●	●	●	●	●	●	●
WASHINGTON																					
1 University of Washington Medical Center, Seattle[20]	●	●	●	●	●	●	–	●	●	●	●	●	●	●	●	●	●	●	●	●	●
2 Providence Sacred Heart Med. Ctr. and Children's Hospital, Spokane	–	–	–	–	–	–	–	–	–	–	–	–	●	●	●	●	●	●	●	●	●
3 Virginia Mason Medical Center, Seattle	–	–	–	–	●	–	–	–	–	–	–	–	●	●	●	●	●	●	●	●	●
4 Providence St. Peter Hospital, Olympia	–	–	–	–	–	–	–	–	–	–	–	–	●	●	●	●	●	●	●	●	●
5 Providence Regional Medical Center Everett	–	–	–	–	–	–	–	–	–	–	–	–	●	●	●	●	●	●	●	●	●
5 Swedish Medical Center-First Hill, Seattle	–	–	–	–	–	–	–	●	–	●	–	–	●	●	–	●	●	●	●	●	●
7 Swedish Medical Center-Cherry Hill, Seattle	–	–	–	–	–	–	●	–	●	–	–	–	●	●	●	●	●	●	–	–	●
8 MultiCare Good Samaritan Hospital, Puyallup	–	–	–	–	–	–	–	–	–	–	–	–	●	●	●	●	–	–	●	●	●
8 UW Medicine/Harborview Medical Center, Seattle	–	–	–	–	–	–	–	●	–	●	–	●	●	–	●	●	–	●	●	●	●
8 UW Medicine/Valley Medical Center, Renton	–	–	–	–	–	–	–	–	–	–	–	–	●	●	●	●	●	●	●	●	●
11 PeaceHealth Southwest Medical Center, Vancouver	–	–	–	–	–	–	–	–	–	–	–	–	●	●	●	●	●	●	●	●	●
WASHINGTON, D.C.																					
1* MedStar Georgetown University Hospital	–	–	●	–	–	●	–	–	–	–	–	●	●	●	●	●	–	●	●	●	●
4* MedStar Washington Hospital Center	–	●	–	–	–	–	–	–	–	–	–	–	●	●	●	●	●	●	●	●	●
WEST VIRGINIA																					
1 Charleston Area Medical Center, Charleston	–	–	●	–	–	–	●	–	●	–	●	–	●	●	●	●	●	●	●	●	●
2 West Virginia University Hospitals, Morgantown	●	–	–	–	–	–	–	–	–	–	●	●	●	●	●	●	●	●	●	●	●
3 St. Mary's Medical Center, Huntington	–	–	–	–	–	–	–	–	–	–	–	–	●	●	●	●	●	●	●	●	●
WISCONSIN																					
1 University of Wisconsin Hospitals, Madison	●	●	●	–	●	●	●	●	●	●	●	●	●	●	●	●	●	●	●	●	●
2 Aurora St. Luke's Medical Center, Milwaukee	●	●	●	–	●	●	●	●	●	●	●	●	●	●	●	●	●	●	●	●	●
3 Froedtert Hospital and the Medical College of Wisconsin, Milwaukee	●	–	–	●	●	–	●	●	●	–	●	●	●	●	●	●	●	●	●	●	●
4 Aspirus Wausau Hospital, Wausau	–	–	–	–	–	–	–	–	–	–	●	–	●	●	●	●	●	●	●	●	●
5 St. Mary's Hospital, Madison	–	–	–	–	–	–	–	–	–	–	–	–	●	●	●	●	●	●	●	●	●
6 Aurora Medical Center Grafton	–	–	–	–	–	–	–	●	–	●	–	–	●	●	●	●	●	●	●	●	●
6 Mercy Hospital and Trauma Center, Janesville	–	–	–	–	–	–	●	–	●	–	●	–	●	●	●	●	●	●	●	●	●
8 Bellin Memorial Hospital, Green Bay	–	–	–	–	–	–	–	–	–	–	–	–	●	●	●	●	●	●	●	●	●
9 Mayo Clinic Eau Claire	–	–	–	–	–	–	–	–	–	–	●	–	●	●	●	●	●	●	●	●	●

In complex care specialties, (-) indicates hospital is not nationally ranked or high performing.
In procedures and conditions, (-) indicates care not offered or hospital has too few Medicare patients to be rated.

A footnote indicates that another hospital's results are included, that the hospital has a different name in one or more areas of care, or both.
[20]Seattle Cancer Care Alliance/University of Washington Medical Center.

*Reflects Best Regional Hospitals rank in D.C. metro area, which includes many hospitals in Maryland and Virginia. These two are located within the District.

▶ More @ usnews.com/bestregionalhospitals

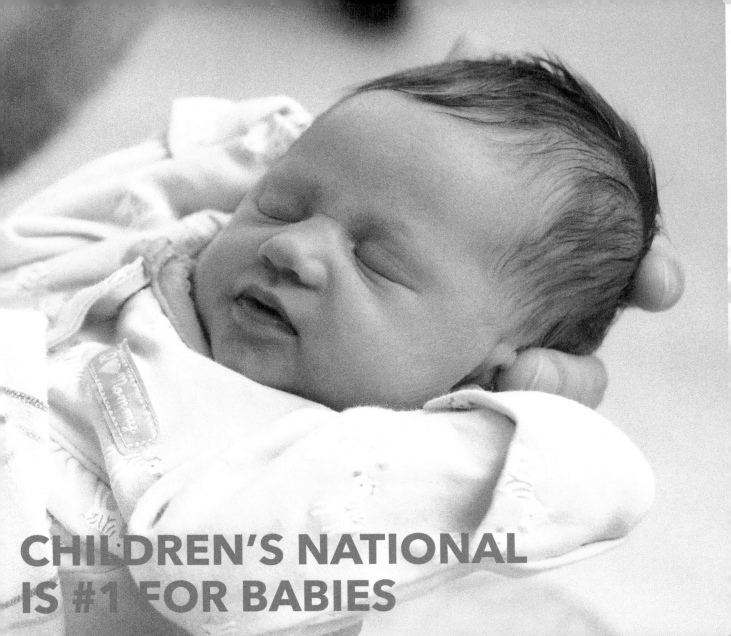

CHILDREN'S NATIONAL IS #1 FOR BABIES

Children's National is proud to be named #1 for newborn intensive care in the *U.S. News & World Report* Best Children's Hospitals survey and ranked among the Top 10 children's hospitals overall. What makes us the best choice for care in the nation's capital? Expertise that's focused on children's unique needs and support for every family. At Children's National, we want every child to **GROW UP STRONGER.**

Learn more about top-ranked care for children at childrensnational.org/usnews

1-888-884-BEAR | childrensnational.org | #GrowUpStronger

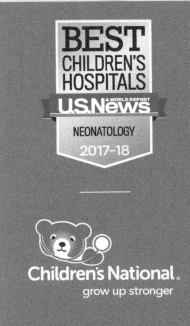

BEST CHILDREN'S HOSPITALS
U.S.News & WORLD REPORT
NEONATOLOGY
2017–18

Children's National®
grow up stronger

CPSIA information can be obtained
at www.ICGtesting.com
Printed in the USA
BVOW05s1504031017
496613BV00001B/1/P